Last Minute

Internal Medicine

Notice

Last Minute

Internal Medicine

REBECCA A. MIKSAD, MD, MPH
Instructor in Medicine
Attending Physician
Division of Hematology and Oncology
Beth Israel Deaconess Medical Center
Harvard Medical School
Boston, Massachusetts

PATRICIA A. DELAMORA, MD
Clinical Instructor of Pediatrics
Attending Physician, Pediatric Infectious Diseases
New York-Presbyterian Hospital
Weill Medical College of Cornell University
New York, New York

GEORGE KEITH MEYER, MD
Attending Physician
Miami Children's Hospital
Division of Critical Care Medicine
Medical Director-LifeFlight®
Section Director-Neuro Intensive Care
Section Director-Patient Safety and Outcomes
Section Director-Clinical Research
Miami, Florida

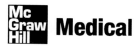

New York   Chicago   San Francisco   Lisbon   London   Madrid   Mexico City   Milan
New Delhi   San Juan   Seoul   Singapore   Sydney   Toronto

The McGraw-Hill Companies

Last Minute Internal Medicine

1 2 3 4 5 6 7 8 9 0   DOC/DOC   0 9 8 7

ISBN 978-0-07-144589-4
MHID 0-07-144589-7

This book was set in Garamond by International Typesetting and Composition.
The editors were James F. Shanahan and Christie Naglieri.
The production supervisor was Thomas Kowalczyk.
Project management was provided by Vastavikta Sharma, International Typesetting and Composition.
The index was prepared by Robert Swanson.
RR Donnelley/Crawfordsville was printer and binder.

This book is printed on acid-free paper.

Library of Congress Cataloging-in-Publication Data

Last minute internal medicine / edited by Rebecca Miksad, Keith Meyer,
    Patricia DeLaMora.—1st ed.
        p. ; cm.
    Includes bibliographical references and index.
    ISBN-13: 978-0-07-144589-4 (pbk. : alk. paper)
    ISBN-10: 0-07-144589-7
    1. Internal medicine—Outlines, syllabi, etc. 2. Internal medicine—
Examinations, questions, etc. I. Miksad, Rebecca. II. Meyer, Keith.
III. DeLaMora, Patricia A.
    [DNLM: 1. Internal Medicine—methods—Outlines. WB 18.2 L349   2007]
RC59.L37   2007
616.0076—dc22

                                                        2007031824

Contents

Authors

Rebecca A. Miksad, MD, MPH
Instructor in Medicine
Attending Physician
Division of Hematology and Oncology
Beth Israel Deaconess Medical Center
Harvard Medical School
Boston, Massachusetts

Patricia A. DeLaMora, MD
Clinical Instructor of Pediatrics
Attending Physician, Pediatric Infectious Diseases
New York-Presbyterian Hospital
Weill Medical College of Cornell University
New York, New York

George Keith Meyer, MD
Miami Children's Hospital
Division of Critical Care Medicine
Medical Director-LifeFlight®
Section Director-Neuro Intensive Care
Section Director-Patient Safety and Outcomes
Section Director-Clinical Research
Miami, Florida

Associate Editors

Suzanne Baumwell, MD
Beth Israel Deaconess Medical Center
Harvard Medical School
Boston, Massachusetts

Stephanie Heon, MD
Beth Israel Deaconess Medical Center
Harvard Medical School
Boston, Massachusetts

Shoshana J. Herzig, MD
Beth Israel Deaconess Medical Center
Harvard Medical School
Boston, Massachusetts

Reyan Ghany, MD
Jackson Memorial Hospital
University of Miami School of Medicine
Miami, Florida

Hilton Gomes, MD
Jackson Memorial Hospital
University of Miami School of Medicine
Miami, Florida

Alina Khan, MD
Jackson Memorial Hospital
University of Miami School of Medicine
Miami, Florida

Contributors

Douglas M. Beach, MD
Beth Israel Deaconess Medical Center
Harvard Medical School
Boston, Massachusetts

Sigall Bell, MD
Beth Israel Deaconess Medical Center
Harvard Medical School
Boston, Massachusetts

Claire Boccia-Liang, MD
New York-Presbyterian Hospital
Weill Medical College of Cornell University
New York, New York

Mariana C. Castells, MD, PhD
Brigham and Women's Hospital
Harvard Medical School
Boston, Massachusetts

Christine M. Choi, MD, MBA
New York-Presbyterian Hospital
Weill Medical College of Cornell University
New York, New York

Sergai N. DeLaMora, MD
New York Orthopaedics
Scarsdale, New York

Sandhya Dhruvakumar, MD
New York-Presbyterian Hospital
Weill Medical College of Cornell University
New York, New York

David P. Dobesh, MD
New York-Presbyterian Hospital
Weill Medical College of Cornell University
New York, New York

Timothy C. Dutta, MD
New York-Presbyterian Hospital
Weill Medical College of Cornell University
New York, New York

Petros Efthimiou, MD
The Hospital for Special Surgery
New York-Presbyterian Hospital
Weill Medical College of Cornell University
New York, New York

Lara Rymarquis Fuchs, MD
Bellevue Hospital
New York University
New York, New York

Victor D. Guardiola, MD
Jackson Memorial Hospital
University of Miami School of Medicine
Miami, Florida

Claudia Ginsberg, MD
Morristown Memorial Hospital
Morristown, New Jersey

Choli Hartono, MD
Massachusetts General Hospital
Harvard Medical School
Boston, Massachusetts

Naomi Hayashi, MD
New York-Presbyterian Hospital
Weill Medical College of Cornell University
New York, New York

Vivian Hernandez-Trujillo, MD
Miami Children's Hospital
Miami, Florida

F. Ida Hsu, MD
Brigham and Women's Hospital
Harvard Medical School
Boston, Massachusetts

Michelle Kang Kim, MD
New York-Presbyterian Hospital
Weill Medical College of Cornell University
New York, New York

Keith LaScalea, MD
New York-Presbyterian Hospital
Weill Medical College of Cornell University
The Hospital for Special Surgery
New York, New York

May C. Lau, MD, MPH
Miami Children's Hospital
Miami, Florida

Thomas C. Lee, MD
New York-Presbyterian Hospital
Weill Medical College of Cornell University
New York, New York

Jonah Licht, MD
New York-Presbyterian Hospital
Weill Medical College of Cornell University
New York, New York

Jacqueline C. Machado, MD
Miami Children's Hospital
Miami, Florida

Joseph A. Markenson, MD
Hospital for Special Surgery
Weill Medical College of Cornell University
New York, New York

Shunda M. McGahee, MD
Massachusetts General Hospital
Harvard Medical School
Boston, Massachusetts

Raymond D. Pastore, MD
New York-Presbyterian Hospital
Weill Medical College of Cornell University
New York, New York

Jay Raman, MD
New York-Presbyterian Hospital
Weill Medical College of Cornell University
New York, New York

Gregory J. Riely, MD, PhD
Memorial Sloan-Kettering Cancer Center
New York, New York

John B. Roseman, MD
McLean Hospital
Harvard Medical School
Boston, Massachusetts

Joseph E. Safdieh, MD
New York-Presbyterian Hospital
Weill Medical College of Cornell University
New York, New York

Robert Schaefer, MD
New York-Presbyterian Hospital
Weill Medical College of Cornell University
New York, New York

Stephen Scheidt, MD
New York-Presbyterian Hospital
Weill Medical College of Cornell University
New York, New York

Douglas S. Scherr, MD
New York-Presbyterian Hospital
Weill Medical College of Cornell University
New York, New York

Jila Senemar, MD
Baptist Hospital of Miami
Miami, Florida

Contributors

Saumil R. Shah, MD
Beth Israel Deaconess Medical Center
Harvard Medical School
Boston, Massachusetts

Abby Siegel, MD
Columbia Presbyterian Hospital
Columbia University
New York, New York

Ann Tilley, MD
New York-Presbyterian Hospital
Weill Medical College of Cornell University
New York, New York

Tiffany Traina, MD
Memorial Sloan-Kettering Cancer Center
New York, New York

Jonathan A. Waitman, MD
New York-Presbyterian Hospital
Weill Medical College of Cornell University
New York, New York

Thomas H. Watson, MD
New York-Presbyterian Hospital
Weill Medical College of Cornell University
New York, New York

Gil Weitzman, MD
New York-Presbyterian Hospital
Weill Medical College of Cornell University
New York, New York

Dana Zappetti, MD
New York-Presbyterian Hospital
Weill Medical College of Cornell University
New York, New York

Preface

We are pleased to introduce a unique concept for internal medicine board preparation. While studying for our boards, we found many review books but none that efficiently provided high-yield information in an easy-to-read table format. Our colleagues, both recent residency graduates and practicing physicians, were similarly frustrated with the options available to study for the boards.

Our goal is to provide the reader with a book that can be picked up to quickly review a focused topic or to study a summary of key concepts. This book provides high-yield, easy-to-read, absolutely-need-to-know information without burdening the reader with extraneous details. This book is designed to arm you with the essential information required to pass the internal medicine board exam. Our philosophy is that it is more important to understand core concepts and the primary distinguishing features of each disease, rather than disparate pieces of detailed information.

We recommend reading this book *before* the initiation of studying for the exam in order to identify your strengths and weaknesses, *during* studying to help you focus on important details, and *at the end* of studying to solidify key concepts.

We would like to thank everyone who contributed their time, expertise, and guidance in writing this book. In particular, we would like to thank the faculty and fellows of New York-Presbyterian Hospital/Weill Medical College of Cornell University for their support and contributions. We would also like to thank Jim Shanahan of McGraw-Hill for his encouragement and guidance during this project.

Rebecca A. Miksad
Patricia A. DeLaMora
George Keith Meyer

Last Minute

Internal Medicine

Chapter 1

Cardiology

Table 1-1

Risk Factors for Cardiovascular Disease and Prevention Goals

CATEGORY	RISK FACTOR	PRIMARY PREVENTION GOAL (DECREASE RISK OF FIRST CARDIOVASCULAR EVENT IN PERSONS WITHOUT KNOWN CARDIOVASCULAR DISEASE)	SECONDARY PREVENTION GOAL (DECREASE RISK OF CARDIOVASCULAR EVENTS IN PERSONS WITH KNOWN CARDIOVASCULAR DISEASE)
Major Risk Factors	Hypertension	<140/90 mm Hg	
		<130/80 mm Hg if renal insufficiency or diabetes	
	Diabetes (CAD equivalent)	Normal fasting plasma glucose (<110 mg/dL)	
		Near normal HbA1c (<7%)	
	Dyslipidemia	LDL-C <160 mg/dL if ≤ 1 risk factor	LDL-C <100 mg/dL
	• Elevated LDL-C	LDL-C <130 mg/dL if ≥ 2 risk factors and 10-year CAD risk* is <20%	
	• Low HDL cholesterol (<40 mg/dL)	LDL-C <100 mg/dL if ≥ 2 risk factors, 10-y CAD risk is ≥ 20% or if diabetes	
	Tobacco use	Complete cessation.	
		No exposure to environmental tobacco smoke.	
	Increasing Age	Not modifiable	
	• Male >45 years		
	• Female >55 years		
	Family history of premature CAD	Not modifiable	
Independent Predisposing Risk Factors	Elevated triglycerides	<150 mg/dL	
	Obesity	Achieve and maintain desirable weight (body mass index 18.5–24.9 kg/m^2)	
	Sedentary lifestyle	At least 30 min of moderate-intensity physical activity on most	

High-fat diet		Consume a variety of fruits, vegetables, grains, low-fat or nonfat dairy products, fish, legumes, poultry, and lean meats.
Protective Factor	Elevated HDL > 60 mg/dL	As above
Associated Risk Factors	C-reactive protein	Unclear if treatment reduces mortality
	Fibrinogen level	
	Apoprotein(a)	Measurement of markers of inflammation such as C-reactive protein currently are not recommended for general population screening
	Homocysteine	
	Impaired fasting glucose	
	Subclinical atherosclerosis	

*The Framingham Risk score can be used to calculate 10-year cardiovascular risk;

CAD = coronary artery disease; HDL = high density lipoprotein; LDL-C = low-density lipoprotein cholesterol.

Metabolic syndrome describes a constellation of cardiovascular risk factors: hypertension, abdominal obesity, dyslipidemia, and insulin resistance.Data adapted from Smith SC, Allen J, Blair SN, Bonow RO, Brass LM, Fonarow GC, Grundy SM, Hiratzka L, Jones D, Krumholz HM, Mosca L, Pasternak RC, Pearson T, Pfeffer MA, Taubert KA. AHA/ACC guidelines for secondary prevention for patients with coronary and other atherosclerotic vascular disease: 2006 update. *J Am Coll Cardiol* 2006;47:2130–9. doi:10.1016/j.jacc.2006.04.026. http://content.onlinejacc.org/cgi/content/full/47/10/2130 Accessed July 10, 2007.

Table 1-2

Other Interventions for Prevention of Cardiovascular Disease

AGENT	PRIMARY PREVENTION	SECONDARY PREVENTION
Aspirin	• Consider if 10-year risk of first cardiovascular event* is ≥10%	• Indicated if known cardiovascular disease
	If at risk for bleeding (gastrointestinal tract bleeding, epistaxis, ecchymosis, hemorrhagic stroke) weigh risks and benefits	
Beta-Blocker	• Consider in peri-operative setting or as indicated for treatment of cardiovascular risk factors	• Consider if status post myocardial infarction/acute coronary syndrome, or if left ventricular dysfunction
Angiotensin-Converting Enzyme (ACE) Inhibitor	• Consider as indicated for treatment of cardiovascular risk factors	• Consider if left ventricular ejection fraction ≤40% or if hypertension, diabetes, or chronic kidney disease • Consider angiotensin receptor blockers if patient cannot tolerate ACE inhibitor
Clopidogrel		• Consider in combination with aspirin for 12 months after acute coronary syndrome • Consider in combination with aspirin after percutaneous coronary intervention with stent placement (duration depends on type of stent)
Influenza Vaccination	• As per routine care	• Consider if known cardiovascular disease

*The Framingham Risk score can be used to calculate 10-year cardiovascular risk; ACE = angiotensin-converting enzyme.

Table 1-3

Suggested Therapeutic Lifestyle Modifications to Reduce Cardiovascular Risk

METHOD	GOAL
Regular Exercise	• 30 minutes daily
Weight Loss	• Achieve and maintain desirable weight (body mass index 18.5–24.9 kg/m^2)
Limit Alcohol Intake	• Men: no more than two drinks per day • Women: no more than one drink per day
Salt Restriction	• Less than 2.4 grams of sodium per day
Dietary Changes	• Diet rich in fruits and vegetables with reduced saturated fat and total cholesterol. • Initial dietary goals: <30% of calories from fat and <300 mg/day of cholesterol • More stringent dietary goals: <30% of calories from fat and <200 mg/day of cholesterol
Fish Oil	• May help lower triglycerides
Dietary Fiber	• Not clearly shown to be helpful
Hormone Replacement Therapy	• Not indicated • May increase risk of cardiovascular events

Table 1-4

Pharmacological Treatment Options for Dyslipidemia

CLASS	EXAMPLE OF AGENT	SELECT TREATMENT BENEFITS	SELECT SIDE EFFECTS

HMG CoA Reductase Inhibitors	Statin	• Lowers LDL by 20–60%
		• Atorvastatin and rosuvastatin most potent for lowering LDL and may lower triglycerides
		• Mortality benefit as primary and secondary prevention of cardiovascular disease
		• Usually first-line choice because generally well tolerated and largest reduction in LDL
			• Headache
			• Myositis/rhabdomyolysis
			  - Less common with pravastatin than other statins
			  - Increased risk if concurrent fibrate use
			• Elevated liver function tests
			• May potentiate warfarin and raise digoxin levels

Fibrates	Fenofibrate Gemfibrozil	• Lowers plasma triglycerides • Raises HDL levels	• Fenofibrate: Nausea, bloating, cramping, and myalgia • Increases risk of muscle side effects if taken concurrently with statin
Nicotinic Acid	Nicotinic acid	• Raises HDL levels at low doses • Lowers LDL and VLDL levels at higher doses	• Cutaneous flushing (Prostaglandin-mediated) • Often poorly tolerated
Cholesterol Absorption Inhibitors	Ezetimibe	• Lowers LDL • Useful in combination with statin because may help avoid need for high doses of a statin	• Elevated liver function tests if concurrent statin use
Bile Acid Sequestrant	Cholestyramine	• Lowers LDL	• Nausea, bloating, and cramping • Elevated liver function tests • Impaired absorption of fat soluble vitamins and some medications • Often poorly tolerated
Other	Neomycin	• Lowers LDL	• Ototoxicity • Nephrotoxicity

Note: Pharmacologic interventions should be combined with life-style modifications when feasible and appropriate.
VLDL = very low density lipoprotein.

Table 1-5

Summary of Hypertension

Type	Definition	Etiology	Presentation	Diagnosis	Long-Term Consequences	Notes
Essential	• Idiopathic (i.e. not caused by another disease)	• Unknown	• Usually Asymptomatic • Generally found on routine physical exam • Symptoms from end organ damage such as headache are possible	• Elevation in systolic and/or diastolic blood pressure • Hypertension = >140/90 mm Hg on two separate visits • Prehypertension= 120 to 139/ 80 to 89 mm Hg	Increased risk of • Left ventricular hypertrophy • Stroke • Renal disease • Peripheral arterial disease	• Prevalence increasing • 50 million individuals in the United States have hypertension
Secondary	• Caused by an underlying disease	• Chronic kidney disease • Renovascular disease • Medication (e.g. Chronic steroid use, oral contraception, nonsteroidal anti-inflamatories, nicotine) • Cushing syndrome • Hyperaldosteronism • Obstructive sleep apnea • Coarctation of the aorta • Hyperthyroidism • Hyperparathyroidism • Pheochromocytoma	• Signs and symptoms of underlying disease or end organ damage	• Rule out secondary hypertension by evaluating for other causes • Rule out white coat hypertension by obtain-ing measurements outside of a medical environment	• Retinopathy • Hypertensive heart disease	

Table 1-6

Pharmacological Treatment Options for Hypertension

Type of Agent	Consider if (Select Conditions)	Select Contraindications/Cautions	Select Side Effects
Thiazide Diuretic	• Untreated, uncompli-cated hypertension	• Gout • Hyponatremia • Renal impairment	• Electrolyte abnormalities
Beta-Blocker	• Ischemic heart disease or stable angina • Acute coronary syn-dromes (unstable angina or myocardial infarction) • Atrial tachyarrythmias/ fibrillation • Patient is peri-operative • Essential tremor	• Asthma • Reactive airway disease • Second or third degree heart block • Bradycardia	• Depression • Bronchospasm • Erectile dysfunction
Inhibitor	• Acute coronary syn-dromes (unstable angina or myocardial infarction) • Heart failure • Diabetes • Chronic kidney disease • Stroke	• Pregnancy • History of angioedema • Renal or hepatic impairment	• Cough (can last months after discontinuation) • Hyperkalemia • Intestinal angioedema
Angiotensin Receptor Blocker	• Intolerant of ACE • Heart failure • Diabetes • Chronic kidney disease	• Pregnancy • History of angioedema • Renal or hepatic impairment	• Hyperkalemia • Rhabdomyolysis
Calcium Channel Blocker	• Raynaud's	• Second or third degree heart block • Atrial fibrillation/flutter asso-ciated with accessory bypass tract (e.g. Wolff-Parkinson-White) • Congestive heart failure • Impaired liver function	• Edema

Note: Pharmacological intervention should be combined with lifestyle modification when feasible and appropriate. Consider adding second antihypertensive agent if blood pressure not controlled with one agent.
If prehypertension, encourage lifestyle modification.

Table 1-7

Summary of Acute Coronary Syndromes (ACS)

Definition	Patients whose clinical presentations cover the following range of diagnoses: • Unstable angina • Non-ST-segment elevation myocardial infarction (MI) • ST-segment elevation MI
Epidemiology	• First manifestation often myocardial infarction or sudden death • Coronary artery disease is the leading cause of death in the United States
Etiology	• Imbalance between myocardial oxygen supply and demand
Treatment	• Symptomatic relief • Reduction of myocardial oxygen demand • Restoration of blood flow to the myocardium

Table 1-8

Causes of Chest Pain

CAUSE	SYMPTOMS	TIMING OF SYMPTOMS	WORK-UP/DIAGNOSIS

Chronic Stable Angina
 	
Unstable Angina
	• Discomfort in the:
	  - Chest
	  - Neck
	  - Jaw
	  - Back
	  - Arm (usually left)
	  - Epigastrium
	
	• Discomfort may be described as:
	  - Dull ache
	  - Sharp pain
	  - Squeezing
	  - Pressure
	  - Heaviness
	  - Burning
	  - Dyspnea
	  - Suffocation/choking
		• Provoked by exertion
		• Relieved by rest
		• Relieved by use of sublingual nitroglycerin
			• A change in the pattern of symptoms warrants further investigation.
			• Noninvasive testing for CAD adds most information when pretest probability is intermediate.
			• Appropriate stress test modality depends on information needed and patient factors.
			• Both the mode of stress and method of evaluation can be modified.

		• A change in the pattern of chronic stable angina symptoms • Chest pain may occur at rest • Chest pain not relieved by normal dose of sublingual nitroglycerin	
Non-ST-segment elevation myocardial infarction (NSTEMI) **ST-segment elevation myocardial infarction (STEMI)**		• May be worse with exertion	
Vasospastic or Prinzmetal's angina		• Unrelated to exertion	• Stress tests usually negative • Diagnosis: transient ST elevations in association with chest pain with benign ECG, telemetry, or Holter monitor.
Noncardiac causes		• May or may not be related to exertion	• Consider evaluation of gastrointestinal tract, chest wall, aorta, and lungs

CAD = coronary artery disease.

Table 1-9

Etiology of Unstable Angina and Myocardial Infarction

TYPE	ETIOLOGY	NOTES
Nonocclusive Thrombus	• Develops on a ruptured atherosclerotic plaque	• Most common etiology
Severe Coronary Artery Narrowing	• Usually caused by chronic calcified plaque	• Less frequent
Dynamic Obstruction	• Vascular and endothelial dysfunction results in intermittent epicardial coronary artery vasospasm (Prinzmetal's angina)	• Less frequent • Rarely causes infarction.
Extrinsic Conditions	• Hypotension • Hypoxemia • Anemia • Tachycardia • Thyrotoxicosis	• Less frequent

Table 1-10

Stress Test Options

MODE FOR INDUCING CARDIAC STRESS	METHOD OF INDUCING STRESS	NOTES
Exercise	• Walking/running on a treadmill	• Exercise goal: increase HR to ≥ 85% of maximum predicted value
Dobutamine	• Mimics catecholamine release with exercise	• Usually used in conjunction with echocardiography
Adenosine or Dipyrimadole (persantine)	• Coronary vasodilation	• Usually used in conjunction with myocardial perfusion imaging

HR = heart rate.

Table 1-11

Summary of Acute Treatment for ST-Segment Elevation Myocardial Infarction (STEMI)

Initial Treatment	• Aspirin • Narcotic analgesics • Intravenous nitroglycerin • Intravenous beta-blockers • Heparin
Immediate reperfusion therapy	• Thrombolysis or percutaneous coronary intervention (PCI) • Thrombolysis should be started within 30 minutes of entry to the hospital • For PCI, the infarct-related artery should be recanalized within 90 minutes • Current recommendations favor primary PCI over thrombolysis if transfer to an experienced cardiac catheterization center is feasible within 90 minutes of presentation
GP IIb/IIIa antibodies and receptor antagonists	• GP IIb/IIIa antibodies and receptor antagonists inhibit the final common pathway of platelet aggregation (the crossbridging of platelets by fibrinogen binding to the GP IIb/IIIa receptor) and may also prevent initial adhesion to the vessel wall. • Consider administration of a GP IIb/IIIa inhibitor "as early as possible" before primary PCI (with or without stenting)

GP = Glycoprotein.

Table 1-12

Anterior Versus Inferior Wall Myocardial Infarction (MI)

	CHARACTERISTIC EKG FINDINGS	**TREATMENT ISSUES**
Anterior Wall MI	ST elevation in leads V1–V6	• Avoid large amounts of fluid, especially if pulmonary edema on chest radiograph
Inferior Wall MI	ST elevation in leads II, III and AVF	• Avoid nitrates • May benefit from fluids if hypotensive

Figure 1-1

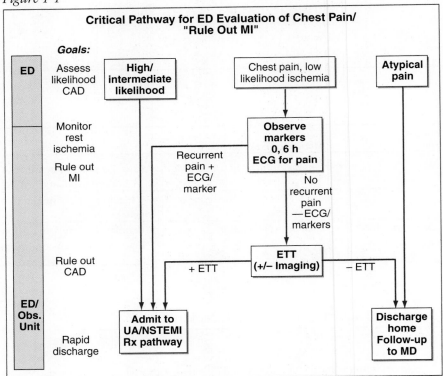

Diagnostic evaluation of patients presenting with suspected UA/NSTEMI. The first step is to assess the likelihood of coronary artery disease. Patients at high or intermediate likelihood are admitted to the hospital. Those with clearly atypical chest pain are discharged home. Patients with a *low* likelihood of ischemia enter the pathway and are observed in a monitored bed in the emergency department (ED) or observation unit over a period of 6 h and 12-lead electrocardiograms are performed if the patient has recurrent chest discomfort. A panel of cardiac markers (e.g., troponin and CK-MB) are drawn at baseline and 6 h later. If the patient develops recurrent pain, has 5T-segment or T-wave changes, or had positive cardiac markers, he/she is admitted to the hospital and treated for UA/NSTEMI. If the patient has negative markers and no recurrence of pain, he/she is sent for exercise treadmill testing, with imaging reserved for patients with abnormal baseline electrocardiograms (e.g., left bundle branch block or left ventricular hypertrophy). If positive, the patient is admitted; if negative, the patient is discharged home with follow-up to his/her primary physician, (CAD, coronary artery disease; ECG, electrocardiogram; E.D., emergency department; ETT, exercise tolerance test; MI, myocardial infarction; OBS, observation unit.) [*Adapted from CP Cannon, E Braunwald, in E Braunwald et al (eds): Heart Disease: A Textbook of Cardiovascular Medicine, 6th ed. Philadelphia, Saunders, 2001.*]

Table 1-13

Etiology of Unstable Angina and Myocardial Infarction

CLINICAL CONDITION	INDICATION FOR CATHETERIZATION
Acute Coronary Syndrome (ACS)	• ST-segment elevation MI • New LBBB in association with chest pain and new wall motion abnormalities on echocardiogram • Dynamic ST depressions • Contraindication to thrombolysis • Persistent symptoms despite anti-ischemic or thrombolytic therapy • Elevated cardiac markers • Stress test with high-risk findings • Prior coronary artery bypass surgery or coronary intervention in previous 6 months and patient presents with chest pain.
ACS with Clinical Instability	• Worsened congestive heart failure • Cardiogenic shock and hemodynamic instability • Recurrent ventricular arrhythmia • Suspicion for papillary muscle rupture
Other Clinical Conditions	• New reduced left ventricular systolic function • Class III or IV angina despite medical therapy • Sudden cardiac death survivor • Sustained ventricular tachycardia • Evaluation of valve areas

LBBB = left bundle branch block.

Table 1-14

Contraindications for Thrombolytic Therapy

Absolute Contraindications	• Hemorrhagic stroke • Nonhemorrhagic stroke or CVA in past year • Intracranial neoplasm • Active internal bleeding or active peptic ulcer disease • Suspected aortic dissection • BP > 180/110 mm Hg despite therapy
Relative Contraindications	• BP > 180/110 mm Hg initially but lowered with medication • History of proliferative diabetic retinopathy • Use of oral anticoagulant with INR ≥ 2 or known bleeding diathesis • Recent trauma or major surgery (within 4 weeks) • Noncompressible vascular puncture • CPR for greater than 10 minutes • Pregnancy • For streptokinase or anistreplase use, previous exposure or allergic reaction

CVA = cerebral vascular accident; BP = blood pressure; INR = international normalized ratio; CPR = cardiopulmonary resuscitation.

Table 1-15

Treatment Options for Angina

TYPE	NOTES
Long-Acting Nitrates	• Dilates coronary arteries
Beta-blockers (BB)	• Reduces myocardial oxygen consumption (decrease HR and BP) • Use BB if HTN, reduced LVEF, or post myocardial infarction
Calcium channel blockers (CCB)	• Avoid short-acting dihydropyridine • CCB have not been shown to reduce mortality
Percutaneous coronary intervention (PCI)	• Patients who undergo stent placement may have clopidogrel bisulfate added to their regimen Consider PCI if: • Symptoms refractory to medical therapy • Single- or double-vessel CAD
Coronary artery bypass graft (CABG)	Consider CABG if: • Severe multivessel disease • Diabetes • Similar benefit from PCI and CABG, except in diabetic patients who do better with CABG

CAD = coronary artery disease; BP = blood pressure; HR = heart rate; LVEF = left ventricular ejection fraction; HTN = hypertension.

Table 1-16

Atrial Fibrillation Versus Atrial Flutter

	CHARACTERISTIC ECG FINDINGS	GOALS OF TREATMENT	ANTICOAGULATION	PHARMACOLOGICAL TREATMENT	NONPHARMACOLOGICAL TREATMENT
Atrial Fibrillation (a-fib)	• Discrete P waves are absent • Undulating fibrillatory waves are present • The ventricular rate typically is irregular	• Goals of treatment: - Decrease risk thrombus formation in the left atria and subsequent thromboembolic events - Prevent tachycardia induced cardiomyopathy - Minimize symptoms from tachycardia - Rhythm control offers no survival advantage over rate control	• If chronic or recurrent a-fib and moderate to high to moderate risk for stroke, anticoagulate with warfarin for goal INR 2.0–3.0 • Risk factors for stroke: age, hypertension, heart failure, low ejection fraction and diabetes • Risk of stroke up to 30% in elderly • Consider aspirin alone if low risk of stroke • If unknown onset or duration >48 hours, three to four weeks of anticoagulation prior to cardioversion and at least four weeks after cardioversion	• Block calcium channel with non-dihydropyridine CCB • Decrease sympathetic tone with beta blockade • Enhancement of parasympathetic tone with vagotonic drugs (e.g. digoxin) • Consider amiodarone (slows AV nodal conduction and increases AV nodal refractoriness)	• Cardioversion may convert rhythm • Ablation may offer a long-term cure • Consider transesophageal echocardiogram (TEE) prior to cardioversion even if anticoagulated
Atrial Flutter	• Sawtooth pattern • Negative flutter waves in leads II, III, and aVF				

Note: Acute a-fib may be precipitated by infection, thyrotoxicosis, pericarditis, congestive heart failure, or pulmonary embolus. These underlying causes should be treated when present.

13

Figure 1-2 A&B

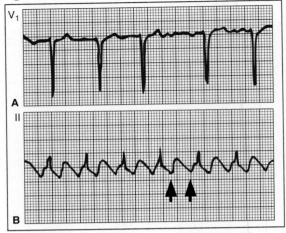

Atrial Fibrillation and Atrial Flutter. (Reproduced, with permission, from Kasper DL, Braunwald, E, Fauci, AS, Hauser SL, Longo DL, Jameson, JL, & Isselbacher KJ, Eds. *Harrison's Principles of Internal Medicine, 16th Edition.* Figure 214-5, page 1345. McGraw-Hill, Inc., 2005.)

Figure 1-3

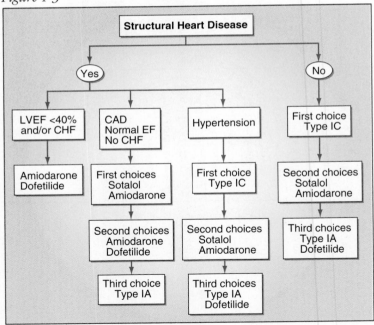

Recommendations for the Selection of Antiarrythmic Medications to Reduce the Recurrence of Atrial Fibrillation. (Reproduced, with permission, from Kasper DL, Braunwald, E, Fauci, AS, Hauser SL, Longo DL, Jameson, JL, & Isselbacher KJ, Eds. *Harrison's Principles of Internal Medicine, 16th Edition.* Figure 214-6, page 1346. McGraw-Hill, Inc., 2005.)

Table 1-17
Tachyarrhythmias

ARRHYTHMIA	ECG	MECHANISM	COMMENTS	TREATMENT
Atrio-ventricular (AV) nodal reentrant tachycardia (AVNRT)	• Regular, 160–180 bpm • Retrograde P wave usually buried in QRS	• Dual pathways in AV node with discrepant conduction velocities and refractory periods • Heart usually structurally normal	• Occurs in all age groups, but more common between 20 and 40 years • More common in women • Episodes more frequent and prolonged in older patients	• Vagal maneuvers (Valsalva, ice water, carotid massage) can terminate the arrhythmia in 80% of cases • Adenosine if vagal maneuvers fail • BB or CCB can prevent recurrence • Antiarrhythmic class IC and III (not preferred treatment) • If refractory AVNRT or drug intolerant, consider curative catheter ablation
Preexcitation syndromes (atrioventricular reentrant tachycardia such as Wolff-Parkinson-White (WPW) syndrome)	• Most with preexcitation seen on ECG (delta wave, short PR) • Most cases are narrow complex (orthodromic reentry with antegrade conduction down AV node)	• Accessory pathway connecting atria to ventricle bypasses the AV node	• Usually presents at younger ages • Increased risk for atrial and ventricular fibrillation	• Avoid AV nodal blocking agents (BB, CCB) if wide complex • If narrow complex (orthodromic), consider adenosine • Direct current (DC) cardioversion if unstable • If WPW with atrial fibrillation consider flecainide, amiodarone, procainamide, ibutilide, propafenone • Consider curative radio-frequency ablation for drug-resistant tachycardia in WPW, drug intolerance, or if patient has high-risk profession (pilots etc)

(*continued*)

Table 1-17

Tachyarrhythmias (continued)

ARRHYTHMIA	ECG	MECHANISM	COMMENTS	TREATMENT
Atrial tachycardia	• 150–250 bpm	• Can be due to reentry (most common), increased automaticity, or triggered by activity	• Consider digoxin toxicity as a cause, especially if AV block also present	• Often resistant to drug treatment • BB, CCB, antiarrhmic class Ia, Ic, and II • Ablation of atrial focus curative
Multifocal atrial tachycardia (MAT)	100–130 bpm • At least 3 different P wave morphologies on ECG	• Form of atrial tachycardia • Unknown mechanism	• Older patients • Consider underlying COPD, theophylline use or CHF	• BB, CCB if tolerated • Antiarrhythmics ineffective
Inappropriate sinus tachycardia	• 100–180 bpm • Elevated resting HR, exaggerated response to activity		• Mostly affects women • Exclude secondary causes	• Consider BB or CCB
Premature atrial contractions (PAC)			• Common, benign • Exclude secondary causes such as atrial enlargement, pressure elevation (HTN, valvular heart disease), stress, or stimulants	• Management of underlying pathology or avoidance of trigger • If symptomatic and desire therapy, BB or CCB can be used

bpm = beats per minute, HR = heart rate; CHF = congestive heart failure; COPD = chronic obstructive pulmonary disease; HTN = hypertension; AV = atrioventricular.

Figure 1-4 A-C

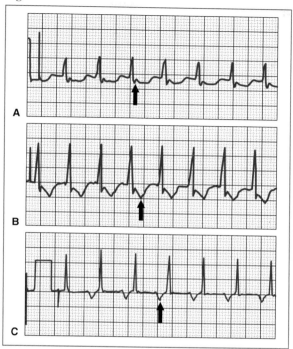

Examples of supraventricular tachycardia (SVT). Arrows indicate P waves. A. AV nodel reentry. Upright P waves are visible at the end of the QRS complex. B. AV reentry using a concealed bypass tract. Inverted retrograde P waves are superimposed on the T waves C. Automatic atrial tachycardia. Inverted P waves follow the T waves and precede the QRS complex. (Reproduced, with permission, from Kasper DL, Braunwald, E, Fauci, AS, Hauser SL, Longo DL, Jameson, JL, & Isselbacher KJ, Eds. *Harrison's Principles of Internal Medicine, 16th Edition*. Figure 214-7, page 1349. McGraw-Hill, Inc., 2005.)

Figure 1-5

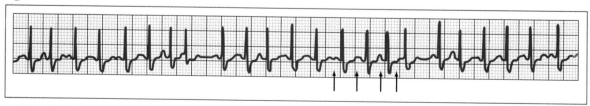

Multifocal atrial tachycardia. A lead I rhythm strip demonstrates a multifocal atrial tachycardia defined by ≥3 consec morphology and rate >100 beats/min (*arrows*). (Reproduced, with permission, from Kasper DL, Braunwald, E, Fauci, AS, Hauser SL, Longo DL, Jameson, JL, & Isselbacher KJ, Eds. *Harrison's Principles of Internal Medicine, 16th Edition*. Figure 214-9, page 1350. McGraw-Hill, Inc., 2005.)

Figure 1-6

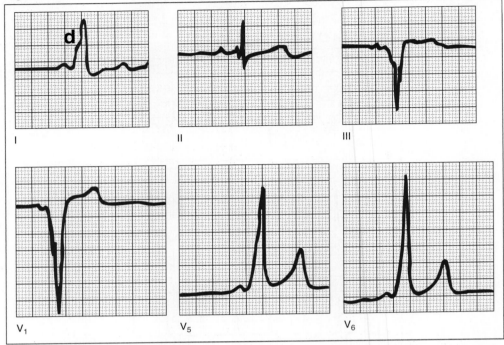

ECG in Wolf-Parkinson-White syndrome. There is a short PR Interval (0.11 s), a wide QRS complex (0.12 s), and sulrring on the upstroke of the QRS produced by early ventricular activation over the bypass tract (delta wave, d in lead I). The negative delta waves in V_1 are diagnostic of a right-sided bypass tract. Note the Q wave (negative delta wave) in lead III, mimicking myocardial infarction. (Reproduced, with permission, from Kasper DL, Braunwald, E, Fauci, AS, Hauser SL, Longo DL, Jameson, JL, & Isselbacher KJ, Eds. *Harrison's Principles of Internal Medicine, 16th Edition.* Figure 214-10, page 1350. McGraw-Hill, Inc., 2005.)

Table 1-18

Ventricular Tachycardia (VT)

TYPE OF VT	DEFINITION	NOTES
Ventricular Tachycardia (VT)	• Three or more beats of ventricular origin in succession at a rate greater than 100 beats per minute • A number of criteria help determine if a wide complex tachycardia is due to VT or SVT with aberrancy (see dedicated table)	• VT is associated with hemodynamic instability and sudden cardiac death • If there is a possibility that rhythm is VT, the arrhythmia should be treated as such because of the high mortality of untreated VT
Nonsustained VT (NSVT)	• Three or more consecutive ventricular beats but less than 30 seconds	• VT in the presence of a structurally normal heart is often catecholamine dependent and is not associated with sudden cardiac death
Sustained VT (SVT)	• Greater than 30 seconds of VT	

Table 1-18

Ventricular Tachycardia (VT) (continued)

TYPE OF VT	DEFINITION	NOTES
Monomorphic VT	• The QRS complexes in an episode of VT are identical	• Reentrant circuit around scar tissue caused by previous MI • If abnormal heart structure, consider ischemic or non-ischemic cardiomyopathy as cause
Polymorphic VT	• During VT, the QRS complexes change from beat to beat and the rhythm appears chaotic	• May be due to myocardial ischemia, electrolyte disturbances, drugs, and long QT syndrome • If normal QT, consider Brugada syndrome as cause

Figure 1-7

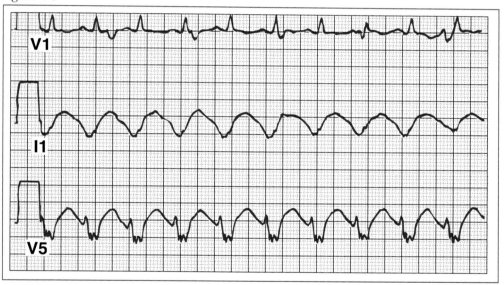

Ventricular tachycardia with AV dissociation. P waves are dissociated from the underlying wide complex rhythm (best seen on lead V₁). (Reproduced, with permission, from Kasper DL, Braunwald, E, Fauci, AS, Hauser SL, Longo DL, Jameson, JL, & Isselbacher KJ, Eds. *Harrison's Principles of Internal Medicine, 16th Edition*. Figure 214-11, page 1352. McGraw-Hill, Inc., 2005.)

Figure 1-8

Second-degree sinoatrial exit block. Surface ECG denoting abrupt absence of P wave during sinus rhythm. Prior to the pause, the sinus rate is regular. The interval of the pause is exactly twice the basal sinus cycle length. The arrow marks the appropriate location for the absent P wave. SA exit block can be 2:1 as above or longer, as shown in Fig. 213-6. (Reproduced, with permission, from Kasper DL, Braunwald, E, Fauci, AS, Hauser SL, Longo DL, Jameson, JL, & Isselbacher KJ, Eds. *Harrison's Principles of Internal Medicine, 16th Edition*. Figure 213-5, page 1335. McGraw-Hill, Inc., 2005.)

Table 1-19

Bradyarrythmias

Type	Clinical Presentation	Causes/Notes
Carotid Sinus Hypersensitivity	• Manifests as sinus arrest with syncope and dizziness	• Typically occurs in older patients with CAD
Sinus Node Dysfunction		
Sinus Bradycardia	• HR <60	• May be normal in youth, healthy adults, or in athletes Excessive vagal tone: • Vasovagal (Spontaneous bradycardia) • Acute MI (usually inferior MI) • Medications • Hypothyroidism • Increased intracranial pressure
Sinus Arrest or Exit Block	• Sinus node stops firing (arrest) or depolarization fails to exit (exit block) • Depending on duration, escape beats or rhythm may occur	• Idiopathic • Medications that suppress sinus node (beta blocker, calcium channel blocker, digitalis)
Chronotrophic Incompetence	• Normal resting HR • Unable to accelerate HR appropriately	
Tachy-brady Syndrome (Sick Sinus Syndrome)	• Bradycardia punctuated by episodes of sustained ventricular tachycardia	• If symptomatic, consider pacemaker to control bradycardia, medications to control tachycardia
Atrioventricular Block (AVB)		
First Degree AVB	• PR interval > 200ms	• Usually no treatment unless symptoms
Second Degree AVB, Mobitz Type I (Wenkebach)	• Progressively longer PR before a blocked beat • QRS narrow	• Usually no treatment unless symptoms
Second Degree AVB, Mobitz Type 2	• Stable PR interval before blocked beat • Usually wide QRS	• Consider pacemaker if symptomatic and/or advanced AVB (2 or more P waves fail to conduct)
Third Degree AVB (Complete Heart Block)	• No relationship between P waves and QRS complexes	• Pacemaker insertion indicated

Figure 1-9

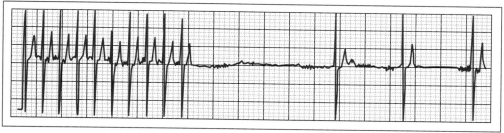

Tachycardia-bradycardia syndrome. Rhythm strip of ECG lead II showing spontaneous cessation of supraventricular tachycardia followed by a 5-s pause prior to resumption of sinus activity. The patient was asymptomatic during Supraventricular tachycardia, but the sinus pause caused severe light-headedness. (Reproduced, with permission, from Kasper DL, Braunwald, E, Fauci, AS, Hauser SL, Longo DL, Jameson, JL, & Isselbacher KJ, Eds. *Harrison's Principles of Internal Medicine, 16th Edition.* Figure 213-4, page 1335. McGraw-Hill, Inc., 2005.)

Figure 1-10 A&B

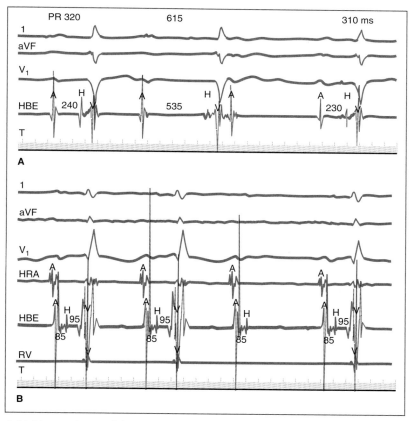

A. Mobitz type I second-degree AV block. Intracardiac recordings demonstrate that the PR prolongation (320, 615 ms) is localized to the AV node (AH 240, 535 ms, respectively). HBE, His bundle electrogram; A, atrium; H, His; V, ventricle. Time lines (T) = 100 ms. B. Mobitz type II second-degree AV block. Intracardiac recordings document block below the His bundle. During sinus rhythm right bundle branch block is present. AV nodal conduction is normal (AH, 85 ms), but His-Purkinje conduction is markedly prolonged (HV, 95 ms). The third sinus P wave suddenly blocks below the recorded His deflection without any preceeding change in AV conduction. *(From ME Josephson, Clinical Cardiac Electrophysiology: Techniques and Interpretations, 3d ed. Philadelphia, Lippincott Williams & Wilkins 2002, with permission.)*

Figure 1-11

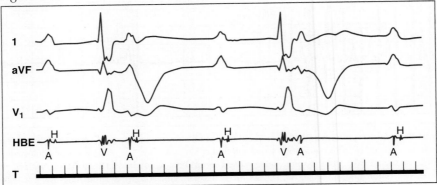

Third-degree AV block. The figure shows surface leads 1, aVF, V₁, and an intracardiac. His bundle recording (HBE). Complete heart block is evident on the surface leads. The intracardiac recording demonstrates an absence of QRS deflection (V) after a His bundle (H) spike. This indicates block below the His bundle. Note that following the second QRS complex (V), there is an atrial (A) deflection indicating retrograde conduction. Retrograde conduction is often present when block is in the His-Purkinje system but is virtually never present when block is in the AV node. *(From ME Josephson, Clinical Cardiac Electrophysiology: Techniques and Interpretations, 3d ed. Philadelphia, Lippincott Williams & Wilkins, 2002, with permission.)*

Table 1-20

Toxicity of Frequently Used Antiarrythmic Agents

DRUG	NONARRHYTHMIC TOXICITY	PROARRHYTHMIC TOXICITY			
		TDP[a]	A FLUTTER 1:1	VT/VF	BRADYCARDIA
Digoxin	Anorexia, nausea, vomiting, visual changes	Atrial tachycardia, VT, AV nodal block, accelerated junctional rhythms, atrial and ventricular prema ture depolarizations; acceleration of ventricular rate during atrial fibrillation or flutter in the presence of preexcitation			
Quinidine[b]	Anorexia, nausea, vomiting, diarrhea, cinchonism, tinnitus, hearing and visual changes, thrombocytopenia, hemolytic anemia, rash, potentiation of digoxin levels	2%	++	++	+
Procainamide[b]	Lupus erythematosus-like syndrome, anorexia, nausea	2%	+	++	+
Disopyramide[b]	Anticholinergic actions: dry mouth, urinary retention, visual disturbances (avoid in narrow-angle glaucoma) constipation, congestive heart failure	2%	+	++	+
Lidocaine	Dizziness, confusion, delirium, seizures, coma; side effects potentiated by liver and heart failure	–	–	–	+[b]
Mexiletine	Ataxia, tremor, gait disturbances, rash, vomiting	–	–	–	–
Flecainide	Dizziness, nausea	Rare	+++	++	++
Propafenone[c]	Taste disturbance, bronchospasm	Rare	+++	++	++

Table 1-20

Toxicity of Frequently Used Antiarrythmic Agents (continued)

DRUG	NONARRHYTHMIC TOXICITY	PROARRHYTHMIC TOXICITY			
		TDPa	A FLUTTER 1:1	VT/VF	BRADYCARDIA
Amiodarone	Pulmonary infiltrates and fibrosis, hepatitis, hypo- and hyperthyroidism, photosensitivity, peripheral neuropathy, tremor	Rare	+++	+++	+++
Sotalol	Bronchospasm	+++	+	+	+++

aTDP (torsades de pointes) occurs most often in the setting of slow heart rates, QT prolongation, and hypokalemia or hypomagnesemia and at the time of conversion from atrial fibrillation to sinus rhythm. OT prolongation and torsades de pointes are not dose-related phenomena. QRS prolongation is a dose-related phenomenon also and will occur at toxic concentrations. QT and WRS intervals should be monitored and dose reductions made for interval prolongations.

bMay suppress sinus node function in patients with underlying sinus node dysfunction. May suppress escape foci in patients with complete heart block.

cAvoid in patients with prior myocardial infarction and depressed left ventricular function. Use in combination with AV nodal blocking agent to limit risk of atrial flutter with 1:1 conduction.

Note: A flutter 1:1, atrial flutter with 1:1 atrioventricular (AV) conduction; VT/VF, ventricular tachycardia/ventricular fibrillation.

(Reproduced, with permission, from Kasper DL, Braunwald, E, Fauci, AS, Hauser SL, Longo DL, Jameson, JL, & Isselbacher KJ, Eds. Harrison's Principles of Internal Medicine, 16th Edition. Table 214-8, page 1356. McGraw-Hill, Inc., 2005.).

Table 1-21

Indications for Pacemaker Insertion for Bradyarrythmias

CATEGORY	INDICATION
Cardiac Evaluation	• Pause >3 seconds during carotid sinus massage in patients with syncope • Heart rate <30 beats per minute while awake • Third degree AVB (complete heart block)
Symptoms • Dizziness • Fatigue • Dyspnea • Presyncope or syncope	• Symptomatic bradycardia at rest • Symptomatic with exercise intolerance

Table 1-22

Summary of Syncope

Definition of Syncope	• Transient loss of consciousness
Etiology	• Neurocardiogenic syncope is a common cause of syncope in the absence of a cardiac arrhythmia or structural heart disease
Diagnosis	• History and physical examination alone identify the probable cause of syncope in about 50% of cases • Pertinent history: triggers, associated symptoms, witness accounts, medical conditions, detailed medication history, and family history • A history of seizure disorder, prolonged confusion after awakening (postictal state) or prolonged seizure-like muscular activity should prompt further neurological work-up
Prognosis	• In the absence of structural heart disease, syncope and near-syncope are generally benign

Table 1-23

Causes of Syncope

ETIOLOGY	TYPE	EXAMPLE
Cardiac	Electrical	• Tachycardia (ventricular tachycardia, Torsades de pointes, supraventricular tachycardia) • Bradycardia (sick sinus syndrome, second or third-degree AV block (Stokes-Adams attack)) • Pacemaker failure

	Mechanical	• Outflow obstruction
		  - Left-sided (atrial stenosis, hypertrophic obstructive cardiomyopathy, mitral stenosis, left atrial myxoma)
		  - Right-sided (pulmonary stenosis, pulmonary embolism, pulmonary HTN)
		  - Myocardial (coronary artery disease, left ventricular dysfunction)
		  - Tamponade

Extra-Cardiac	Neurocardiogenic	• Vasovagal (50%) • Situational/visceral (micturition, defecation, cough, ocular pressure) • Carotid sinus syncope • Psychiatric (somatization, anxiety, panic) • Other (exercise, high-altitude, drug-induced) • Cervical spondylosis
	Vascular	• Vertebrobasilar TIA/stroke • Subarachnoid hemorrhage • Subclavian steal syndrome
	Metabolic	• Hypoxia • Hypoglycemia • Hypocapnia
	Orthostatic hypotension	• Drug-induced (e.g. antihypertensives) • Venous pooling (postural, pregnancy) • Autonomic neuropathy (primary: Shy-Drager, secondary: Diabetes mellitus) • Hypovolemia (blood loss, diuresis) • Pheochromocytoma

AV = atrioventricular; LV = left ventricular; HTN = hypertension; TIA = transient ischemic attack.

Table 1-24

Heart Failure

Definition	• A clinical syndrome caused by either a structural or functional cardiac disorder that impairs ventricular filling and/or ejection such that the metabolic demands of the tissue are unmet
Epidemiology	• Single largest cardiovascular health care expenditure in the United States • Affects approximately 5 million people • 30–50% of patients with heart failure die of sudden cardiac death due to arrhythmia
Etiology	• Up to 70% of all heart failure is caused by coronary artery disease and resultant ischemic cardiomyopathy. This category of heart failure portends the poorest prognosis
Symptoms	• Dyspnea on exertion • Orthopnea • Paroxysmal nocturnal dyspnea • Cough • Fatigue • Decreased mental acuity • Orthopnea • Paroxysmal nocturnal dyspnea
Diagnosis	• Evaluation should focus upon determination of volume status and functional capacity • Echocardiogram to determine left ventricular ejection fraction, presence of valvular disease, and to classify the patient as having either systolic or diastolic dysfunction • 12-lead ECG may reveal evidence of prior MI, ischemia, conduction disturbances, or arrhythmias • Screening for diabetes and hypertension should be considered • Radionuclide stress testing to determine whether reversible ischemia exists • Consider coronary angiography/percutaneous coronary intervention if atherosclerotic cardiovascular disease is suspected as a cause of heart failure

Table 1-25
Heart Failure: Clinical Presentation and Treatment

TYPE	ETIOLOGY	CLINICAL NOTES	TREATMENT

Systolic Dysfunction	Coronary artery disease/ischemic cardiomyopathy	• Symptoms of heart failure
		• Pulmonary and/or peripheral edema
		• Right ventricular heave if right-sided heart failure present
		• S3 gallop
		• Laterally displaced PMI (point of maximal impulse)
		• Elevated jugular venous pressure
		• Increased left ventricular cavity size on echocardiogram with segmental or global hypokinesis
			• Primary Therapeutic Interventions:
			  - Decrease sodium intake
			  - Fluid restriction (<2 L/day)
			  - Beta blockers (carvedilol or metoprolol)
			  - ACE inhibitor (first choice) or ARB for EF <40% or post-myocardial infarction
			  - Diuretics to achieve euvolemia (e.g. loop diuretics)
			  - Beta blockers (carvedilol or metoprolol)
			  - Consider digoxin
			  - Hydralazine/long-acting nitrate for those unable to tolerate ACE inhibitors
			  - Secondary prevention, including aspirin and lipid-lowering therapy
			  - Consider empiric ICD if prior MI and EF ≤30%
			• Acute treatment for severe heart failure:
			  - Intravenous ionotropes (dopamine, dobutamine, milrinone)
			  - Nesiritide (intravenous B-type natriuretic peptide)
			• Other treatment considerations
			  - Consider biventricular pacing for refractory symptoms, EF <35% or QRS >120 ms
			  - Cardiac transplantation
			  - Anticoagulation controversial for low EF

Table 1-25

Heart Failure: Clinical Presentation and Treatment (continued)

TYPE	ETIOLOGY	CLINICAL NOTES	TREATMENT
Systolic Dysfunction (cont.)	Nonischemic (30%) • Valvular disease • Viral • Hypertension • Alcohol • Inherited • Drug-induced • Autoimmune disease • Connective tissue diseases (amyloidosis/sarcoidosis) • Hemochromatosis • Hypo- or hyper-thyroidism • Idiopathic	• As above	• Correct underlying disease • Abstain from alcohol • Frequent spontaneous resolution if viral etiology • Pharmacotherapy same as ischemic cardiomyopathy

Diastolic Dysfunction (30–50% of All Cases)	• HTN
	• Valvular disease (e.g. atrial stenosis)
	• Hypertrophic cardiomyopathy
	• Infiltrative cardiomyopathy
		• Symptoms of heart failure
		• Elevated JVP
		• S4 gallop common
		• S3 less common
		• Pulmonary vascular congestion
		• Pulmonary vascular congestion
		• EF > 40% with normal contractility on echocardiogram and normal left ventricular cavity size
		• Symptoms of heart failure
		• Other findings depend on underlying cause
			• Increase LV filling time with negative chronotropes (e.g. beta-blockers)
			• Other antihypertensives:
			  - ACE inhibitors
			  - HCTZ
			  - Spironolactone
			  - Rule out CAD with ischemia work-up

High Output	• Large peripheral shunts • Hyperthyroidism • Beri beri • Carcinoid Syndrome • Anemia	• Symptoms of heart failure • Anorexia • Nausea • Right ventricular heave • Elevated JVP • Peripheral edema • Edema of visceral organs (liver)	• Treatment of underlying cause

(continued)

Table 1-25

Heart Failure: Clinical Presentation and Treatment (continued)

Type	Etiology	Clinical Notes	Treatment
Right Ventricular Failure	• Pulmonary HTN (cor pulmonale) • Pulmonic stenosis • Prior right ventricular infarct • Right ventricular dysplasia • Often secondary to left-sided hear failure	• Presentation depends on underlying etiology	• Goal: euvolemia (usually achieved with diuretics) • Nitrates • Calcium channel blockers • If secondary to pulmonary hypertension, consider oxygen therapy to relieve cor pulmonale, if present

MI = myocardial infarction; CAD = coronary artery disease; EF = ejection fraction; ICD = implantable cardiac-defibrillator; JVP = jugular venous pressure; HTN = hypertension; ACE = angiotensin-converting enzyme (ACE) inhibitors; ARB = Angiotensin II Receptor Blockers; HCTZ = hydrochlorothiazide.

Table 1-26

Acute Heart Failure and Shock

Definition	Acute heart failure associated with hypoxemia and hypotension	
Treatment Options	**General**	• May require intubation and intravenous vasopressors (norepineph rine, dobutamine, dopamine) to maintain oxygenation and cardiac output
	Intra-aortic balloon pump	**Indications:** • Imminent or frank pump failure (systolic blood pressure cannot be adequately maintained despite the use of vasopressors) • Acute mitral regurgitation • Unstable angina refractory to medications **Contraindications:** • Moderate to severe aortic insufficiency • Presence of aortic dissection or a prosthetic aortic graft • Severe aortic or iliac atherosclerotic disease **Mechanism:** • The balloon pump is inserted into the thoracic aorta • Balloon fills during diastole, thereby increasing coronary blood flow by "backfilling" • Balloon deflates during systole, decreasing afterload and prompting forward flow • The overall effect reduces myocardial work and oxygen consumption

Table 1-27

Acute Heart Failure and Shock

World-Wide Epidemiology	• Rheumatic heart disease remains a major cause of valvular heart disease throughout the underdeveloped world • Rheumatic heart disease (usually mitral stenosis or aortic stenosis) is preventable • For patients with a history of rheumatic fever, every episode of streptococcal pharyngitis increases risk for further valve damage. Treat with prophylactic antibiotics (benzathine penicillin G IM every 4 weeks or penicillin V twice a day) for 10 years after the last episode or until age 40 years
Medical Management	• Monitor disease progression • Relieve symptoms • Appropriate timing of surgical intervention • Infective endocarditis prophylaxis for procedures with a high risk of bacteremia as per current guidelines
Valve Surgery	General indications: • Symptomatic patients • Evidence of systolic dysfunction • Increased LV dimension • Pulmonary hypertension • Surgery should be done before disease progression makes operative risks too high and before irreversible heart damage. However, performing surgery too early can expose the patient to unnecessary risks and may require reoperation to replace worn-out prosthetic valve. Optimal timing of surgery can be difficult to determine
Prognosis	• Gradually developing chronic lesions may be well tolerated for years • Acute valve failure due to dissection, endocarditis, or papillary muscle rupture can be rapidly fatal and often requires emergent surgery (left ventricle does not have time to compensate)

Table 1-28

Choice of Prosthetic Valve for Valve Replacement

Type of Valve	Disadvantage	Advantage	Notes
Mechanical	• Requires anticoagulation • Similar risk of endocarditis compared to bioprosthetic	• Increased durability compared to bioprosthetic	• Often implanted in younger patients to delay reoperation as long as possible and in older patients who require anticoagulation for another condition • Infective endocarditis prophylaxis for procedures with a high risk of bacteremia as per current guidelines
Bioprosthetic	• Shorter lifespan than mechanical valves • Similar risk of endocarditis compared to mechanical	• Does not require anticoagulation	• Implanted when anticoagulation is contraindicated or in older patients with a relatively short life expectancy • Infective endocarditis prophylaxis for procedures with a high risk of bacteremia as per current guidelines

Table 1-29

Types of Valvular Disease, Symptoms, Murmur Characteristics, Etiology, and Treatment

Type	Symptoms	Murmur		Associated Findings	Etiology	Treatment
		Character and Timing	Maneuvers to Highlight Murmur			
Innocent Flow Murmur	• None	• Soft • Ejection • Mid-systolic • Beats heard at base or mid-LSB	• None	• None	• Advanced age • High flow state (anemia, pregnancy)	• None

Aortic Stenosis (AS)	• May be asymptomatic
	• Angina
	• Exertional syncope
	• Dyspnea
		• Harsh
		• Mid-systolic
		• Crescendo-decrescendo (diamond shaped)
		• Late-peaking if more severe
		• Radiation to carotids
		• Best heard at right 2nd ICS
		• High-pitched, blowing
			• Decreases with handgrip or standing	• Paradoxical split S2
				• Pulsus parvuset tardus (the pulse wave comes much later than the heartbeat)
				• Sustained apical impulse
				• ECG:
				  - LVH
				• Echocardiogram:
				  - Shows obstructed orifice
					• Degenerative calcification of the aortic cusps
					• Age related degeneration most common cause
					• Congenital
						• Surgery when valve area < 1.0 cm², symptomatic or LV dysfunction (age and decreased EF are not contraindications).
						• Noncardiac surgery on AS patients requires careful hemodynamic monitoring.

Aortic Regurgitation (AR)	• DOE • Fatigue • PND	• Diastolic • Decrescendo • Austin-Flint murmur (low-pitched mid-systolic murmur at apex) • Best heard at LSB	• Loudest at end-expiration with patient leaning forward • Increase in left lateral decubitus position and with exercise	• Apical impulse forceful and displaced downward and laterally • Wide pulse pressure • "Water-hammer pulse" • ECG: - LVH	• Rheumatic disease • Congenital bicuspid valve • May be secondary to endocarditis or trauma • Connective tissue disease (Marfan) • More frequent in men	• Vasodilators (nifedipine, ACE inhibitor, hydralazine) • AVR if symptomatic (after onset of LV dysfunction but before severe symptoms)

(continued)

Table 1-29

Types of Valvular Disease, Symptoms, Murmur Characteristics, Etiology, and Treatment (continued)

| TYPE | SYMPTOMS | MURMUR | | ASSOCIATED FINDINGS | ETIOLOGY | TREATMENT |
		CHARACTER AND TIMING	MANEUVERS TO HIGHLIGHT MURMUR			
Mitral Stenosis (MS)	• Dyspnea • Cough • Pulmonary edema • Symptoms exacerbated by: - Exercise - Stress - Fever - Pregnancy	• Diastolic • Low-pitched rumbling • Best heard at apex • Opening snap	• Increase in left lateral decubitus position and with exercise	• Valves are "fish-mouthed" • Echocardiogram: - Evaluate mitral orifice size • ECG: - LAA ("P-mitrale") - Atrial fibrillation - RVH if pulmonary HTN present (Right ventricular systolic pressure >40 mm Hg)	• 40% of patients with rheumatic disease • Valves are diffusely thickened • More frequent in women	• Diuretics may improve symptoms • Beta-blockers and digoxin to slow heart rate if AF • Valvotomy if symptomatic and no contraindications • MVR if significant associated mitral regurgitation
Mitral Regurgitation (MR)	• DOE • Fatigue • PND • Pulmonary edema if acute	• Blowing • Holosystolic • Radiates to axilla • Best heard at apex		• Hyperdynamic apical impulse • S3 • ECG: - LAA - Atrial fibrillation, especially if chronic	• Often results from ischemia • May be secondary to mitral valve prolapse (most common cause requiring MR surgery) • May be congenital • Often progressive	• Limit exertion • Diuretics and vasodilators to relieve symptoms • MV repair or replacement if severe symptoms and no contraindications

LSB = left sternal boarder; ICS = Intercostal Space; CHF = congestive heart failure; LVH = Left ventricular hypertrophy; CAD = coronary artery disease; EF = ejection fraction; LA = left atrial; MR = mitral regurgitation; AVR = Atrial valve replacement; MVR = mitral valve replacement; HTN = hypertension; MV = mitral valve, LV = left ventricular; PND = paroxysmal nocturnal dyspnea; DOE = dyspnea on exertion; MVP = mitral valve prolapse; ACE = angiotensin-converting enzyme; ARB = Angiotensin II Receptor Blockers; LAA = Left atrial abnormality.

Table 1-30

Less Common Valvular Diseases and Murmurs

Type	Symptoms	Murmur		Associated Findings	Etiology	Treatment
		Character and Timing	Maneuvers to Highlight Murmur			
Tricuspid Regurgitation	• RHF • Usually occurs secondary to LHF	• Holosystolic • Blowing • Best heard at LLSB	• Increases with inspiration (Carvallo's sign)	• Atrial fibrillation • Hepatic pulsation	• Usually occurs secondary to pulmonary HTN and LHF • Dilation of tricuspid annulus	• Diuretics • Treatment of left-sided heart disease if present
Tricuspid Stenosis (TS)	• Symptoms of mitral stenosis (usually develops before TS) • Pulmonary congestion	• Diastolic • Low-pitched rumble	• Increases with inspiration • Reduced with valsalva	• RV heave • Giant jugular a-wave (a-wave is produced by atrial contraction) • EKG: - Right atrial enlargement - No RVH (if isolated TS)	• Associated with mitral stenosis	• Diuretics • Valvotomy or valve replacement
Ventricular Septal Defect (VSD)		• Murmur of aortic regurgitation			• Post MI • Endocarditis • Congenital	• Emergent surgery caused by myocardial infarction or endocarditis • See congenital VSD
Pulmonic Regurgitation		• High pitched • Diastolic • Decrescendo			• Secondary to pulmonary HTN (dilation of pulmonary annulus)	• Treatment rarely indicated

ICS = intercostal space; LLSB = Left lower sternal border' LUSB = Left upper sternal border' RLSB = Right lower sternal border; LAA = Left atrial abnormality; LVH = Left ventricular hypertrophy; RAA = Right atrial abnormality; RHF = right heart failure; LHF = left heart failure; MI = myocardial infarction; HTN = hypertension.

Table 1-31

Summary of Adult Congenital Heart Disease (CHD)

ISSUE	NOTES
Uncorrected CHD in Adults	• Usually less severe because the patient has either been asymptomatic and undiagnosed throughout childhood or was diagnosed but has not required intervention
Eisenmenger's Syndrome	• Congenital left-to-right shunt causing pulmonary hypertension resulting in shunt reversal, right-to-left shunt and cyanosis
Management	• The most important decision is deciding if and when repair is needed • Infective endocarditis prophylaxis for procedures with a high risk of bacteremia as per current guidelines • Management of cardiac complications and pulmonary hypertension • Cyanotic patients may develop erythrocytosis. Can be treated with phlebotomy if symptoms of hyperviscosity or hematocrit >65%
Prognosis	• After right-to-left shunting occurs, lesions are generally inoperable and carry a poor prognosis • Patients who have undergone repair before the development of pulmonary hypertension usually have a good prognosis and can lead normal lives • Risks following surgical repair are repair failure, pulmonary hypertension, heart failure, endocarditis, and arrhythmias

Table 1-32
Uncorrected Acyanotic Congenital Heart Disease (CHD) in Adulthood

DISEASE	CLINICAL PRESENTATION		NOTES
	SYSTEMIC FINDINGS	CARDIAC FINDINGS	
Atrial Septal Defect (ASD)	• Pulmonary hypertension (HTN) • Paradoxical embolus if reversal of shunt • Cyanosis and clubbing if right-to-left shunt	• Fixed, widely split S2 • Atrial arrhythmias and first degree heart block • Bidirectional, then right-to-left shunting of blood • Right ventricular dilation • Heart failure	• 2nd most common CHD in adults after bicuspid aortic valve • Occurs more often in women • Patients usually asymptomatic until 4th decade of life • Consider repair if significant shunt
Ventricular Septal Defect (VSD)	• Pulmonary HTN • Eisenmenger syndrome (pulmonary vascular obstruction) • Cyanosis and clubbing if right-to-left shunt	• Wide spectrum of findings • Aortic regurgitation • Heart failure	• Functional compromise depends on size of VSD • Most large defects found (and repaired) in childhood • The degree to which pulmonary vascular resistance is elevated before VSD repair determines postoperative outcome • Consider repair if significant shunt
Patent Ductus Arteriosus (PDA)	• Pulmonary HTN • Eisenmenger syndrome • Differential cyanosis (toes, but not fingers, are cyanotic)	• Continuous machine-like murmur	Associated causes of mortality in adults: • Cardiac failure • Endocarditis • Consider repair if significant shunt
Aortic Coarctation (Narrowing of Lumen)	• Radial to femoral pulse delay (any appreciable delay in the femoral pulse compared to the radial pulse when both are palpated simultaneously) • Headache • Cold extremities • Notching of the ribs on CXR due to erosion by dilated collateral vessels	• ECG: - Left ventricular hypertrophy	• Associated with gonadal dysgenesis • Most adults with isolated coarctation are asymptomatic • Consider repair
Pulmonary Stenosis (PS)	• Usually asymptomatic • Right heart failure if severe • Dyspnea on exertion • Fatigue	• Systolic high-pitched crescendo-decrescendo murmur best heard at left 2nd intercostals space • Valve opening click • ECG: - Right ventricular hypertrophy	• May present in pregnancy • PS complicated by other abnormalities may lead to cyanosis

HTN = hypertension; ECG = electrocardiogram; CXR = chest radiograph.

Table 1-33
Aortic Disease

TYPE	PATHOPHYSIOLOGY/ RISK FACTORS	CLINICAL PRESENTATION		DIAGNOSIS	MANAGEMENT
		SYMPTOMS	SIGNS		
Aortic Dissection • **Type A: ascending aorta involved** • **Type B: only descending aorta involved**	• Hypertension (in 70%) • Cystic medial necrosis (collagen and elastic fiber degeneration in the tunica media of the aorta) • Male • Blunt chest trauma	• Acute chest pain • Tearing upper back pain	• Hypotension • Blood pressure and pulse differential (Differences in the blood pressure and pulse between the right and left arms, or between the arms and the legs). • Atrial regurgitation if proximal dissection	• Wide mediastinum on CXR • To visualize intimal flap: - TEE (TTE with poorer sensitivity) - CT angiogram/MRI	• Aggressive antihypertensive therapy with beta-blocker or calcium channel blocker • Type A: Emergency surgery • Type B: Medical management unless complicated or progressive
Thoracic Aortic Aneurysm	• Atherosclerosis (most common) • Cystic medial necrosis • Hypertension	• Usually none • Compression of local structures may cause pain, cough, hoarseness	• Unequal pulses and BP in upper extremities	• CT • MRI • TEE (TTE has poor sensitivity)	• Surgery if diameter > 6.0 cm or increasing at > 1 cm/year

Abdominal Aortic Aneurysm	• Male • Risk factors for atherosclerosis (age, smoking etc.) • Family history	• Usually none • Abdominal pain may signal impending rupture • Palpable, pulsatile mass in abdomen	• Ultrasound • CT or MRA	• Risk of rupture low if less than 5 cm in diameter • Operate/percutaneous stenting if > 5.5 cm diameter • Mortality of acute rupture (even with surgical intervention) is >50%
Marfan's Syndrome	• Autosomal dominant genetic disease of fibrillin • Family history	Clinical Triad • Aortic aneurysm (typically begins at aortic base) • Lens dislocation (reduced vision) • Long, thin extremities with loose joints and arachnodactyly (long spider-like fingers and toes) • Rate of dilatation of aneurysm unpredictable • Often have mitral and tricuspid prolapse	• DNA gene testing • Echocardiogram	• Beta-blockers to reduce blood pressure may delay aortic dilatation • Follow with echocardiogram for aneurysm • Consider surgical repair of cardiovascular manifestations • Screen first-degree relatives

CT = computed tomography; MRI = magnetic resonance imaging; TEE = transesophageal echocardiogram; TTE = transthoracic echocardiogram; mm = millimeter; CXR = chest radiograph; DNA = Deoxyribonucleic acid.

Table 1-34

Pericarditis and Cardiac Tamponade

The pericardial sac surrounds the heart. It allows the heart to move during contraction and accommodates enlargement of the cardiac chambers during diastolic filling.

DIAGNOSIS	PATHOPHYSIOLOGY	ETIOLOGY	SIGNS/SYMPTOMS	FINDINGS	TREATMENT
Acute Pericarditis	• Inflammation or irritation of the pericardium	• For both pericarditis and temponade Infection: - Viral (Coxsackie A, B) - Bacterial (staph, strep) - Fungal (histoplasmosis, blastomycosis) - Tuberculosis - Neoplasm • Postmyocardial infarction - Acute: occurs 1–7 days after MI and is result of extension of inflammation - Dressler's: occurs 2–8 days after MI and has autoimmune etiology	• Pleuritic chest pain that improves with leaning forward • Tachypnea and tachycardia • Malaise • Diaphoresis • Mild troponin elevation if myocarditis also present • Pericardial rub (A rubbing sound heard on auscultation of the heart due to the friction between visceral and parietal pericardial layers)	• Diffuse ST elevation, PR depression	• Echo within first 24 hours to assess for effusion (occurs in 50% of patients) • Risk of tamponade in 15% of acute cases • NSAIDs for 2–4 weeks • Steroids as second-line (may experience recurrence of pericarditis after rapid discontinuation) • Outpatient treatment if no effusion

Cardiac Tamponade				

• Clinical diagnosis
• Pericardial pressure > cardiac filling pressure
• Large volumes of pericardial fluid can be tolerated if they accumulate slowly
	• Metabolic (uremia, hypothyroidism)
	• Collagen vascular disease (SLE, scleroderma)
	• For tamponade, additional etiologies:
	  - Trauma
	  - Aortic dissection
		• Pulsus paradoxus (drop in systolic blood pressure during inspiration > 10 mm Hg)
		• Tachycardia and tachypnea
		Beck's triad:
		• Hypotension
		• Muffled heart sounds
		• JVD
			• ECG:
			  - Low-voltage
			  - Electrical alternans
			• Echocardiogram:
			  - Right atrium and ventricle diastolic collapse
			  - Dilated inferior vena cava
			• CXR:
			  - Water bottle silhouette
			  - Right heart catheterization:
			  - Equalization of diastolic pressures
				• Pericardiocentesis with or without pericardiotomy
				• Avoid diuretics and vasodilators
				• Treat underlying cause
				• Fluid administration

Table 1-34

Pericarditis and Cardiac Tamponade (continued)

Diagnosis	Pathophysiology	Etiology	Signs/Symptoms	Findings	Treatment
Constrictive Pericarditis	• Fibrosed, thickened, adherent and/or calcified pericardium	• Any cause of acute pericarditis may result in constrictive pericarditis Major causes: • Tuberculosis • Radiation-induced • Post-cardiotomy • Idiopathic	• May mimic CHF (hepatosplenomegaly, edema, ascites) • Dyspnea • Fatigue • Palpitations • Kussmaul's sign (paradoxical increase in JVP with inspiration)	ECG: • Low voltage • Flat T wave CXR: • Pericardial calcification • Effusions CT/MRI/TEE: • Pericardial thickening Cardiac catheterization: • Equalization of diastolic pressures	• Pericardiectomy is the treatment of choice

CXR = chest radiograph; EKG = electrocardiogram; CT = computed tomography; MRI = magnetic resonance imaging; TEE = transesophageal echocardiogram; CHF=congestive heart failure; JVP = jugular venous pressure; SLE = Systemic Lupus Erythematosus; Staph = Staphylococcus; Strep = Streptococcal.

Table 1-35

Restrictive and Hypertrophic Cardiomyopathy

DIAGNOSIS	PATHOPHYSIOLOGY	ETIOLOGY	CLINICAL PRESENTATION	FINDINGS	TREATMENT
Restrictive Cardiomyopathy	• Reduction in ventricular compliance • Usually due to infiltrative process • Reduced filling of heart chambers • Pulmonary and venous congestion	• Amyloidosis • Sarcoidosis • Hemochromatosis • Scleroderma	• Dyspnea • Exercise intolerance • Fatigue • JVD • Hepatosplenomegaly • Ascites • Edema	ECG: • Low voltage Echocardiogram: • Nondilated, nonhypertrophied ventricles with preserved ejection fraction • Biatrial enlargement • Diastolic dysfunction Catheterization: • Elevated pulmonary artery pressures • Ventricular pressures do not equalize during diastole	• Diuretics as tolerated (patients require high preload to maintain cardiac output) • Conduction abnormalities frequent (especially in amyloid cardiomyopathy) and often preclude use of nodal blocking agents such as digitalis and calcium channel blocker • Stroke volume small and fixed, and adequate cardiac output depends on fast enough heart rate

(continued)

Table 1-35

Restrictive and Hypertrophic Cardiomyopathy (continued)

Diagnosis	Pathophysiology	Etiology	Clinical Presentation	Findings	Treatment
Hypertrophic obstructive cardiomyopathy (HOCM)	• Hypertrophic cardiomyopathy subtype • Thickening of myocardium decreases chamber size and reduces filling of chamber • Septal thickening causes obstruction with left ventricular outflow tract (LVOT) obstruction • Obstruction variable and exacerbated when decreased preload brings the septum closer into the LVOT	• Genetic disease of the cardiac sarcomere	• Dyspnea and chest pain on exertion • Postexertional syncope • Sudden cardiac death (1%/y) • Prominent apical impulse • S4 Murmur: • Late-peaking systolic crescendo murmur • Best heard at apex and lower left sternal border • Radiation to axilla and base • Louder with decreased preload (valsalva) and softer with hand-grip	ECG: • LVH Echocardiogram: • LVOT obstruction	Medications with negative inotropic and negative chrono-tropic properties • Beta-blockers • Nondihydropiridine calcium channel blockers • Disopyra Other: • Surgical septal myomectomy • Percutaneous septal ablation with alcohol • Consider AICD if syncope, VT or family history of sudden cardiac death • Avoid intense exercise

AICD = automatic implantable cardioverter defibrillators; VT = ventricular tachycardia; LVH = left ventricular hypertrophy; JVD = jugular venous distension; ECG = electrocardiogram.

Table 1-36

Summary of Peripheral Vascular Disease (PVD)

ISSUE	NOTES
Epidemiology/Risk Factors	• Similar to those for coronary artery disease
Clinical Presentation	• Asymptomatic (>50%) • Claudication (pain in the legs with walking (primarily in the calves) that is relieved by rest) in about 1/3 • Critical leg ischemia (ischemic pain in the distal foot at rest, ischemic ulceration, or gangrene) in 5–10%
Diagnosis	• Diagnostic of PVD: Ankle-brachial index (ABI) ≤ 0.9 • Advanced ischemia: ABI ratio < 0.4 • Evaluate for PVD if patient at increased risk: age or presence of atherosclerotic risk factors, leg symptoms on exertion, or distal limb ulceration without obvious explanation

Table 1-37

Treatment of Peripheral Vascular Disease (PVD)

TYPE OF INTERVENTION	INTERVENTION SPECIFICS	PURPOSE
Cardiovascular Risk Factors	Risk factor modification goals: • Smoking cessation • LDL < 100 mg/dL • HgbA1c < 7.0% • BP < 130/85 • ACE inhibitor • Antiplatelet therapy	• Slower progression of PVD • Reduction of cardiac events • Helps prevent ischemic events independent of BP • At least one agent recommended in all suitable patients Agents: • Aspirin • Clopidogrel Bisulfate irreversible blocks the adenosine diphosphate (ADP) receptor on platelet cell membrane • Contraindicated if bleeding risk
Claudication Therapy	• Supervised exercise	• Improvement of walking distance
	• Cilostazol	• Improvement of walking distance • Cilostazol is an inhibitor of phosphodiesterase III • Contraindicated in patients with CHF and bleeding disorders
Revascularization: **(If critical leg ischemia or disabling symptoms despite medical therapy)**	• Angioplasty • Bypass surgery	• Improves symptoms by restoring blood flow • Less morbidity than bypass surgery • Proximal lesions have better patency rates
		• Improves symptoms by restoring blood flow • Use of prosthetic material reduces 5-year patency rates

BP = blood pressure, LDL = low density lipoprotein; CHF = congestive heart failure; ACE = angiotensin-converting enzyme; HgbA1c = glycosylated hemoglobin.

Chapter 2

Pulmonology

Table 2-1

Pulmonary Function Tests (PFTS)

NAME	DESCRIPTION	USE
PFTs	Differentiate between obstructive and restrictive lung physiologies • Results reported as absolute values and as predicted percentages of normal values (adjusted for age and gender) • Bronchodilators used to identify reversible airway disease	• Diagnosis • Monitor disease progression and response to treatment
Modalities of PFT Measurements		
Spirometry	• Measures the volume and flow of air exhaled from maximally inflated lungs	• Assesses physiologic performance of the lungs using a volume-time curve
Lung Volume	• Measured by body plethysmography or helium dilution	• Measurement independent of airflow velocity

Table 2-2

Lung Function Test Terminology

MEASUREMENT	DESCRIPTION
Forced Residual Capacity (FRC)	• Volume of air in the lung following normal exhalation
Vital Capacity (VC)	• Volume change that occurs between maximal inhalation and maximal exhalation • Measured as the amount of air exhaled (maximal effort, no time limit)
Total Lung Capacity (TLC)	• Total volume of air the lungs can hold at maximal inhalation. • Often very diminished in restrictive lung disease
Tidal Volume (TV)	• Volume of air inhaled or exhaled during each respiratory cycle
Forced Vital Capacity (FVC)	• Total amount of air that can be exhaled as fast as possible following a deep breath
Forced Expiration Volume in 1 sec (FEV1)	• The volume of air exhaled during the first second of forced exhalation
FEV1/FVC ratio	• Expressed as a percentage of the FVC • A useful index to evaluate airflow limitation: decreased in obstructive lung disease • May remain normal in restrictive lung disease if both FEV1 and FVC decline
Residual Volume (RV)	• Amount of air remaining in the lungs after maximal exhalation • A calculated value: RV= TLC-VC • This volume is not exhaled and therefore is not measured by spirometry • Measured by Helium dilution or body plethysmography • Increased during asthma exacerbations and obstructive lung disease due to air trapping
Forced Expiratory Flow 25–75% (FEF 25–75%)	• Flow of forced air during mid-exhalation • Often decreased in obstructive lung disease

Figure 2-1

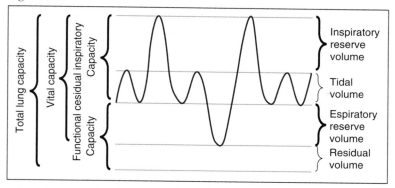

Spirometry. (Reproduced, with permission, from Meyer GK, DeLaMora PA, eds. *Last Minute Pediatrics*, 1st ed. Figure 5-1. Page 76. McGraw-Hill, Inc., 2004.)

FRC = functional residual capacity; VC = vital capacity; TLC = total lung capacity; TV = tidal volume; FVC = forced vital capacity; FEV1 = forced expiratory volume in 1 second; RV = residual volume; FEF = forced expiratory flow.

Figure 2-2

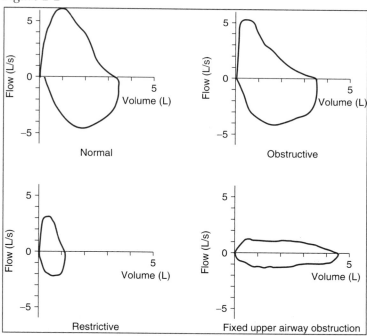

Flow-volume Loops. (Reproduced, with permission, from Meyer GK, DeLaMora PA, eds. *Last Minute Pediatrics*, 1st ed. Figure 5-2. Page 76. McGraw-Hill, Inc., 2004.)

Note: Flow-volume loops measure the volume dynamics of the respiratory cycle and its shape can aid in diagnosis. For example, obstructive lung disease has a characteristic downward scooping on the expiratory flow-volume curve.

Table 2-3

Obstructive vs. Restrictive Lung Disease

	OBSTRUCTIVE	RESTRICTIVE
Tidal Volume	↓	↓
Residual Volume	↑	↓
Total Lung Capacity	↔ ↑	↔↓
Functional Residual Capacity	↑	↓
Vital Capacity	↔ ↓	↓
FEV1	↓	↔ ↓
FEV1/FVC Ratio	↓	↔ ↑
Forced Vital Capacity	↓	↔ ↓
FEF 25–75	↓	↔ ↓

Table 2-4

Summary of Obstructive and Restrictive Lung Disease

CATEGORY	DESCRIPTION	CAUSES
Obstructive Lung Disease	• Obstruction of small airways resulting in increased resistance to airflow • FEV1/FVC ratio less than 70% on spirometry	• Asthma • Bronchiolitis • Pneumonia (viral, mycoplasma) • Cystic fibrosis • Emphysema • Foreign body • Tumors • COPD
Restrictive Lung Disease	• Decreased lung volumes due to parenchymal, pleural, or chest wall disease	• ARDS • Pneumonia (lobar, bacterial) • Pulmonary fibrosis • ILD • Scoliosis • Pleural effusion • Pulmonary edema

FEV1 = Forced expiratory volume in 1 second; FVC = Forced vital capacity; COPD = chronic obstructive lung disease; ARDS = acute respiratory distress syndrome; ILD = interstitial lung disease; FEF = Forced expiratory flow.

Disorders of the Respiratory System

Table 2-5
Obstructive Lung Disease

DISEASE	DEFINITION	ETIOLOGY	EPIDEMIOLOGY	CLINICAL PRESENTATION	DIAGNOSIS	TREATMENT
Asthma	• Obstructive airway disease that is partially or fully reversible when a bronchodilator is administered	• Airway hyper-responsiveness and chronic inflammation in the presence of inflammatory mediators Triggers: • Allergens (dust mites, cockroaches) • Irritants (air pollution, smoke, cold) • Infections (viral upper respiratory infections) • Other (exercise, aspirin, emotional stress, beta-blockers)	• Incidence, morbidity and mortality are all increasing in the United States	• Nighttime cough • Exercise induced cough • Wheezing • Nasal flaring • Intercostal retractions Signs of distress: • Cyanosis • Hypoxemia • Lactic acidosis • Limited or absent air movement	• History, physical and spirometry • Reversibility of airway disease shown with bronchodilator on pulmonary function test • Note that wheezing may be due to other causes, including anterior mediastinal mass and cardiac etiologies Associated with: • Family history of asthma • Atopy • Nasal polyps • Smoke exposure (passive) • Chronic lung disease	• Regulation of chronic airway inflammation • Not clear if anti-inflammatory treatment prevents progressive decline in lung function • Patient education and action plan key to control • Antibiotics generally not indicated • Control triggers • PFTs are sometimes useful to monitor disease progression

(*continued*)

Table 2-5

Obstructive Lung Disease (continued)

DISEASE	DEFINITION	ETIOLOGY	EPIDEMIOLOGY	CLINICAL PRESENTATION	DIAGNOSIS	TREATMENT
Cystic Fibrosis	• Deficient chloride transport regulation resulting in abnormal mucous accumulation	• Autosomal recessive disorder found on the long arm of chromosome 7 • Over 1000 gene mutations • Most common mutation is ΔF508, cystic fibrosis transmembrane conductance regulator (CFTR), an integral membrane protein that functions as a cyclic adenosine monophosphate activated chloride channel in epithelial cells • This mutation is expressed as a deficient chloride transport mechanism in epithelial cells, predominantly in the lungs and exocrine pancreas, resulting in abnormal mucous accumulation	• Most common in Caucasians (1/25,000 live births) • Affects approximately 30,000 children and adults in the United States • Most common life-shortening genetic disease in whites (median life expectancy = 33 years) • Most common cause of death is end-stage bronchiectasis • More than 4% diagnosed as adults (usually have milder symptoms)	• Chronic sinopulmonary disease and infections • Progressive lung dysfunction • Pancreatic insufficiency (diabetes, fat malabsorption, fat-soluble vitamins deficiency and weight loss) • Pancreatitis • Osteoporosis	• History and physical • Gold standard: Sweat testing to measure sweat chloride concentration • False positive sweat test possible with inadequate sample (most common), hypothyroidism, adrenal insufficiency, and nephrogenic diabetes • Genetic DNA testing is available, however can only detect approximately 100 of the more than 1000 mutations	• Improve and maintain pulmonary function and mucociliary clearance • Nebulized recombinant human DNase, which degrades extracellular DNA to reduce sputum viscosity • Airway clearance with physical therapy • Bronchodilators and anti-inflammatory agents • Infections difficult to control with antibiotics (*Staphylococcus aureus* and *Pseudomonas aeruginosa* common) • Optimize nutrition and pancreatic function

Bronchiolitis	• An acute or chronic cellular inflammation of the bronchioles	• Smokers • Viral pneumonia (RSV, influenza)	• All ages	• Cough with or without airflow obstruction • Wheezing may be present	• History and physical • Spirometry reveals reversible airway obstruction	• Good prognosis • Cough suppressant • Bronchodilators • Corticosteroids rarely indicated
Bronchiolitis Obliterans	• Severe form of bronchiolitis (not BOOP) • A chronic scarring process involving granulation tissue of the respiratory bronchioles	• Toxic fumes (popcorn, potato chips) • Infection—Viral/mycoplasma • Systemic disease—ulcerative colitis, rheumatoid arthritis • Bone marrow transplant—preceded by graft versus host disease • Lung transplant (up to 50% of transplants) • Idiopathic		• Cough with or without airflow obstruction • Usually no wheezing	• History and physical • Spirometry reveals fixed airway obstruction	• Poor prognosis • Corticosteroids

Boop = Bronchiolitis obliterans organizing pneumonia; RSV = Respiratory syncytial virus.

Table 2-6

Classification and Treatment of Asthma

CLASSIFICATION	CLINICAL SYMPTOMS	TREATMENT
• **Exercise Induced** • **Cough Variant** • **Mild Intermittent**	• Daytime symptoms two times a week or less • Infrequent nighttime symptoms	• Inhaled short-acting β2-agonist or cromolyn sodium 30 minutes before sports activity • Histamine antagonist if allergic symptoms are present • Consider daily leukotriene modification during sports season
Mild Persistent	• Daytime symptoms more than two times a week • Nighttime symptoms three to four times a month	• Daily inhaled anti-inflammatories (steroids, cromolyn) • Short-acting β2-agonists as needed for exacerbations • Oral steroids for acute exacerbations • Consider trial of daily leukotriene modification
Moderate Persistent	• Daily daytime symptoms • Weekly nighttime symptoms (≥ five times a month)	• Same as for mild persistent • Oral steroids as needed for acute exacerbations
Severe Persistent	• Daily daytime symptoms • Frequent nighttime symptoms	• Same as for moderate persistent • May need frequent short-acting β2-agonists and oral steroid courses
Status Asthmaticus	• Symptoms refractory to initial bronchodilator therapy • Medical emergency • Risk factors include recent increase in β-agonist use, recurrent hospitalizations, large fluctuations in peak flow readings • Mortality high if respiratory failure (5–10%)	• Oxygen supplementation • Intravenous steroids • Continuous inhaled or intravenous β-agonists (terbutaline) • Magnesium sulfate • May need mechanical ventilation

Modified from National Institutes of Health: *Practical Guide for the Diagnosis and Management of Asthma.* NIH Publication number 97-4053, October 1997.

Table 2-7

Asthma Syndromes

SYNDROME	ETIOLOGY	CHARACTERISTICS	TREATMENT
Exercise Induced Asthma (EIA)	• Due to environmental activation of bronchial hyper reactivity	• May be present without resting symptoms • Most asthmatics have EIA • Airways dilate during exercise. Therefore, symptoms start 10–15 minutes post exercise • Cool air and dry mucosa trigger bronchospasm	• Pretreatment with a β-agonist can prevent 90% of exacerbations
Aspirin Induced Asthma	• Cross-reactivity with all inhibitors of cyclo-oxygenase pathway	• Adults and nonatopics • Associated with rhinitis, nasal polyps and recurrent sinusitis • Syndrome: bronchospasm, facial flushing and nasal congestion	• Leukotriene modulators • Avoidance of aspirin and NSAIDs
Cough Variant Asthma		• Cough without bronchoconstriction • Common underdiagnosed cause of chronic cough • Cough after irritant or trigger	• β-agonist • Inhaled steroid as needed
Allergic Bronchopulmonary Aspergillosis (ABPA)	• Immunologic response to *Aspergillus* antigen	• Wheeze, fleeting pulmonary infiltrates and brown mucus plugs in patients with severe asthma or cystic fibrosis	• Oral corticosteroids • Antifungal therapy

Table 2-8

Hypersensitivity Pneumonitis (Extrinsic Allergic Alveolitis)

CATEGORY AGENTS	CLINICAL SYNDROME EXAMPLE	SOURCE OF ANTIGEN
• Animals	• Bird fancier's, breeders or handler's lung	• Bird feathers • Bird droppings
• Plants	• Tobacco worker's disease	• Mold on tobacco
• Low molecular weight chemicals	• Chemical hypersensitivity pnuemonitis	• Polyurethane foam • Varnish

• Clinical syndrome due to allergic reaction to inhaled low-molecular weight antigens deposited in the lower respiratory tract
- Acute: fever, cough, dyspnea, crackles after antigen exposure
- Chronic: indolent, constitutional symptoms of weight loss, fever, and fatigue
• Diagnosis: Clinical symptoms, demonstration of immune response to antigen and resolution with removal of antigen (usually within 48 hours)
• Treatment: Removal of antigen

Table 2-9
Chronic Obstructive Pulmonary Disease (COPD)

	EMPHYSEMA	CHRONIC BRONCHITIS
	• There are two types of chronic obstructive pulmonary disease (COPD): emphysema and chronic bronchitis • COPD is progressive and is characterized by airflow obstruction without complete reversibility	
Description	• Abnormal permanent enlargement of the airspaces distal to the terminal bronchioles, accompanied by destruction of their walls without obvious fibrosis	• Presence of chronic productive cough for 3 months in each of two successive years in a patient in whom other causes of chronic cough have been excluded
Risk Factors	• Cigarette smoking is a major risk factor (20% of regular smokers develop progressive airflow obstruction) • Up to 10% of COPD patients never smoked • α-1-antitrypsin deficiency is a risk factor for emphysema • Patients at risk should be screened with spirometry	
Epidemiology	COPD is the fourth leading cause of mortality in the United States	
Symptoms	• Shortness of breath • Dyspnea on exertion • Wheeze if airway hyper-responsiveness present	• Productive cough • Shortness of breath • Dyspnea on exertion
Radiographic Evidence	• CXR is not sensitive or specific for the presence or the severity of COPD • CXR may show a flattened diaphragm and hyper-inflated lung fields • Computed tomography may show cystic changes but extent of changes does not correlate with the degree of airflow obstruction	• CXR often normal • "Ring shadows"—thickened airways in cross section • "Dirty chest"—increased bronchial markings at lung bases
α-1-Antitripsin Deficiency	• Z allele causes production of the AT protein that does not readily leave the hepatocyte • ZZ: serum AT levels 10–15% of normal • MZ: AT levels 50% of normal. Not predisposed to emphysema • Emphysema (lower lobe predominance) • Cirrhosis • Suspect if young and no history of smoking or family history of early emphysema	

CXR = chest radiograph; AT = antitrypsin; ZZ = homozygotes; MZ = heterozygotes.

Table 2-10

Treatment of COPD

AGENT	INDICATION
Bronchodilators	• Mainstay of therapy, even if no response to bronchodilators on PFT • Anticholinergic (Ipratroprium or tiotropium) + selective β2-agonist has additive effect (better response and improvement in FEV1 than if either drug used alone) • Long-acting salmeterol
Glucocorticoids	• Generally makes patients feel better • However, short course (prednisone 40 mg/d × 2 weeks) does not tend to improve lung function (improves in less then 25% of patients) • If frequent use, monitor for osteopenia/osteoporosis
Antibiotics	• Empiric antibiotics are recommended for exacerbation • Common organisms: *Haemophilus influenzae, streptococcus pneumoniae and Moraxella catarrhalis* • Consider *Pseudomonas aeruginosa* if severe lung dysfunsion
Vaccination	• Yearly influenza vaccination; pneumococcal vaccination

Supplemental O₂	• 24 hour O$_2$ therapy prolongs survival if patient is hypoxemic
	• Indications for O$_2$ therapy:
	  - PaO$_2$<55 mm Hg
	  - PaO$_2$<60 mm Hg if: pulmonary hypertension, right heart failure

Smoking Cessation	• Slows rate of FEV1 decline • Nonsmoker: FEV1 declines 20–30 mL/year • Smoker: FEV1 declines 50–60 mL/year
Pulmonary Rehabilitation	• Does not improve lung function or survival • Increases quality of life and may increase exercise performance
Lung-Volume Reduction Surgery	• In selected patients (upper lobe disease) with moderate/severe COPD, may improve functional status
Transplantation	• Long waiting time (> 18 months) • Half of lung transplants performed for severe COPD and 20% for cystic fibrosis • Median survival after transplant is 4 years and course complicated by rejection and immunosuppression
A1AT protein	• Weekly infusion of purified A1AT protein may slow rate of lung decline in patients with α-1-Antitrypsin deficiency

PFT = Pulmonary Function Test; FEVI = Forced expiratory volume in 1 second; A1AT = α-1 antitrypsin; COPD = Chronic Obstructive Pulmonary Disease; O$_2$ = Oxygen; Hg = Mercury; ML = Milliliters.

Restrictive Lung Disease

Table 2-11
Pneumothorax

	PNEUMOTHORAX	PRIMARY SPONTANEOUS PNEUMOTHORAX	SECONDARY SPONTANEOUS PNEUMOTHORAX
Definition	• Accumulation of air in the pleural space	• Pneumothorax *without* presence of underlying lung disease	• Pneumothorax *with* presence of underlying lung disease
Etiology	• Traumatic (blunt or penetrating force) • Spontaneous (primary or secondary) • Iatrogenic (e.g. mechanical ventilation)		
Incidence		• Men: 7–18 per 100,000/yr • Women: 1–6 per 100,000/yr	
Clinical	• Decreased breath sounds on the affected side • Respiratory distress • Hypoxemia • Cardiovascular collapse	• Tall/thin males aged 10–30 • Smoking increases risk 20x • Acute, pleuritic chest pain and shortness of breath	• May be more symptomatic and more hypoxic because have less lung reserve due to underlying disease
Diagnosis	• CXR	• CXR	• CXR/CT scan
ABG		• Mild-moderate hypoxemia • Respiratory alkalosis	• Significant hypoxemia • Hypercapnea (in COPD)
Treatment	• 100% oxygen (helps shrink pneumothorax via nitrogen washout.) • Small pneumothorax (<10%) may resolve spontaneously • If a larger pneumothorax or if signs of respiratory distress consider emergent chest tube placement or needle decompression	• Observe if less than 15% of lung • If recurrent consider surgical exploration to treat persistent air leaks or blebs	• Generally need chest tube drainage +/− pleurodesis (sclerosing agents instilled through the chest tube) • More difficult than primary pneumothorax to manage over long term
Risk of Recurrence		• 30%	• 39–47%

CXR = Chest radiograph; CT = Contrast computed tomography; COPD = Chronic Obstructive Pulmonary Disease; x = times.

Table 2-12

Causes of Secondary Pneumothorax

CATEGORY	EXAMPLE
Airway Disease	• COPD • CF
Interstitial Lung Disease	• Sarcoidosis • Rheumatoid associated disease • Idiopathic pulmonary fibrosis • Radiation fibrosis
Infectious Disease	• *P. jiroveci* • *M. tuberculosis* • Necrotizing gram-negative pneumonia • Anaerobic pneumonia

COPD = Chronic Obstructive Pulmonary Disease; CF = cystic fibrosis.
Note: Pneumocystis Carinii (PCP) recently renamed Pneumocystis jiroveci.

Table 2-13

Measurement of Pulmonary Gas Exchange

TEST	DESCRIPTION	NOTES
Pulse Oximetry	• Noninvasive method of measuring arterial oxygen saturation • Measures percentage of hemoglobin sites bound by available oxygen	Factors limiting accuracy: • Carboxyhemoglobin • Methemoglobin • Sickle cell anemia • Hypothermia • Diminished peripheral perfusion • Jaundice/increased serum bilirubin • Painted fingernails if measurement probe placed on finger
Diffusion	• Measures exchange of gas in the lung • Performed during pulmonary function test	• Results adjusted for hemoglobin level • Accuracy limited by fibrosis and inflammatory disorders

Table 2-14

Oxyhemoglobin Dissociation Curve

PHYSIOLOGIC EFFECT	NORMAL CAUSE	NORMAL EFFECT	PATHOLOGIC CAUSES	AFFECT ON DISSOCIATION CURVE
Increased attraction between hemoglobin and oxygen	• Increased partial pressure of oxygen • Normal state in lung	• Oxygen transferred from the air to hemoglobin in the lung	• Increased pH • Decreased temperature • Decreased 2–3 DPG • Fetal hemoglobin • Decreased PCO_2	• Shift to the left
Decreased attraction of oxygen to hemoglobin	• Decreased partial pressure of oxygen • Normal state in tissue	• Oxygen delivered to tissue	• Decreased pH • Increased temperature • Increased 2–3 DPG • Increased PCO_2	• Shift to the right

Note: The oxyhemoglobin dissociation curve describes the relationship of oxygen saturation to the partial pressure of oxygen, the "force" that attracts or releases oxygen from hemoglobin. The S shape is due to cooperative binding: hemoglobin is most attracted to oxygen when three of polypeptide chains already bound to oxygen.
DPG = diphosphoglycerate; PCO_2 = partial pressure carbon dioxide.

Figure 2-3

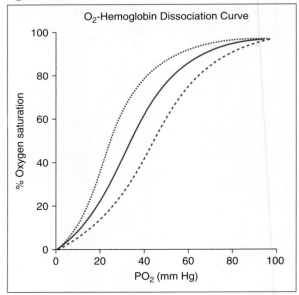

Oxyhemoglobin Dissociation Curve. (Reproduced, with permission, from Meyer GK, DeLaMora PA, eds. *Last Minute Pediatrics*, 1st ed. Figure 5-3. Page 78. McGraw-Hill, Inc., 2004.)

Inflammatory Lung Disease

Inflammatory Lung Disease

	IDIOPATHIC PULMONARY FIBROSIS	CRYPTOGENIC ORGANIZING PNEUMONIA (COP)	SARCOIDOSIS
	TYPES OF IDIOPATHIC INTERSTITIAL PNEUMONIA		
Definition	• The most common form of idiopathic interstitial pneumonia • A chronic, progressive interstitial lung disease of unknown etiology	• Interstitial lung disease of uncertain etiology. Also called BOOP, which is different from bronchiolitis obliterans (see obstructive lung disease)	• A chronic multisystem disorder characterized by accumulation of T lymphocytes, mononuclear phagocytes, and noncaseating epithelioid granulomas
Epidemiology	• Affects patients in the fifth to seventh decades of life • Affects men more than women • Slowly progressive over months to years	• Affects patients in the fifth and sixth decades of life • Affects men and women equally	• Worldwide, affects all races and sexes equally • In the United States, more common in African Americans • Most patients present between the ages of 20–40 years
Etiology	• Cause/risk factors unknown • Chronic aspiration from GE reflux has been implicated	• 80% idiopathic • Many patients have a preexisting chronic systemic inflammatory disease (Rheumatoid arthritis) • Drugs (amiodirone, methotrexate) • Infections (viruses, malaria) • Connective tissue disorders • Post transplant	• Cause/risk factors unknown
Clinical Presentation	Chronic, progressive: • Dyspnea on exertion • Nonproductive cough • Bilateral inspiratory crackles at bases • Hypoxemia • Clubbing • Pulmonary hypertension • Right ventricular failure	• Flu-like symptoms are frequently manifested within 2 months of diagnosis • Fever • Cough • Dyspnea • Inspiratory crackles	• May be asymptomatic • 90% have pulmonary symptoms • Dyspnea on exertion • Nonproductive cough • Constitutional symptoms • Other organs involved: skin, bone, liver, eye, and spleen

(continued)

Table 2-15

Inflammatory Lung Disease (continued)

	IDIOPATHIC PULMONARY FIBROSIS	CRYPTOGENIC ORGANIZING PNEUMONIA (COP)	SARCOIDOSIS
	TYPES OF IDIOPATHIC INTERSTITIAL PNEUMONIA		
Diagnosis	• History and physical examination • PFTs • Lung biopsy	• History and physical examination • PFTs • Lung biopsy	• Diagnosis of exclusion: clinical history and evidence of noncaseating granuloma in two separate organs • Gallium scan and angiotensin converting enzyme (ACE) level not reliable • Must exclude lymphoma as etiology
PFTs	• Restrictive abnormality • Decreased diffusing capacity	• Restrictive abnormality	• Restrictive, obstructive, or mixed abnormalities
Radiographic Evidence	• Chest radiograph (CXR): - Bilateral diffuse fine reticular opacities, usually in lower lung zones • High resolution Computed tomography (CT): - Pleural honeycomb changes - Lower lobe interstitial infiltrates with increased septal markings, and traction bronchiectasis	• Unilateral or bilateral focal consolidations with air bronchograms • High resolution CT: dense infiltrates on a background of fine ground glass changes. Small nodular opacities	• CXR: - Stage I: hilar adenopathy - Stage II: hilar adenopathy and parenchymal opacities - Stage III: parenchymal opacities - Stage IV: fibrosis • CT: - Ground glass or nodular opacities are likely reversible - Cystic air spaces and parenchymal distortion are likely irreversible
Pathology	• Usual interstitial pneumonia (UIP): - Cellular thickening and fibrosis of alveolar wall	• Peribronchial inflammation • Granulation tissue plugging in distal airspaces • Ratio of lymphocytes to CD8$^+$ cells is significantly increased • CD4$^+$/CD8$^+$ ratio is significantly decreased	• Compact noncaseating granuloma

Manifestations	• Progressive hypoxemia and respiratory failure	• Progressive dyspnea and hypoxemia	• 90% have hilar adenopathy • 25% have skin manifestations (erythema nodosum) • 25% have ophthalmic lesions (uveitis) • 40–70% have liver granulomas (dysfunction is rare) • 10% have cardiac involvement (arrhythmias)
Course	• Usually fatal and rarely responds to therapy	• Majority of patients have some degree of long term clinical recovery with treatment • Relapse is common	• Spontaneous remission - Stage I—60–80% - Stage II—50–60% - Stage III—< 30% • Factors that portend a poor prognosis - Age of onset > 40 years old - Symptoms present for > 6 months - > three organs involved
Treatment	• Smoking cessation • Control infections • Oxygen as needed • Early referral to lung transplant • Limited benefit of systemic glucocorticoids, colchicine, and immunosuppressives	• High dose prednisone with a long taper • Smoking cessation • Control infections • Oxygen as needed	• Most do not require therapy as the disease will clear spontaneously in 50% of patients • If symptomatic, consider oral corticosteroids and methotrexate

BOOP = bronchiolitis obliterans organizing pneumonia.

Disorders of Respiration

Table 2-16
Apnea Disorders

	DEFINITION	ETIOLOGY	CLINICAL PRESENTATION	DIAGNOSIS	COMPLICATIONS	TREATMENT
OSA	• Upper airway obstruction during sleep and subsequent apnea despite continued chest wall effort	• Anatomical obstruction to the upper airway • Enlarged tonsils and adenoids frequent cause in otherwise healthy people • Risk factors: - Obesity - Muscular dystrophies - Down syndrome - Neuromuscular disease	• Nighttime snoring with episodic airway obstruction (silent periods) • Abnormal sleep patterns • Daytime hypersomnolence • Behavioral changes	• Clinical history and presentation • Gold standard: Polysomnography (sleep study)	• Polycythemia • Right ventricular hypertrophy • Pulmonary hypertension • Chronic carbon dioxide retention • Chronic hypoxemia • Chronic sleep deprivation • Poor work/ school performance	• If severe, ECG to rule out pulmonary hypertension • CPAP or BiPAP • Surgical removal of the enlarged tonsils and adenoids
Central Apnea	• Respiratory pauses with lack of respiratory effort usually lasting 10 seconds or more	• Nervous system dysfunction • Brain tumors • Arnold Chiari malformation	• Can occur anytime	Differential diagnosis: • Narcotic use • Seizures • Brain tumors	• Hypoxemia • Hypercarbia • Headache • Behavioral changes	• Based on etiology

OSA = obstructive sleep apnea; CPAP = continuous positive airway pressure; BiPAP = bilevel positive airway pressure.

Pulmonary Vascular Disease

Pulmonary Hypertension

	DEFINITION	CLINICAL PRESENTATION	DIAGNOSIS	TREATMENT

Pulmonary Hypertension	• Mean PAP greater than 25 mm Hg at rest or greater than 30 mm Hg with exertion	• Progressive dyspnea, dizziness and syncope
		• Increased right ventricular hypertrophy
		  - Elevated jugular venous pressure (increased P2, audible S4)
		  - Hepatomegaly
		  - Hoarse voice from impinged recurrent laryngeal nerve
		  - Progressive disease can cause severe functional limitations and death
			• Must rule out secondary causes
			• Right heart catheterization to exclude intracardiac shunt, pulmonary emboli, to measure PAP and PCWP and to assess response to pharmacologic interventions
				• If secondary pulmonary hypertension, treat underlying cause
				• If stable, endothelin receptor antagonist (bosentan)
				• If less stable, prostaglandin analogue (continuous intravenous infusion of epoprostenol)
				• Anticoagulation
				• Diuresis
				• Digoxin
				• Goal: decrease PAP and peripheral vascular resistance without decreasing cardiac output or causing hypotension

Primary Pulmonary Hypertension		• Usually idiopathic • Rare		
Secondary Pulmonary Hypertension		• Associated with infections, rheumatologic diseases, immune system diseases, and diseases causing organ dysfunction		

PAP = pulmonary artery pressure; PCWP = pulmonary capillary wedge pressure.

Table 2-18

Causes of Secondary Pulmonary Hypertension

CATEGORY	EXAMPLE
Volume and Pressure Overload	• Atrial or ventricular septal defects • Left atrial hypertension • Mitral stenosis or regurgitation • Left ventricular systolic or diastolic dysfunction • Constrictive pericarditis • Pulmonary venous obstruction: pulmonary veno-occlusive disease
Decreased Area of the Pulmonary Vascular Bed	• Chronic thromboembolic disease • Obstruction/obliteration of the pulmonary artery • Collagen vascular disease [systemic lupus erythematosus, scleroderma, rheumatoid arthritis, CREST syndrome (limited systemic sclerosis: Calcinosis, Raynaud disease, Esophageal dysmotility, Sclerodactyly and Telangiectasia)] • Vasculitis (Wegener's, polyarteritis nodosum) • Miscellaneous (sarcoidosis, carcinomatosis, parasitic or HIV infection, fibrosis)
Hypoxic Vasoconstriction	• Chronic obstructive pulmonary disease • Hypoventilation disorders • Obstructive or central sleep apnea • Kyphoscoliosis • High altitude
Drugs	• Anorexigenic agents • Cocaine abuse

Table 2-19

Microbial Pathogens by Type of Pneumonia

Type of Pneumonia	Common Microbial Pathogens	Notes
Community Acquired	• *Mycoplasma pneumoniae* • *Streptococcus pneumoniae* • *Haemophilus influenzae* • *Chlamydia pneumoniae* • *Legionella pneumophila*	• Diagnosis: Chest radiograph • Sensitivity of gram stain and culture poor, but may provide information about resistance patterns
	• Oral anaerobes • *Moraxella catarrhalis* • *Staphylococcus aureus* • *Nocardia* spp.	• Treatment: Empiric therapy based on severity of pulmonary disease, patient comorbidities and local resistance patterns
	• Viruses[a]	
	• Fungi[b]	
	• M. tuberculosis	
	• *Chlamydia psittaci*	
Hospital Acquired	• Enteric aerobic gram-negative bacilli • *Pseudomonas aeruginosa* • *S. aureus*	
	• Oral anaerobes	
HIV Infection Associated	• *P. jiroveci* • *M. tuberculosis* • *S. pneumoniae* • *H. influenzae* • Fungi[b]	
	• Atypical mycobacterium • All microorganisms affecting nonimmunocompromised hosts as above	

[a] Influenza virus, cytomegalovirus, respiratory syncytial virus, measles virus, varicella zoster virus, and hantavirus.
[b] *Histoplasma, Coccidioides,* and *Blastomyces* species.

Table 2-20

Pulmonary Vasculidities

	WEGENER GRANULOMATOSIS	**CHURG–STRAUS**	**DIFFUSE ALVEOLAR HEMORRHAGE**
Disease Characteristics	• Vasculitis with necrotizing granulomas • Upper airway, lung and kidney involvement • Severity varies from mild organ dysfunction to organ failure	• Systemic vasculitis with extravascular granulomas in patients with asthma - peripheral eosinophilia > 10% • Presents with pulmonary infiltrates, myocarditis, peripheral neuropathy, and skin rash • Can occur occasionally in asthmatics who are on tapering prednisone and starting leukotriene inhibitors	• Capillaritis with diffuse alveolar hemorrhage • Cough and shortness of breath • Occasional hemoptysis • Can progress rapidly to respiratory failure

Diagnosis	• Serology suggests diagnosis:
	  - +ANA
	  - +ELISA for proteinase 3
	  - +ANCA
	  - There are two types of ANCA, c-ANCA (granular), and p-ANCA (perinuclear)
	  - c-ANCA most specific for Wegener's
		• ARA Criteria:
		Need ≥ four criteria (85% sensitivity and 100% specificity)
		  - Asthma
		  - Peripheral blood eosinophilia > 10%
		  - Mono or polyneuropathy
		  - Nonfixed pulmonary infiltrates
		  - Paranasal sinus abnormality
		  - Extravascular eosinophils
			• CXR with diffuse alveolar infiltrates
			• ANCA negative
			• Necrosis of capillary wall and occlusion of capillary lumen with fibrin thrombin

Treatment	• Start with prednisone and cyclophosphamide • Maintenance prednisone or prednisone plus methotrexate	• Systemic glucocorticoids	• Cyclophosphamide and glucocorticoids

ANA = antinuclear antibody; ARA = American Rheumatologic Association; ANCA = antineutrophil cytoplasmic antibodies; CXR = Chest radiograph.

Table 2-21

Pulmonary Symptoms

	DEFINITION	ETIOLOGY	NOTES
Hemoptysis	• Coughing or expectorating blood from the airways	• Multiple: See Table 2-22 • Source of blood usually from airways or lungs. However blood from GI tract or sinuses can also be expectorated	• If hemoptysis lasts > 1 week, patient is > 40 years old who is a current or former smoker consider evaluation for occult lung cancer, even if CXR is normal

Massive Hemoptysis	• Greater then 600 cc of blood per 24 hours	• Common causes:
		  - Bronchiectasis
		  - Tuberculosis
		  - Cancer
		  - Aspergilloma
		  - Pneumonia
			• Position patient with the bleeding lung dependent (down) to avoid blood spilling into the healthy lung

Acute Cough	• Sudden onset of cough	• Common cold • Bacterial sinusitis • Exacerbation of COPD • Allergic rhinitis • Pertussis	

Chronic Cough	• Cough that lasts for 3 weeks or longer	Most common:
		• Asthma
		• Postnasal drip
		• GERD
		• Congestive heart failure
		• Chronic bronchitis
		• Medications:
		  - ACE inhibitor
		  - β-blockers
		  - Smoking
		  - Postviral airway hyper-responsiveness
			• Only manifestation of GERD 75% of time
			• Only manifestation of asthma up to 57% of time
			• Often due to more than one condition
			• Smoking cessation and discontinuation of ACE inhibitor may result in relief

Chronic Dyspnea	• Chronic shortness of breath	• Most common:
		  - Asthma
		  - COPD
		  - Interstitial lung disease
		  - Congestive heart failure
		• Other:
		  - Cardiac disease
		  - Psychogenic disorders (diagnosis of exclusion)
		  - Deconditioning (diagnosis of exclusion)
		  - Neuromuscular disorders	

GERD = Gastroesophageal reflux disease; CXR = Chest radiograph; COPD = Chronic Obstructive Pulmonary Disease.

Table 2-22

Frequent Causes of Hemoptysis

CATEGORY	EXAMPLE
Parenchymal Infections	• Tuberculosis • Pneumonia • Lung abscess • Aspergilloma
Airway Disorders and Infections	• Bronchitis • Bronchiectasis • Cancer (primary or metastatic) • Foreign body/airway trauma
Vasculidities	• Wegener's granulomatosis • Goodpasture's syndrome
Other Vascular Disorders	• Pulmonary emboli • Pulmonary arteriovenous malformation • Bronchovascular fistula • Left atrial hypertension
Other	• Iatrogenic • Coagulopathy (liver failure) • Cocaine • Catamenial hemoptysis (pulmonary endometriosis)

Table 2-23

Bronchiectasis

DEFINITION	CAUSES	COMMON ORGANISMS	NOTES
• Persistent inflammation in the airways, often leading to destruction	• Host defense dysfunction (genetic or acquired) • Pneumonia (bacterial, viral or atypical) • Cystic fibrosis	• *Moraxella catarrhalis* • *Haemophilus influenza* • *Pseudomonas* • Tuberculosis	• Common cause of hemoptysis • Abnormal mucous production

Table 2-24

Pleural Effusions

	TRANSUDATIVE	**EXUDATIVE**		
Etiology	• Congestive heart failure • Cirrhosis • Myxedema • Acute renal failure • Uremia • Nephrotic syndrome • Manifestation of PE	• Infection (parapneumonic) • Malignancy • Inflammatory • Collagen vascular disease		
Labs	• Fluid protein: serum protein < 0.5 • Fluid LDH: serum LDH < 0.6 • Fluid LDH < 2/3 upper limit of normal for serum	• Fluid protein: serum protein > 0.5 • Fluid LDH: serum LDH > 0.6 • Fluid LDH > 2/3 upper limit of normal for serum		
Other Pleural Fluid Characteristics		**Fluid Characteristic**		**Etiology**
		• Pus		• Empyema
		• Positive cytology		• Malignancy
		• High triglycerides and chylomicrons		• Chylothorax (lymphoma most common cause)
		• Lymphocyte-predominant (90–95% lymphocytes)		• Tuberculous pleurisy
		• Occurs > 2 months after surgery		• Postcoronary artery bypass graft
Treatment	• Treatment should be directed at underlying cause • Drain if free-flowing (demonstrate on lateral decubitus chest radiograph) and symptomatic. To minimize risk of reexpansion pulmonary edema do not drain more than 1.5 L • Drain parapneumonic effusion if free-flowing and pH < 7.3 • Recurrent pleural effusions difficult to treat (often due to malignancy) • May need pleurodesis or semipermanent indwelling catheter			

Table 2-25

Lung Imaging

MODALITY	USEFUL TO
CT	• *Visualize* nodules • Visualize mediastinal structures • Diagnose pulmonary embolism (in conjunction with spiral images)
High-Resolution CT	• Improve visualization of parenchyma • Directly visualize of emphysema and bronchiectasis
Bronchoscopy	• Directly visualize of proximal airways • Obtain samples and biopsies for cytology, microbiology, and pathology
PET Scan	• Distinguish between malignant (brighter) and benign (less bright) lesions if mass greater than 1 cm
MRI	• Limited utility • Improve visualization of paraspinal masses and mass lesions in the pleura

CT = contrast computed tomography; PET = positron emission tomography; MRI = magnetic resonance imaging.

Chapter 3

Critical Care

Table 3-1

Intensive Care Unit/Assessment of Severity of Illness

REASONS FOR ADMISSION	CATEGORIZATION OF SEVERITY OF ILLNESS	NOTES
Acute organ failure **Impending organ failure**	• Categorization of severity of illness is frequently employed upon a patient's admission to the ICU • The APACHE score is the most frequently used system in the United States	• Precision with which APACHE scores predict patient outcomes is not clear • Admission to ICU often due to respiratory or cardiac dysfunction • Additional uses of these scores include clinical research, demographics, allocation of hospital resources, and quality assurance oversight

APACHE = Acute Physiology and Chronic Health Evaluation; ICU = intensive care unit.

Table 3-2

Summary of Shock Syndromes

	DEFINITION	CLINICAL PRESENTATION	TREATMENT
Shock syndrome	• Inadequate delivery of sufficient oxygen and other nutrients/ substrates to meet the metabolic demands of the tissues	• Signs and symptoms depend on functional category and phase Usually include: • Tachycardia • Tachypnea • Altered mental status • Decreased urine output • Prolonged capillary refill • Lactic acidosis secondary to low tissue perfusion • May occur with a low, normal, or elevated blood pressure	• ABCs • Oxygen supplementation • Obtain adequate venous access • Fluid resuscitation • Cardio-respiratory monitoring • Assessment of cardiac output to help direct therapy • Early and aggressive goal directed therapy • Vasoactive medications (epinephrine, dopamine, norepinephrine, dobutamine, milrinone, vasopressin, etc.) • Treat underlying cause

Table 3-2
Summary of Shock Syndromes (continued)

	DEFINITION	CLINICAL PRESENTATION	TREATMENT
Phases of Shock			
Compensated	• Normal or elevated blood pressure with vital organ function maintained	• Shock signs and symptoms	• Primary treatment goal is prevention of uncompensated and irreversible shock
Uncompensated	• Compromised blood pressure and tissue perfusion with early organ dysfunction	• Shock signs and symptoms plus evidence of early organ dysfunction	• Primary treatment goal is prevention of irreversible shock
Irreversible	• Severe and multiple end organ damage	• Shock signs and symptoms plus evidence of severe damage to multiple end organs	

ABCs = airway control, breathing, and circulation.

Table 3-3
Assessment of Cardiac Output

TYPE	METHOD	PARAMETERS ASSESSED	NOTES
Noninvasive	• Clinical	Evidence of adequate end organ perfusion: • Adequate urine output • Appropriate mental status/ level of consciousness • Blood pressure • Skin perfusion	• Cardiac output helps to direct treatment strategy based on underlying physiology
Invasive	• Arterial catheter	• Continuous monitoring of arterial blood pressure • Estimation of end organ function	

(continued)

Table 3-3

Assessment of Cardiac Output (continued)

TYPE	METHOD	PARAMETERS ASSESSED	NOTES
PAC	• PAC (Swan-Ganz catheter) is inserted percutaneously via the subclavian or jugular vein • Once the catheter is advanced into the superior or inferior vena cava (location known by characteristic pressure wave readouts), a small balloon at the end of the catheter is inflated and floated through the right atrium, the right ventricle, and into the pulmonary artery	• Cardiac output: measured via thermodilution (change in temperature between the right atrium and pulmonary artery after injection of cold sterile saline through the proximal catheter port) • Tissue perfusion: oximetry (indirect measurement) • Intravascular volume status: pulmonary capillary wedge pressure (indirect estimate of the left atrial pressure)	• Utility of PAC is unclear

PAC = pulmonary artery catheter.

Table 3-4

Shock Syndromes by Functional Classification

FUNCTIONAL CLASSIFICATION	EXAMPLE	ETIOLOGY	PRESENTATION	TREATMENT
Hypovolemic	• Profuse vomiting, diarrhea • Dehydration • Adrenal crisis • Diabetic keto-acidosis • Diabetes insipidus • Burns • Capillary leak syndromes • Trauma • Fractures (pelvis, long bones) • Great vessel injury	• Sudden decrease in intravascular volume • Inadequate volume to maintain cardiac output (CO)	• Tachycardia • Tachypnea • Decreased CO • Hypotension • Oliguria • Cool extremities • Narrow pulse pressure • Lethargy	• Fluid resuscitation • Blood factor replacement • Surgical intervention • Dexamethasone for adrenal crisis
Distributive	• Early septic shock • Anaphylaxis • Neurogenic (spinal cord trauma) • Thyrotoxicosis	• Vasodilatation and shunting of blood from vital organs	• Tachycardia • Tachypnea • Maldistribution of blood flow • Hypotension • Wide pulse pressure	• Fluid resuscitation • Epinephrine (for anaphylaxis) • Vasoactive medications • Antihistamines • Corticosteroids (for spinal cord injury)
Obstructive	• Pneumothorax • Pericardial tamponade • Massive pulmonary embolus • Pulmonary hypertension • Congenital heart disease (coarctation)	• Mechanical obstruction of ventricular filling and/or cardiac output	• Tachycardia • Tachypnea • Cool extremities • Oliguria • Metabolic acidosis • Decreased CO	• Relief of obstruction

(continued)

Table 3-4

Shock Syndromes by Functional Classification (continued)

FUNCTIONAL CLASSIFICATION	EXAMPLE	ETIOLOGY	PRESENTATION	TREATMENT
Cardiogenic	• Weak or stunned heart • Recent myocardial infarction • Late septic shock	• Inadequate cardiac output	• Tachycardia • Tachypnea • Cool extremities • Oliguria • Metabolic acidosis	• Monitored fluid resuscitation • Mechanical ventilation (may exacerbate preload and improve afterload) • Vasoactive medications • Afterload reduction may exacerbate myocardial ischemia • During MI, rapid reestablishment of blood flow results in the best chance for survival

CO = cardiac output; MI = myocardial infarction.

Table 3-5
The Sepsis Syndromes

CATEGORY	DEFINITION	TREATMENT (GENERAL)	PROBLEM DIRECTED TREATMENT FOR SEPSIS SYNDROMES		
			ISSUE	POTENTIAL TREATMENT	
SIRS	Two or more of: • Temperature >38.0°C (100.4°F) or <36.0°C (96.8°F) • Heart rate >90 beats/min • Resp rate >20 breaths/min or Paco$_2$ <32 mm Hg • WBC >12 or <4, or with 10% bands	• Antibiotics • Fluids • Supportive care			
Sepsis	• SIRS and • Documented or suspected source of infection	EGDT: • Rapid diagnosis • Rapid initiation of frequent hemodynamic monitoring (blood pressure, tissue and organ function: central venous oxygen saturation monitoring and urine output) • Assessment of oxygen carrying capacity of the blood (hemoglobin concentration) • EGDT improves survival; delays in diagnosis of sepsis syndromes contribute to morbidity and mortality	• Infection	• Early initiation of broad spectrum antibiotics based on suspected site of infection and the risk of resistant bacteria (e.g., nosocomial infections)	

(continued)

Table 3-5
The Sepsis Syndromes (continued)

Category	Definition	Treatment (General)	Problem Directed Treatment for Sepsis Syndromes	
			Issue	Potential Treatment
Severe Sepsis	• Sepsis and • End organ and dysfunction or hypotension that responds to volume resuscitation	EGDT: • Rapid diagnosis • Rapid initiation of frequent hemodynamic monitoring (blood pressure, tissue and organ function: central venous oxygen saturation monitoring and urine output) • Assessment of oxygen carrying capacity of the blood (hemoglobin concentration) • EGDT improves survival; delays in diagnosis of sepsis syndromes contribute to morbidity and mortality	• Refractory hypotension	• Frequent administration of crystalloid (isotonic normal saline) in adequate volume (500 mL) every 30 minutes • Initiation of vasoactive medications • Consider norepinephrine for early septic shock • Consider epinephrine for late septic shock
Septic Shock	• Severe sepsis that is refractory to volume resuscitation and requires vasoactive medication therapy		• Mean arterial pressures <60 mm Hg	• Vasoactive medications • Optimize oxygen delivery
			• Central venous oxygen saturation <70%	
			• Relative adrenal insufficiency based on a high-dose cortcotropin stimulation test and severe septic shock	• Low dose corticosteroids may improve survival
			• Severe sepsis (APACHE II scores >25 on ICU admission)	• rhAPC (or drotrecogin alpha) may improve outcomes • rhAPC, has significant risk of life-threatening or fatal bleeding in high-risk patients

SIRS = systemic inflammatory response syndrome; WBC = white blood cells; EGDT = early goal directed therapy; rhAPC = anticoagulant recombinant human activated protein C.

Table 3-6

Summary of Cardiogenic Shock

ETIOLOGY	PRESENTATION	DIAGNOSIS	MECHANISM FOR POST MI CARDIOGENIC SHOCK	NOTES
Left ventricular dysfunction following MI (most common) Myocardial injury resulting in sustained systemic hypoperfusion • **Myocarditis** • **Cardiomyopathy** • **Late septic shock**	"Pump failure" results in: • Pulmonary edema (most frequent) • Hypoxemia • Lactic acidosis • Pallor/cool extremities • Cyanosis • Dyspnea/tachypnea • Altered mental status • Tachycardia • Oliguria Risk factors: • Anterior wall MI • Female • Older age • Previous MI • If post-MI, occurs within 6 hours of acute MI event	• Clinical presentation • ECG: Q waves and ST segment elevations in multiple leads • Echocardiogram: depressed function	• MI → localized ischemia → depressed contractility and function → depressed stroke volume → systemic hypotension and hypoperfusion → elevated left atrial and pulmonary capillary wedge pressure → diastolic dysfunction → reduced coronary perfusion → further myocardial ischemia	• Leading cause of death following MI

ECG = electrocardiogram; MI = myocardial infarction.

Table 3-7
Critical Care Terminology and Formulas to Remember

MEASURE	ABBREVIATION	UNITS	DEFINITION/FORMULA
Chronotropy			= HR
Dromotropy			= Conduction velocity
Inotropy			= Contractility
Cardiac output	CO	L/min	= SV × HR
Cardiac index	CI	L/min/m²	= CO/BSA
Stroke volume	SV	mL/beat	= CO/HR
Oxygen delivery	DO_2	$L\ O_2$/min	= CO × CaO_2 × 10
Arterial O_2 content	CaO_2	mL O_2/dL blood	= (1.34 × Hgb × Sao_2) + (0.003 × Pao_2)
Body surface area	BSA	m²	= Square root (weight × height/3600)
Minute ventilation	MV		= TV × BR
Hemoglobin	Hgb	g/dL blood	
Partial pressure of oxygen in arterial blood	Pao_2	mm Hg	
Arterial oxygen saturation	Sao_2	%	

HR = heart rate; TV = tidal volume; BR = breath rate.

Table 3-8
Hemodynamic Variables of Shock States

	CO	SVR	MAP	PAOP	CVP
Hypovolemic	↓	↑	↔ or ↓	↓	↓
Distributive	↑	↓	↔ or ↓	↔ or ↓	↔ or ↓
Septic (early)	↑	↓	↔ or ↓	↓	↓
Septic (late)	↓	↓	↓	↑	↑ or ↔
Obstructive	↓	↑	↔ or ↓	↑	↑
Cardiogenic	↓	↑	↔ or ↓	↑	↑

CVP = central venous pressure; MAP = mean arterial blood pressure; PAOP = pulmonary artery occlusion pressure (wedge pressure); SVR = systemic vascular resistance.

Table 3-9
Summary of Vasoactive Medication Physiology*

Vasoactive medications are used to manipulate the cardiovascular responses to shock syndromes.

AGENT	RECEPTOR	COMMON DOSE (μG/KG/MIN)*	EFFECT/NOTES	CONSIDER USE IF:
Dopamine	Dopaminergic	Low dose = 0–4	• Splanchnic and renal vasodilatation	• Renal dysfunction associated with multisystem organ failure
	$\beta_{1,2}$	Moderate dose = 5–10	• ↑ Inotropy	• Cardiogenic shock
	$\alpha_1 > \beta_{1,2}$	High dose = 10–50	• Peripheral vasoconstriction	• Distributive and septic shock
Dobutamine	$\beta_{1,2}$	1–20	• ↑ Inotropy • ↑ Chronotropy • ↑ Dromotropy • Peripheral vasodilatation • Pulmonary vasodilatation	• Cardiogenic shock • Postoperative myocardial dysfunction • May cause excessive tachycardia
Epinephrine	$\beta_{1,2}$	Low/moderate dose = 0.05–0.5	• ↑ Inotropy • ↑ Chronotropy • ↑ Dromotropy • Peripheral vasodilatation • Pulmonary vasodilatation	• Cardiogenic shock • Postoperative myocardial dysfunction • Myocardial dysfunction
	$\alpha_{1,2} > \beta_{1,2}$	High dose = 0.5–2	• ↑ Inotropy • ↑ Dromotropy • Peripheral vasoconstriction • Pulmonary vasoconstriction	• Cardiogenic shock • Septic shock (late) • Cardiovascular collapse
Norepinephrine	$\alpha_{1,2} > \beta_{1,2}$	8–12 μg/min	• Peripheral vasoconstriction • Pulmonary vasoconstriction • ↑ Inotropy (weak)	• Distributive and septic shock (early)

(continued)

Table 3-9

Summary of Vasoactive Medication Physiology* (continued)

Agent	Receptor	Common Dose (μG/KG/MIN)*	Effect/Notes	Consider Use If:
Sodium Nitroprusside	Arterial > venous	0.3–10	• Rapid onset • Short duration • $\uparrow$ ICP • V/Q mismatch • Causes cyanide toxicity in patients with renal failure	• Hypertensive crisis • Afterload reduction in congestive heart failure
Nitroglycerin	Venous > arterial	5–200 µg/min	• Peripheral vasodilatation • $\uparrow$ ICP	• Myocardial ischemia • Preload reduction in congestive heart failure
Alprostadil (PGE-1)	Prostaglandin	0.05–0.1	• Maintains patency of ductus arteriosus • Peripheral vasodilatation • Causes fever, apnea	• Ductal dependent congenital heart disease • Intravenous use typically only in pediatric patients • Injectable and transurethral preparations used for erectile dysfunction
Milrinone	Selective phosphodiesterase inhibitor	0.5 (loading dose often required)	• Afterload reduction • $\uparrow$ Inotropy • $\uparrow$ Dromotropy	• Myocardial dysfunction

PVR = peripheral vascular resistance, SVR = systemic vascular resistance, V/Q = ventilation/perfusion, ICP = intracranial pressure

* This table is not intended for clinical reference, as dosages may vary.

82

Table 3-10

Respiratory Distress and Failure

	DEFINITION	ETIOLOGY	PATHOPHYSIOLOGY	PRESENTATION	TREATMENT
Acute Hypoxemic Respiratory Failure (Type I Respiratory Failure)	• Blood gas criteria: PaO_2 <60, PCO_2 >45 in patients without preexisting lung disease	• Pneumonia • Cardiogenic or noncardiogenic pulmonary edema	• Alveolar infiltrates typically due to infection or pulmonary edema	• Tachypnea • Tachycardia • Accessory muscle use • Abnormal breathing pattern • Hypoxemia, hypercarbia, and acidosis from impaired gas exchange • Respiratory distress first sign of impending respiratory failure	• Prompt management of the airway and control of breathing (endotracheal intubation and mechanical ventilation or bag, valve, and mask/noninvasive ventilation) • Prolonged hypoxemia may lead to cardiac arrest
Noncardiogenic Severe Hypoxemic Respiratory Failure					
ARDS	• Bilateral, patchy pulmonary infiltrates on chest x-ray • No clinical evidence of congestive heart failure, or a PCWP of <18 • Ratio of arterial oxygen pressure (PaO_2) to fraction of inspired oxygen (FiO_2), (P/F ratio) <200	• Insufficient oxygenation and/or ventilation due to direct or indirect lung injury Direct lung injury: • Pneumonia • Aspiration • Pulmonary contusion due to trauma	• Alveolar inflammation and edema • Airway collapse • Localized intrapulmonary shunting of blood to more functional areas of lung	• As above	Treatment goals: • Treat underlying etiology • Reinflate the alveoli • Reestablishing gas exchange, without causing additional volutrauma • Limit volutrauma to alveoli from positive pressure ventilation (likely results from cytokine release, contributing to and exacerbating systemic inflammatory response and further lung damage)

(continued)

Table 3-10

Respiratory Distress and Failure (continued)

	DEFINITION	ETIOLOGY	PATHOPHYSIOLOGY	PRESENTATION	TREATMENT
ALI	• As above, except P/F ratio, between 200 and 300	Indirect lung injury from systemic inflammatory states: • Sepsis • Massive blood transfusions • Pancreatitis		• As above	• Potential degree of volutrauma: "S"-shaped pressure-volume relationship, with a lower and upper "inflection point" representing the opening of alveoli and the overdistention of alveoli, respectively • If treated with mechanical ventilation, low TV may significantly improve survival. Titrate to maintain low airway pressures and metabolic homeostasis (arterial pH >7.25)
Acute Hypercarbic Respiratory Failure (Type 2 Respiratory Failure)	• Alveolar hypoventilation from obstructed airways or impaired neurological and/or musculoskeletal systems	Obstruction: • COPD • Asthma Neurological/ musculoskeletal dysfunction: • Drug overdose • Head trauma • Hypothyroidism • Myasthenia gravis • Guillain-Barre • Amyotrophic lateral sclerosis		Frequent signs of respiratory muscle fatigue: • Difficulty speaking • Altered mental status	• Intubation if signs of respiratory muscle fatigue • For asthma or COPD: bronchodilator therapy (nebulized albuterol and ipratropium bromide) and consider intravenous corticosteroids • See chapter 2

ARDS = acute respiratory distress syndrome; ALI = acute lung injury; COPD = chronic obstructive pulmonary disease; PCWP = pulmonary capillary wedge pressure.

Note: Causes of increased metabolic and oxygen demand of tissues: fever, infection, shock syndromes.

Ventilator Basic Principles

(continued)

Table 3-11

Types of Mechanical Ventilation Settings

Type	Description	Benefit	Potential Downsides	Weaning/Notes
Controlled	• Preset number of breaths delivered per minute at a preset volume or pressure		• Patient must be deeply sedated and paralyzed	
Assist-Controlled	• Preset number of breaths delivered per minute at a preset volume or pressure • Patient can overbreathe the set rate and receive additional, patient initiated breaths at preset volume or pressure	• Low work of breathing • Each breath (machine or patient initiated) has same pressure support (if pressure controlled) or TV (if volume cycled)	• May be uncomfortable for patients • Hemodynamic compromise possible	• Periodic spontaneous breathing trial when sedation lifted • Volume cycled, assist controlled often preferred as initial choice if patient unstable
Pressure Controlled	• Spontaneous breathing supported by ventilator using pressure delivered for a preset time (i.e., patient initiates, but does not control cessation of breath)	• Minimizes risk of barotrauma because peak airway pressure can be limited		• Used with assist-controlled
Pressure Support	• Spontaneous breathing supported by ventilator using pressure delivered until flow rate achieved (i.e., patient controls initiation and cessation of breath)	• Useful during weaning • Relatively comfortable for patients • Hemodynamic compromise unlikely	• Work of breathing inversely related to pressure setting	• For weaning, decrease amount of pressure support provided • Used alone (for weaning) or added to SIMV

Table 3-11

Types of Mechanical Ventilation Settings (continued)

Type	Description	Benefit	Potential Downsides	Weaning/Notes
SIMV	• Preset number of breaths delivered per minute at a preset volume or pressure • Patient can overbreathe the set rate and receive additional, patient initiated breaths at patient determined volume and pressure		• Least comfortable for patients • Work may be greater	• For weaning, decrease breath rate as tolerated
PEEP	• Maintains a preset level of pressure in the airways throughout respiratory cycle	• Prevents atelectasis in distal airways • Minimizes oxygen toxicity • May improve oxygenation in patients with ARDS	• May reduce CO by reducing venous return	• Used in any ventilator assisted setting
HFOV	• A piston driven at 3–10 Hz to actively and continuously move small volumes of inhaled and exhaled gases • Ventilation controlled by amplitude and frequency of the oscillations around the mean airway pressure	• Useful for severe hypoxemic respiratory failure/ARDS • Reduces cytokine production by limiting barotrauma	• May reduce cardiac output by reducing venous return	• Main benefit is the control of the mean airway pressure, potentially limiting barotrauma to the lungs in severe illness

| NIPV | • Ventilation support without need for intubation
• Oral/nasal mask, nasal mask or mouthpiece used to deliver positive pressure support
• Level of support adjusted by changing the ratio between inspiratory and expiratory pressure settings
• Expiratory pressure is similar to PEEP and allows treatment of hypoxemia | • May help avoid intubation in patients with COPD, congestive heart failure, and muscular dystrophy | • Contraindicated if
• Patient unstable
• Patient unable to protect airway
• Excessive secretions
• Adequate mask fit not obtained
• Patient unable to tolerate
• Relative contraindication in patients willing to be intubated | • Pressure support most common, but all modes of ventilation can be used for NIPV
• Complications:
- Gastric distension
- Aspiration if patient vomits into mask
- Dry eyes
- Skin breakdown under mask |

SIM V = synchronized intermittent mandatory ventilation; HFOV = high frequency oscillating ventilation; PEEP = positive end expiratory pressure; NIPV = noninvasive positive pressure.

Table 3-12

Summary of Mechanical Ventilation Goals

PURPOSE OF MECHANICAL VENTILATION	FUNCTIONAL COMPONENTS	CONTROL MECHANISMS	MONITORING EFFECTIVENESS	
Control of Oxygenation	(1) Fio_2 (2) Mean airway pressure (MAP)	Conventional (pressure or volume controlled) Ventilation: • Fio_2 • PEEP • Inspiratory time HFOV: • Fio_2 • MAP	• ABG	• Most accurate method of determining metabolic homeostasis (pH), ventilation, and oxygenation
			• Pulse oximetry	• Determines oxygen-hemoglobin saturation by photoelectric measurements through the skin of the fingers, toes, ears, or forehead
			• $ETCO_2$ measurement	• Measures exhaled carbon dioxide and minute ventilation from a direct connection to the ventilator tubing or with small probe placed in the nose or mouth
Control of Ventilation	(1) TV (2) BR • MV = TV × BR	Conventional (pressure or volume controlled) Ventilation: • Respiration rate • TV HFOV ventilation: • Fewer oscillations allows greater gas exchange (Hertz or frequency) • Amplitude	• Same as above	

ABG = arterial blood gas; $ETCO_2$ = end tidal carbon dioxide; MAP = mean airway pressure; MV = minute ventilation.

Table 3-13

Ventilator Troubleshooting

	CONVENTIONAL	HFOV
To ↑ Oxygenation	• ↑ PEEP • ↑ Fio_2 • ↑ Inspiratory time	• ↑ MAP • ↑ Fio_2
To ↓ Oxygenation	• ↓ PEEP • ↓ Fio_2	• ↓ MAP • ↓ Fio_2
To ↑ Ventilation	• ↑ Tidal volume • ↑ Respiratory rate • ↑ Expiratory time	• ↑ Amplitude • ↓ Frequency
To ↓ Ventilation	• ↓ Tidal volume • ↓ Respiratory rate	• ↓ Amplitude • ↑ Frequency

conventional = pressure or volume controlled ventilation.

Table 3-14

Common Causes of Hypoxemia/Decompensation while on a Ventilator

D	• Disconnection
O	• Tube obstruction
P	• Pneumothorax
E	• Equipment failure

Table 3-15

Prevention of Complications Associated with Mechanical Ventilation

Prevention Strategies	• Venous thromboembolism prophylaxis • Stress ulcer prophylaxis • Daily sedation weaning • Elevation of the head of bed • Oral care

Table 3-16

Summary of Common Acute Poisonings

Toxin	Presentation	Diagnosis	Antidote/Treatment
General	• Consider poisoning for patient who presents with an altered mental status, respiratory distress, seizures, lethargy, coma, unexplained acidosis or unexplained bizarre symptoms		
Acetaminophen	• Anorexia, nausea, and vomiting • Vital signs, mental status normal	• Abnormal liver function tests • Acetaminophen level 4 hours after ingestion • Fulminant liver failure is a late finding	• N-acetylcysteine (within 8 hours if possible)
Anticholinergics (Belladonna Alkaloids)	• "Hot as a hare, mad as a hatter, dry as a bone, red as a beet, blind as a bat": - Hyperthermia - Agitation - Dry skin and mucous membranes - Flushed skin - Dilated pupils	• History • Wide QRS complex on ECG	• Cholinesterase inhibitor (physostigmine) • Gastric lavage (if oral ingestion)
Beta-Blockers	• Bradycardia • Hypotension • Hypoglycemia • Bronchospasm	• History • ↑ PR interval on ECG • Atrioventricular block	• Supportive • Glucagon • Beta-agonists • Dialysis
Carbon Monoxide	• Headache • Dizziness, confusion • Nausea • Delayed neuropsychatric symptoms	• Cherry red lips (classic but rare) • Cutaneous pulse oxygen saturation measurements are falsely normal; patient is actually hypoxemic • ↑ Carboxyhemoglobin	• Oxygen (reduces half-life of carboxyhemoglobin) • Hyperbaric oxygen therapy • Most common cause of death in house fires

Cocaine	• Tachycardia • Mydriasis (dilated pupils) • Hypertension • Agitation • Seizures • Chest pain and myocardial ischemia • Rhabdomyolysis exacerbated in presence of warm environment or exercise	• ↑ CPK • Urine toxicology	• Supportive care • Benzodiazepines for agitation and seizures • Aspirin and nitroglycerin for chest pain. May need cardiac reperfusion interventions • Avoid beta-blockers as alpha-vasoconstriction may be unopposed
Digitalis (may be found in herbal teas and laxatives)	• Hypotension • Dysrhythmias • Nausea • Visual changes • Confusion	• Digoxin level • T-wave depression • Prolonged PR interval	• Antidigoxin antibody
Ethylene Glycol (Antifreeze)/ Methanol	• Tachypnea • Lethargy • Blindness (methanol)	• High anion gap acidosis • Osmolar gap	• Immediate treatment • Ethanol to prevent further metabolism to toxic metabolites • Hemodialysis (definitive) • Fomepizole (antidote)
Isoniazid (INH)	• Nausea, vomiting • Seizures	• Anion gap acidosis • Abnormal LFTs • Eosinophilia • Hyperglycemia	*INH:* "Injures **N**eurons and **H**epatocytes" • Pyridoxine
Isopropyl Alcohol (Rubbing Alcohol)	• Lethargy • Coma • Acetone odor • Hemorrhagic tracheobronchitis	• Absent acidosis • Normal glucose • Increased serum osmolarity	• Supportive • Hemodialysis

(continued)

Table 3-16

Summary of Common Acute Poisonings (continued)

Toxin	Presentation	Diagnosis	Antidote/Treatment
Lithium (Narrow Therapeutic Index)	• Altered mental status • Myoclonus • Hyper-reflexia • Ataxia • Seizures	• Lithium level (may not correlate with symptoms)	• Hydration • Hemodialysis
Opioids	• Hypotension • Miosis (constricted pupils) • Altered mental status • Ileus • Respiratory depression	• Urine toxicology • Respiratory acidosis • Hypoxemia	• Naloxone (repeat doses usually required due to short half-life)
Salicylates	• Mental status changes • Seizures • Coagulopathy • Hepatotoxicity • Hypoglycemia	• Mixed primary respiratory alkalosis and metabolic acidosis (anion gap) • Abnormal LFTs and coagulation studies • Serum toxicology • Chronic salicylate users may manifest symptoms at lower levels	• Urine alkalinization (bicarbonate) • Hemodialysis • Suspect overdose with patients who have rheumatologic disease or arthritis
Sedatives (Barbiturates, Benzodiazepines)	• Hypothermia • Hypotension • Respiratory depression	• Elevated Pco_2 • Urine toxicology	• Supportive care • Flumazenil for benzodiazepines • Use care in those with seizure disorders as Flumazenil may precipitate a seizure • Significant overdose can mimic brain death

CPK = creatine phosphokinase; LFTs = liver function test.

Table 3-17

Anaphylaxis

Common Causes	Example	Etiology	Clinical	Treatment
Drugs	• Beta-lactam antibiotics	• IgE-mediated allergen interaction triggers release of mediators from mast cells and basophils • "Anaphylactoid" response is not IgE mediated, but the clinical presentation and treatment are the same as anaphylaxis (hypotension less common in anaphylactoid)	• Symptoms develop shortly after exposure (usually <1 hour) • Urticaria • Angioedema with laryngeal edema • Bronchospasm • Respiratory failure secondary to upper airway obstruction • Vasodilation and increased vascular permeability → hypotension → shock in up to 30% of cases	• Epinephrine (IM or sub Q) • Delay in administration may increase morbidity and mortality • Beta-agonist inhaler for bronchospasm • H1- and H2-receptor blockers (often diphenhydramine and cimetidine) • Corticosteroids
Venoms	• Bee sting			
Foods	• Seafood • Peanuts			
Other	• Latex			

Note: Sensitive individuals should carry and be trained to use an emergency epinephrine kit.

Chapter 4

Gastroenterology

Table 4-1

Disorders of the Esophagus

	DEFINITION	ETIOLOGY	CLINICAL PRESENTATION	DIAGNOSIS	ENDOSCOPY AND BIOPSY RESULTS	TREATMENT/NOTES
GERD	• The passage of gastric contents into the esophagus	• Transient lower esophageal sphincter relaxation causes a reflux of food and/or acid into the esophagus Contributing factors: • Foods that lower esophageal sphincter (chocolate, fatty foods, caffeine) • Esophageal and/or stomach dysmotility • Hiatal hernia (displacement of gastroesophageal junction into the thorax)	• Most commonly presents with heartburn (retrosternal burning discomfort, radiating toward the neck, and most commonly experienced in the postprandial period) • Regurgitation less common • Hoarseness • Chronic cough • Aspiration pneumonia • Asthma • Esophagitis symptoms	• Clinical diagnosis. • A pH probe is most specific for diagnosis of reflux disease, but is rarely performed • Other diagnostic tests include upper GI series, esophageal manometry, and upper endoscopy	• Depends on the esophageal manifestation: may be normal or show signs of esophagitis or Barrett esophagus (see below)	• See Table 4-2
Esophagitis	• Inflammation of any part of the esophagus	• GERD • Pills (potassium chloride, NSAIDS, Fosamax) • Infection (*Candida*, Herpes simplex, CMV)	• Heartburn is primary manifestation of reflux esophagitis • Odynophagia (pain with swallowing food) if esophagitis is severe and/or ulcers are present • Dysphagia (difficulty swallowing food) if lower esophagus narrowed due to stricture	• Endoscopy • Consider barium swallow if symptoms of dysphagia	• Inflamed mucosa with possible ulcerations • Biopsy can identify specific infectious etiology	• Reflux esophagitis: acid antisecretory therapy • Infectious esophagitis: antimicrobials • Pill esophagitis: avoid culprit pill

(continued)

95

Table 4-1
Disorders of the Esophagus (continued)

	DEFINITION	ETIOLOGY	CLINICAL PRESENTATION	DIAGNOSIS	ENDOSCOPY AND BIOPSY RESULTS	TREATMENT/NOTES
Barrett Esophagus	• Intestinal-type columnar epithelium replaces the stratified squamous epithelium normally lining the distal esophagus	• GERD • Risk factors: young age at onset of heartburn and long duration of GERD	• Does not cause symptoms on its own • Often associated with symptoms of GERD, as above	• Endoscopy	• Abnormal tissue visualized • Biopsy confirms intestinal type epithelium (1) cardia type, (2) fundic type, or (3) intestinal metaplasia type	• High dose proton pump inhibitor therapy • Low-grade dysplasia: routine surveillance endoscopy • High-grade dysplasia: esophagectomy or local endoscopic resection • Cancer risk: increased risk of developing adenocarcinoma of the esophagus and gastroesophageal junction with intestinal type metaplasia. Dysplasia is an early pathologic finding prior to cancer formation

GERD = gastroesphageal reflux disease; NSAID = nonsteroidal anti-inflammatory drug; CMV = cytomegalovirus; GI = gastrointestinal.

Table 4-2

Treatment of Gastroesophageal Reflux Disease

TREATMENT MODALITY	EXAMPLES
DIETARY MODIFICATION	• Part of first-line therapy • Avoidance of fatty foods, caffeine, chocolate, alcohol • Reduce meal size
Lifestyle Modification	• Part of first-line therapy • Stop smoking • Weight loss
Reflux Precautions	• Part of first-line therapy • Elevate head of bed when sleeping • Avoid lying down for 3 hours after eating
Medications	• Antacids (magnesium/aluminum salts) • Histamine blockers (ranitidine) • Proton pump inhibitors (omeprazole, pantoprazole)
Barrier	• Sucralfate
Prokinetics	• Metoclopramide • Erythromycin
Surgical Intervention	• If lifestyle/diet modifications and medications do not help • Nissen fundoplication • Endoscopic fundoplication

Table 4-3
Esophageal and Gastric Cancer

	ESOPHAGEAL CANCER		GASTRIC CANCER
	ADENOCARCINOMA	**SQUAMOUS CELL CARCINOMA**	**ADENOCARCINOMA**
EPIDEMIOLOGY	• 50% of all cases and growing in proportion • Primarily white males >40 years old	• 50% of all cases • Blacks five times greater than whites • Males three times greater than females	• Higher incidence in Asian countries • Incidence in second generation Asian immigrants to the United States decline toward U.S. rates • Overall, incidence has declined in past few decades. Theories for this decline include treatment of *Helicobacter pylori* and refrigeration
Etiology/Risk Factors	• Barrett esophagus (intestinal metaplasia with columnar cells and goblet cells)	• Alcohol • Tobacco • Achalasia	• Antral and gastric body adenocarcinoma are linked to *H. pylori* infection • Atrophic gastritis • Intestinal metaplasia • Diets high in nitrates
Clinical Presentation	• History of GERD • Dysphagia to solids > liquids • Chest pain • Odynophagia • Usually diagnosed in advanced stage	• Dysphagia to solids > liquids • Chest pain • Odynophagia • Usually diagnosed in advanced stage	• Often asymptomatic until tumor advanced • Abdominal pain • Early satiety • Nausea • Vomiting • Iron deficiency anemia • Gastric ulcers may have underlying gastric cancer • Usually diagnosed in advanced stage
Diagnosis	• EGD with biopsy and brushings • All suggestive ulcers need to be reevaluated to confirm healing • Persistent mucosal abnormalities require biopsy • Staging with CT scan to evaluate distant metastases • If no distant metastasis, presurgical evaluation with endoscopic ultrasound to evaluate for resectability		
Treatment	• Surgical resection if limited disease • Chemotherapy +/− radiation for advanced disease • Poor prognosis		

CT = computed tomography; EGD = esophagogastroduodenoscopy.

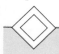

Cholangiocarcinoma

Definition: Cancer of the biliary tract.
Epidemiology: Rare.
Clinical presentation: Presents with painless jaundice and pruritus.
Diagnosis: Ultrasound and magnetic resonance cholangiopancreatography (MRCP) can localize abnormalities of the biliary system. Endoscopic retrograde cholangiopancreatography (ERCP) with brushings of a stricture can also aid in making the diagnosis.
Treatment: Surgery is rarely curative. Percutaneous drainage and stenting by ERCP can palliate biliary obstruction symptoms.

Table 4-4

Gastrointestinal Motility Disorders

	DEFINITION	ETIOLOGY	CLINICAL PRESENTATION	DIAGNOSIS	RADIOLOGIC FEATURES	TREATMENT
Achalasia	• Lack of peristalsis of esophagus with an associated failure to relax a hypertonic lower esophageal sphincter	• Neuromuscular disorder of the esophagus • Loss of esophageal ganglion cells and degeneration of neuromuscular fibers result in loss of the natural rhythmic movement of the esophagus	• Dysphagia to solids and liquids	• Barium swallow: dilated proximal esophagus and narrowed distal esophagus • Manometry	• "Bird Beak" on barium swallow	• Short-term: calcium channel blockers or endoscopic injection of botulinum toxin • Long-term: pneumatic dilation or surgical myotomy
Esophageal Spasm	• Dysmotility of the esophagus with spastic contraction of multiple areas in the esophagus	• Unknown	• Severe noncardiac chest pain	• Manometry: simultaneous onset of esophageal contractions at two or more adjacent recording sites (>20% of esophagus simultaneously contracting)	• "Corkscrew esophagus" on x-ray	• Trial of nitrates or calcium channel blocker (limited data)
Gastroparesis	• Impairment of gastric emptying due to neuromuscular dysfunction	• Systemic disease - Diabetes - Scleroderma - Hypothyroidism • Medication effect - Narcotics - Anticholinergic agents - Calcium channel blockers • Viral illness • Idiopathic causes	• Chronic or intermittent nausea and vomiting • Early satiety • Postprandial dyspepsia • May have significant weight loss in severe cases	• EGD to rule out structural obstruction • Gastric emptying study is the gold standard • Can also perform electrogastrography	• Delayed emptying on gastric emptying study	• Dietary modifications such as small, frequent meals, low fat diet • Prokinetic agents (metoclopramide, erythromycin) • May need jejunal tube for feedings in severe cases

Table 4-5

Peptic Ulcer Disease and Dyspepsia

	DEFINITION	CLINICAL PRESENTATION	NOTES
Peptic Ulcer Disease	• Ulceration of the gastric or duodenal mucosa	• Burning epigastric pain (dyspepsia) with or without upper GI bleeding	• EGD with biopsy for *H. pylori* • Other diagnostic tests for *H. pylori* include urea breath test, fecal antigen, and serologic antibody testing
Dyspepsia	• Pain or discomfort in the upper abdomen • Clinical diagnosis prior to investigation to rule out peptic ulcer disease (above) • No structural lesions are often identified, although work-up needs to rule out peptic ulcer disease • May be related to gallstones, gastroparesis, and gastric cancer • Role of *H. pylori* is controversial	• Postprandial fullness • Early satiety • Epigastric abdominal pain • Bloating and/or nausea	• Treatment: Consider acid antisecretory therapy, *H. pylori* eradication, prokinetic agents such as metoclopramide or erythromycin
NonUlcer Dyspepsia	• Diagnosis of exclusion after ruling out peptic ulcer disease (above) as the cause of dyspepsia		• EGD • Unclear role for *H. pylori* testing

Table 4-6

Etiology and Risk Factors for Peptic Ulcer Disease

ETIOLOGIES	RISK FACTORS
• *H. pylori* infection • NSAIDS • Burns (Curling ulcer) • Head trauma/surgery (Cushing ulcer) • Chronic gastritis • Zollinger-Ellison syndrome (hypergastrinemia)	• Advanced age • Multiple NSAIDS • Anticoagulant therapy • Glucocorticoid treatment

Table 4-7

Peptic Ulcer Disease by Disease Site

ULCER SITE	*H. PYLORI* ASSOCIATED	CLINICAL
Gastric	• Less common	• Pain after eating
Duodenal	• More common	• Pain before eating • Pain relieved with food • Can penetrate through muscularis and perforate, causing pancreatitis

Table 4-8
Celiac and Tropical Sprue

	DEFINITION	ETIOLOGY	CLINICAL PRESENTATION	DIAGNOSIS	TREATMENT	COMPLICATIONS	ASSOCIATED DISEASES
Celiac Sprue	• Gluten-sensitive enteropathy	• Gluten allergy and hypersensitivity cause small bowel mucosal damage and villous atrophy • Gluten is a protein found in wheat, barley, rye, and oats	• Can present at any age • Weight loss • Flatulence • Diarrhea • Mild disease may have no GI symptoms • Affects proximal small bowel first • May have malabsorption of iron and calcium • In one study, celiac found in 10% of patients with asymptomatic AST/ALT elevation	• Small bowel biopsy shows flattening of villi and infiltration with lympho-cytes and plasma cells (may be normal if already on gluten free diet) • Serologic testing a useful adjunct - tissue transglu-taminase (most specific) - serum antigliadin - antiendomysial antibody	• Lifelong gluten free diet • May need to supplement vitamins if malabsorption occurs.	• Iron defi-ciency anemia • Osteopenic bone disease • Hypocalcemia	• Dermatitis herpetaformis • Intestinal lymphoma • Small bowel adenocarci-noma • Elevated liver function tests • HLA DQ2/DR3
Tropical Sprue	• Overgrowth of coliform bacteria and folic acid deficiency	• Infection • More common in those living in or traveling to the tropics	• Similar to celiac sprue	• Biopsy similar to celiac sprue	• Antibiotics • Folic acid sup-plementation		

AST/ALT = aspartate aminotransferase/alanine aminotranferease.

Table 4-9

Acute Diarrhea: Causes and Diagnosis

Type of Diarrhea	Definition	Etiology	Clinical Presentation	Diagnostic Tests	Treatment
Infectious	• Diarrhea is defined by the production of more than 250 g of stool daily, often with increased stool frequency and watery consistency • History reveals sudden onset	**Bacteria:** *Campylobacter jejuni,* nontyphoid *Salmonella,* enteropathic *Escherichia coli, Shigella, Yersinia enterocolitica* **Viruses:** rotavirus, Norwalk virus **Parasites:** *Giardia, Cryptosporidium, Entamoeba histolytica*	• *Y. enterocolitica* may present with signs mimicking appendicitis • *E. coli* O157:H7 may present with hemolytic-uremic syndrome	• Stool tests—culture, Gram stain, ova, and parasites • Hemoccult positive	• Intravenous resuscitation if severely dehydrated • Depends on underlying cause • Antibiotics are controversial • Antidiarrheal agents (loperamide, kaolin, and pectin, diphenoxylate with atropine) for refractory disease
Toxin Mediated		*Staph Aureus, Clostridium perfringens, Vibrio cholerae,* enterotoxigenic *E. coli, Clostridium difficile*	• Nausea and vomiting possible	• Stool test for *C. difficile* toxin A, B	

104

Table 4-10

Chronic Diarrhea: Causes and Diagnosis

Type of Diarrhea	Diagnostic Tests	Etiology
Osmotic	• Fecal osmotic gap >50 Gap = [280 − 2*([Na]+[K])] (measure stool electrolytes) • Improvement of diarrhea with fasting • D-xylose test (rule out small bowel malabsoprtion)	• Lactase deficiency • Nonabsorbed sugars (sorbitol, fructose) • Magnesium intake (magnesium citrate) • Sprue (celiac or tropical) • Pancreatic insufficiency • Laxative abuse
Secretory	• Fecal osmotic gap <50 • No improvement of diarrhea with fasting • Colonoscopy with biopsy • 72-hour fecal fat quantification (rule out fat malabsorption)	• Infectious diarrhea • Bile salt malabsoption • Bacterial overgrowth, postcholecystectomy) • Secreting villous adenoma • VIPoma • Fat malabsorption • Microscopic colitis (collegenous or lymphocytic)
Inflammatory	• Can see ulcers and inflammation on endoscopy • Colonoscopy with biopsy	• Inflammatory bowel disease • Enteroinvasive infections (*Entamoeba histolytica*) • Diversion colitis
Other	• Clinical history • TSH	• Diabetic enteropathy • Irritable bowel syndrome • Hyperthyroidism • HIV (often improves remarkably with antiretroviral therapy if CD4 counts increase by at least 40/μL)

TSH = thyroid stimulating hormone; VIP = vasoactive intestinal peptide.

Table 4-11

Fat Malabsorption

- Patients typically complain of weight loss and diarrhea (bulky, foul-smelling, greasy stools). May have fat-soluble vitamin deficiency (vitamin A, D, E, K) and a low serum calcium. May have complications including nephrolithiasis from calcium oxalate stones and prolonged prothrombin time from vitamin K deficiency

TYPE	CLINICAL PRESENTATION	CAUSES	DIAGNOSIS	TREATMENT
Pancreatic Insufficiency	• Weight loss • Diarrhea: bulky, foul-smelling, greasy stools	• Chronic pancreatitis • Pancreatic resection • Cystic fibrosis	• Clinical history	• Pancreatic enzyme replacement
Bile Salt Deficiency	• Deficiency of fat-soluble vitamins (vitamin A, D, E, K) • Low serum calcium • Complications include: - Calcium oxalate nephrolithiasis - Prolonged prothrombin time	• Cholestasis • Crohn disease • Cholecystocolonic fistula • Short bowel syndrome (>100 cm ileal resection)	• Clinical history • Small bowel series if length of residual bowel unknown after resection (short bowel syndrome)	• Limit fat intake • Supplement with medium-chain triglycerides
Bile Salt Diarrhea		• Ileal resection (<100 cm resected)	• Empiric treatment • Quantification of fecal bile acids	• Cholestyramine
Small Bowel Disease		• Bacterial overgrowth • Celiac sprue • Tropical sprue • Whipple disease • Crohn disease • Eosinophilic enteritis	• Endoscopy with small bowel biopsy • Lactulose breath test shows bacterial over-growth	• Antibiotics for bacterial overgrowth, Tropical sprue, and Whipple disease • Immunosuppresives for Crohn disease, eosinophilic enteritis

Table 4-12

Inflammatory Bowel Disease

	CROHN DISEASE	ULCERATIVE COLITIS
Etiology	• In genetically predisposed individuals, environmental triggers may induce an inflammatory response • Incidence is bimodal with a peak in adolescence and young adulthood and again in later in life (>50 years old) • Classically presents with abdominal pain and bloody stools • May present with only fever, weight loss, or any extraintestinal manifestation listed below	
Location of Involvement	• Mouth to anus	• Colon and rectum
Type of Involvement	• Skip lesions • Transmural inflammation	• Continuous lesions • Mucosal inflammation
Histology	• Granulomas • Fissures • Fistulas • Strictures • Apthous ulcers	• Crypt abscesses
Clinical Features	• Fever • Weight loss • Crampy abdominal pain • Diarrhea • Abscess formation	• Fever • Weight loss • Rectal bleeding • Tenesmus • Abscess formation
Extraintestinal Manifestations (More Common in Crohn Disease)	• Erythema nodosum • Arthritis • Kidney stones • Oral ulcers • Digital clubbing	• Erythema nodosum • Arthritis • Pyoderma gangrenosum • Sclerosing cholangitis • Ankylosing spondylitis • Episcleritis/uveitis
Cancer Risk	• Low	• High
Diagnosis	• EGD/colonoscopy with biopsy • Serology: ASCA	• Colonoscopy with biopsy • Serology: ANCA

(continued)

Table 4-12

Inflammatory Bowel Disease (continued)

	CROHN DISEASE	ULCERATIVE COLITIS
TREATMENT	• Corticosteroids • 5-ASA medications • 6-Mercaptopurine/azathioprine • Methotrexate • Anti-TNF therapy (infliximab) • Antibiotics for suspected abscess • Surveillance for malignancy • Surgery only useful for treatment of complications	• Corticosteroids (enemas or oral) • 5-ASA medications • 6-Mercaptopurine/Azathioprine • Cyclosporine • Methotrexate • Surveillance for malignancy • Colectomy is curative

ANCA = serum antineutrophil cytoplasmic antibody; ASCA = serum anti-*Saccharomyces cervisiae* antibody; TNF = tumor necrosis factor.

Table 4-13

Irritable Bowel Syndrome

	IRRITABLE BOWEL SYNDROME
Definition	• Functional disorder characterized by altered bowel habits with or without abdominal pain in the absence of organic disease
Etiology	• Unknown • Often have visceral hypersensitivity to noxious stimuli
Epidemiology	• Affects all people, but younger women more likely to be diagnosed. Incidence estimated to be 10–15% in North America
Histology	• Normal
Clinical Features	• Patients fall into one of three categories: (1) constipation predominant (2) diarrhea predominant (3) pain predominant
Extra-intestinal Manifestations	• None
Cancer Risk	• None
Diagnosis	• Diagnosis of exclusion • Laboratory tests negative (e.g., CBC, ESR) • Endoscopy negative
Treatment	• Reassurance • Dietary modification (lactose restriction, fiber supplementation) • Symptom based medication treatment (antimotility agents for diarrhea, anticholinergic agents for colonic spasm) • Consider psychotherapy or antidepressants if evidence of symptom exacerbation from psychiatric etiology

CBC = complete blood count; ESR = erythrocyte sedimentation rate.

Table 4-14

Diverticulitis and Diverticular Bleeding

	DIVERTICULITIS	DIVERTICULAR BLEEDING
Etiology	• Micro or macrosopic perforation leading to inflammation of a diverticulum	• Bleeding from a diverticulum (usually right-sided)
Notes about Underlying Diverticular Disease	• A diverticulum is a sac-like protrusion of the colonic wall • Diverticulosis describes the presence of diverticula • Prevalence increases with age: about 5% at 40 years to 65% at 85 years • Higher prevalence in Western countries where it tends to occurs in the left colon • Risk factor: low fiber diet • 70% of patients with diverticular disease are asymptomatic	
Epidemiology	• 15–20% of patients with diverticulular disease	• 5–15% of patients with diverticular disease • Most common cause of lower GI bleed
Clinical Features	• Left lower quadrant abdominal pain • Nausea • Vomiting • Recent obstipation • Diarrhea • Fever • Leukocytosis	• Massive bleeding in one-third of patients • Spontaneously stops in 75% of cases • High risk of rebleeding
Diagnosis	• CT scan shows pericolic stranding and bowel wall thickening • Colonoscopy and barium enema contraindicated because of the risk of rupture	• Radionuclide scan may localize bleeding • Angiogram most accurate for detection of the site of bleeding, but higher risk of complications • Colonoscopy less accurate than angiography in localizing source of bleeding
Diagnosis	• Colonoscopy • CT	• Colonoscopy • CT
Treatment	• Bowel rest • Intravenous fluids • Broad spectrum antibiotics should produce improvement in 48–72 hours • 25% of first time patients develop complicated diverticultitis (localized perforation, colonic obstruction, pericolonic abscess or fistula formation)	• Colonoscopic evaluation allows epinephrine injection near bleeding diverticulum or coagulation of visibly bleeding vessels • If bleeding uncontrolled, may need segmental colonic resection • Lower rates of postoperative rebleeding if source of bleeding localized preoperatively

Table 4-15

Colon Cancer

	COLON CANCER
Definition	• Invasive or noninvasive cancer arising in the colon
Etiology	• Nearly all colon cancers arise from adenomatous polyps of the colon (tubular, tubulovillous, or villous) • Malignant transformation of adenomas may take 5 or more years • Only 5–10% of sporadic adenomas progress to cancer
Epidemiology	• Third most common cancer in men and women and third most common cause of cancer death in men and women • 70% of cases are sporadic • Increased incidence after age 50
Risk Factors	• Western diet (high fat, low fiber) • Tobacco use • Advanced age • Family history of colon cancer • IBD
Genetics	• Carcinogenesis involves accumulation of genetic mutations and epigenetic alternations • Mutations in APC gene occur early in malignancy process in both sporadic and inherited tumors • Mutations in the p53 suppressor gene occur late in malignancy process • See Table 14-6
Protective Factors	• Aspirin and COX-2 inhibitors may protect against colon cancer • Folic acid may protect against colon cancer, especially in those who drink moderate amounts of alcohol • Calcium may also be protective, as are diets high in fiber, low in fats • Avoidance of tobacco products and moderate alcohol intake • Removal of adenomas
Clinical Features	• Precancerous polyps rarely symptomatic • Hematochezia • Altered bowel habits • Abdominal pain • Iron-deficiency anemia
Screening	• Fecal occult blood testing every year • Various guidelines for screening with colonoscopy or sigmoidoscopy • Frequent screening colonoscopies if history of inflammatory bowel disease, genetic predisposition or strong family history
Diagnosis	• Colonoscopy is diagnostic test of choice because biopsies are needed for pathologic examination • Once diagnosis made, CT scan of abdomen can evaluate the extent of the disease and show evidence of liver metastases • Baseline CEA levels should be obtained

(continued)

Table 4-15
Colon Cancer (continued)

	COLON CANCER
Treatment	• Polypectomy is curative if not a invasive tumor • For localized disease, hemicolectomy with lymph node sampling may offer cure • Adjuvant chemotherapy with 5-fluorouracil based combination chemotherapy after resection if high-risk disease • Isolated liver metastases may be resectable • Metastatic disease treated with 5-fluorouracil based combination chemotherapy and may include bevacizumab, an anti-VEGF (vascular endothelial growth factor) antibody

COX-2 = cyclooxygenase 2; IBD = inflammatory bowel disease; VEGF = vascular endothelial growth factor.

Table 4-16
Colon Cancer Genetics

	IMPORTANT RESPONSIBLE GENES	MODE OF ACQUISITION
FAP	• APC	• Germline (inherited)
HNPCC or Lynch Syndrome	• MMR • MMR mutations can be identified by the presence of MSI • MSI associated with longer survival	• Germline (inherited)
Sporadic Tumors	• Tumor suppressor genes (p53, APC and others) • Oncogenes (c-myc, ras, and others) • MMR genes defects (15–20% of sporadic tumors) • In contrast to HNPCC, epigenetic hyper-methylation of promoter region and/or loss of imprinting of MMR genes lead to MSI in sporadic cancers	• Somatic (acquired)

FAP = familial adenomatous polyposis; APC = adenomatous polyposis coli; MMR = mismatch repair genes; MSI = microsatellite instability; HNPCC = hereditary nonpolyposis colorectal cancer.

Table 4-17

Gastrointestinal Bleeding

	UPPER GI BLEEDING	LOWER GI BLEEDING

Blood from Oropharynx	• Bright red blood (hematemesis)
	  - suggests active or rapid bleed
	• Black clots/"coffee grounds"
	  - suggests an old or slow bleed
		• None

Blood from Rectum	• Bright red blood is very *rare* and indicates a very rapid bleed • Melena (thick, black, foul-smelling stool)	• Bright red blood (hematochezia) • Melena - Distal colonic or slow bleed
Etiology	• Esophageal/gastric variceal bleeding (suspect if chronic liver disease) • Swallowed epistaxis • Gastritis • Erosive esophagitis • Peptic ulcer disease • Vascular malformation • Mallory-Weiss tear • Cancer • Hypertensive portal gastropathy • Foreign body/trauma • Aorto-enteric fistula	• Hemorrhoids • Anal fissure • Infectious colitis • Ischemic colitis • Inflammatory bowel disease • Colon cancer • Polyps • Diverticulosis • Vascular malformation • Colonic ulcers

Treatment	• Supportive
	  - IV fluid resuscitation
	  - Blood transfusion if needed
	  - Reversal of any coagulopathy
	• Localized treatment as indicated: for variceal bleeding may need emergent endoscopy with sclerotherapy and banding, as well as octreotide infusion
	• Consider arterial embolization if massive bleeding
	• May cause life threatening cardio-pulmonary complications	

IV = intravenous.

Table 4-18

Ischemic Bowel

	ACUTE MESENTERIC ISCHEMIA	CHRONIC MESENTERIC ISCHEMIA (INTESTINAL ANGINA)	ISCHEMIC COLITIS
Etiology	• Thrombosis/embolism in the celiac trunk or SMA	• Decreased blood flow from atherosclerosis of mesenteric vessels	• Decreased blood flow in nonproximal vessels such as the IMA
Location	• Primarily affects small bowel	• Affects stomach and proximal small bowel	• Primarily affects "watershed" areas of colon (left side)
Risk Factors	• Atrial fibrillation • Valvular heart disease • Hypercoagulability	• Diabetes • Atherosclerotic vascular disease	• Hypotension • Aortic bypass surgery • Hypercoagulability
Clinical Presentation	• Severe abdominal pain • Pain out of proportion to physical exam	• Postprandial abdominal pain • Weight loss • Fear of eating	• Hematochezia • Diarrhea • Crampy abdominal pain
Diagnosis	• Angiography • CT scan • Abdominal x-ray ("Thumb printing")	• Duplex doppler ultrasound • Angiography	• Flexible sigmoidoscopy or colonoscopy (rarely affects rectum)
Treatment	• Thrombolysis/vasodilation therapy during angiography • Surgery if evidence of necrotic bowel	• Surgery • Angioplasty	• IV fluids +/– antibiotics • Rare need for surgery

SMA = superior mesenteric artery; IMA = inferior mesenteric artery.

Table 4-19

Etiologies and Clinical Manifestations of AST and ALT Elevation

DISEASE	PHYSICAL EXAM FINDINGS	DEGREE OF AST/ALT ELEVATION SEVERE: >1000 MODERATE: >250 AND <1000 MILD: <250 NORMAL: <40
Chronic Liver Disease or Cirrhosis	• Spider nevi • Palmar erythema • Gynecomastia • Caput medusae	• Mild • If severe can be associated with thrombocytopenia, hypoalbuminemia, and elevated prothrombin
Cirrhosis	• Palpable left hepatic lobe • Splenomegaly	• Mild
Hepatic Congestion	• Jugular venous distension • Hepato-jugular reflex • Right heart failure	• Mild
Cholecystitis	• Murphy's sign (sudden arrest of inspiration while palpating right upper quadrant) • Fevers	• Mild
Alcoholic Hepatitis	• Painful hepatomegaly	• Moderate (frequently >2:1 AST:ALT ratio)
Viral Hepatitis	• Painful hepatomegaly	• Moderate or severe
Drug-Induced Hepatitis	• Painful hepatomegaly	• Severe
Wilson Disease	• See Table 4-25	• Usually <2000 • AST often greater than ALT
Others (Hemochromatosis, Autoimmune, 1-Antitrypsin Deficiency)	• See Table 4-25	• Variable

Note: Aspartate aminotransferase (AST) and alanine aminotransferase (ALT) are hepatocyte intracellular transaminating enzymes and are detected in the serum after hepatocyte injury or death.

Serum alkaline phosphatase (AP) elevation may be due to production in the liver (glutamyltransferase level [GGT] is also elevated in liver production), bone, intestine, and placenta.

Table 4-20

Disorders Causing Hyperbilirubinemia

| INDIRECT HYPERBILIRUBINEMIA | | DIRECT HYPERBILIRUBINEMIA | |
ETIOLOGY	DESCRIPTION/NOTES	ETIOLOGY	SOURCE OF CHOLESTASTASIS
Gilbert syndrome	• Decreased glucuronyl transferase enzyme activity • Description: mild jaundice during illness or fasting • Treatment: supportive	• **Sepsis**	• Intrahepatic
Crigler-Najjar syndrome	• Autosomal recessive • Treatment: phototherapy and exchange transfusion	• **Postoperative**	• Intrahepatic
Dubin-Johnson syndrome	• Autosomal recessive. Defect in conjugated bilirubin transfer • Clinical: causes the liver to turn black	• **Drug-induced**	• Intrahepatic
Liver disease (cirrhosis)	• See Table 4–27	• **Hepatitis**	• Intrahepatic • See Table 4–21
Hemolysis	• See Chapter 9	• **Primary biliary cirrhosis**	• Intrahepatic • See Table 4–26
		• **Choledocholithiasis**	• Extrahepatic
		• **Neoplasm**	• Extrahepatic
		• **Primary sclerosing cholangitis**	• Extrahepatic • See Table 4–26

AMA = antimitochondrial antibody; ANA = antinuclear antibody; ERCP = endoscopic retrograde cholangiopancreatography; MRCP = magnetic resonance cholangiopancreatography.

Table 4-21

Overview of the Hepatitis Viruses

	Hepatitis Virus				
	A	**E**	**B**	**C**	**D**
Transmission	• Fecal-oral	• Fecal-oral	• Body fluids - Perinatal in Asia - IV drug abuse - Pre-1980s transfusions	• Body fluids • Percutaneous transmission (IV drug use), most common	• Body fluids • Percutaneous transmission (IV drug use), most common
Acute or Chronic	• Acute only	• Acute only	• Acute or chronic	• Acute or chronic	• Acute or chronic
Clinical Details	• Generally self-limited • Can present as fulminant hepatic failure if have chronic liver disease	• Young adults/pregnant women at increased risk for fulminant hepatic failure • More common in developing countries	• Chronic carriers who receive chemotherapy or radiation therapy may have reactivation	• Acute: usually asymptomatic and rarely diagnosed • Chronic: fatigue and vague abdominal discomfort	• Requires coinfection with HBV • Endemic in Africa and the Mediterranean
Diagnosis	• Anti-HAV IgM	• Anti-HEV antibody	• See Table 4-22	• Anti-HCV antibody	• Anti-HDV antibody
Risk for Chronic Hepatitis and Hepatocellular Carcinoma	• No	• No	• Yes	• Yes	• Yes
Prevention	• Pre-/postexposure immunization • Good hygiene	• Safe drinking water	• Pre-/postexposure immunization	• Behavior modification	• Pre-/postexposure HBV immunization

(continued)

Table 4-21
Overview of the Hepatitis Viruses (continued)

	HEPATITIS VIRUS				
	A	E	B	C	D
Vaccination	• Universal recommendation to general population as well as: - Travelers to endemic regions - Intravenous drug abusers - Homosexuals	• None available	• Universal recommendation to general population as well as: - Health care workers - IV drug abusers - Hemodialysis patients - Close contacts of HBV carriers	• None available	• None available
Immunoglobulin	• Travelers • Household/sexual contacts of patients with hepatitis A	• None available	• Perinatal • Sexual exposure to partner with acute disease • Nonimmune rape victim • Nonimmune with blood exposure whose source cannot be assessed	• None available	• None available
Treatment	• Supportive	• Supportive	• Adefovir • Lamivudine	• Pegylated interferon and ribavirin	• Supportive • Prevention and treatment of HBV
Notes for Acute Hepatitis	• Hepatitis A is by far the most common cause of acute viral hepatitis, followed by Hepatitis B • Presentation ranges from asymptomatic elevation in aminotransferase to severe hepatitis • Frequent prodrome of nonspecific symptoms with anorexia and fatigue • Nausea and right upper quadrant discomfort • Later, jaundice with dark urine and light stools may occur • Liver biopsy is rarely necessary in diagnosing acute hepatitis				
Notes for Chronic Hepatitis	• Liver biopsy is the gold standard for diagnosis and staging of chronic hepatitis • Presentation of chronic hepatitis: often asymptomatic elevation of aminotransferase. May also report fatigue, fever, and jaundice				

HAV = hepatitis A virus; HBV = hepatitis B virus; HCV = hepatitis C virus; HDV = hepatitis D virus; HEV = hepatitis E virus.

Table 4-22
Hepatitis B Serologies

INTERPRETATION	HBsAg	HBeAg	IgM ANTI-HBc	IgG ANTI-HBc	ANTI-HBs	ANTI-HBe	HBV DNA
Acute HBV infection	+	+	+				+
Window phase			+				+/−
Resolved infection				+	+	+	−
Chronic HBV infection	+	+		+			+
HBV reactivation	+	+/−	+				+
Precore mutant	+					+	+
Vaccinated					+		

Table 4-23
Alcoholic Hepatitis and Nonalcoholic Fatty Liver Disease

	ALCOHOLIC HEPATITIS	NAFLD
Definition	• Alcohol-induced injury includes fatty liver, alcoholic hepatitis, and cirrhosis	• Biopsy findings similar to alcoholic hepatitis, but patients lack significant alcohol consumption history
Etiology/Risk Factors	• Alcohol	Risk factors: • Diabetes • Hyperlipidemia • Hypertension • Obesity
Clinical	• Right upper quadrant pain • Jaundice • Fever	• Typically asymptomatic
Laboratory	• Leukocytosis • Anemia • Elevation of aminotransferases with AST:ALT ratio > 2:1	• Elevated transaminases
Diagnosis	• Based on the clinical history and laboratory features	• Diagnosis of exclusion
Liver Biopsy	• Necrosis • Inflammatory infiltrate • Mallory bodies	• Similar to alcoholic hepatitis
Treatment	• Steroids may be helpful if severe • Contraindicated if viral infection	• Treatment of the underlying risk factors • Ursodeoxycholic acid and vitamin E have been used

NAFLD = nonalcoholic fatty liver disease.

Table 4-24

Autoimmune Hepatitis

	TYPE I	TYPE II
Percent of Autoimmune Hepatitis Cases	70–80%	
Female Predominance	Yes	No
Age of Onset	Bimodal: 10–20 years of age and around menopause	Adolescence
Clinical Presentation	• Jaundice • Fatigue • May be asymptomatic • May present with fulminant hepatic failure	
Liver Biopsy	• Dense mononuclear infiltrate (lymphocytes and plasma cells) in the portal triad	
ANA Positive	Yes	No
ASMA Positive	Yes	No
Liver-Kidney Microsomal Antibody Positive	No	Yes
Treatment	• Steroids, azathioprine, cyclosporine, tacrolimus, and mycophenolate mofetil	
Responsiveness to Steroid Treatment	Responsive	Less responsive
Liver Treatment	• Liver transplant for end-stage disease • 25% have recurrence in the graft	
Prognosis	• If untreated, 40% die within 6 months and survivors develop cirrhosis • If treated, prognosis excellent	

ASMA = antismooth muscle antibody.

Table 4-25
Inherited Disorders of the Liver

	Wilson Disease	**AAT**	**Hemochromatosis**
Definition	• Disorder of copper metabolism	• Decreased secretion of alpha1-antitrypsin	• Iron overload
Genetics	• Autosomal recessive • Mutation in ATP7B protein that transports copper in the hepatocyte	• Autosomal recessive • Homozygous most common type (phenotype ZZ) • AAT is an inhibitor of the proteolytic enzyme elastase	• Autosomal recessive • Mutations in the HFE gene • HLA linked
Etiology	• Copper deposits in the liver and other organs (eye, central nervous system)	• AAT is required to protect the liver and lung from proteolytic damage	• Increased intestinal iron absorption • HFE mutation may interact with the transferrin receptor • Iron absorption not regulated by content of iron stores • Iron deposits in the liver, pancreas, heart, joints, and pituitary
Epidemiology	• Presents in childhood and young adulthood	• Likely under-recognized • Studies suggest that prevalence of 1 in 1500 to 1 in 5000 people	• Prevalence in Caucasians: heterozygous state = 10%, homozygous state = 5% • Rare in African Americans
Hepatic Findings	• Acute or chronic hepatitis • Cirrhosis	• Hepatitis or cirrhosis	• Hepatomegaly
Extra-Hepatic Findings	• Kayser-Fleischer rings • Hemolytic anemia • Neuropathy • Neuropsychiatric abnormalities • Arrhythmias	• Emphysema in young (less than 45 years), nonsmokers • Panniculitis (not common)	• Diabetes • Cardiomegaly • Arthralgias • Impotence • "Bronze diabetes" (cirrhosis, diabetes, and skin pigmentation), occurs late in the disease
Diagnosis	• Clinical • Laboratory	• Isolectric focusing or PCR techniques to determine deficient genotype	• Definitive test is liver biopsy • Laboratory

(continued)

Table 4-25

Inherited Disorders of the Liver (continued)

	Wilson Disease	AAT	Hemochromatosis
Laboratory	• Increased transaminases and bilirubin • Decreased ceruloplasmin • Increased urinary copper and hepatic copper concentration	• Low AAT level	• Increased LFTs • Elevated transferrin • Decreased unsaturated iron binding capacity • Elevated ferritin • Transferrin saturation (serum iron divided by transferrin) of >60% in men and >50% in women is frequently diagnosed • Hepatic iron index • Genetic testing for the C282Y mutation of the HFE gene is available
Treatment	• Copper restricted diet • Copper chelation: D-penicillamine and trientine	• Liver transplantation only definitive treatment	• Phlebotomy is the mainstay of treatment • Iron chelation: Deferoxamine

AAT = alpha1-antitrypsin.

Table 4-26
Primary Biliary Cirrhosis and Primary Sclerosing Cholangitis

	PBC	PSC
Etiology	• Destruction of smaller bile ducts	• Destruction of larger bile ducts
Epidemiology	• 95% female • Age 30–65	• 70% male • Mean age 40
Clinical Presentation	• Pruritus • Fatigue • Asymptomatic	• Asymptomatic cholangitis
Laboratory	• Increased alkaline phosphatase	• Increased alkaline phosphatase • Mildly elevated transaminases
Serology	• Antimitochondrial antibody	• No specific antibody • Frequently ANCA positive
Diagnosis	• Liver biopsy	• ERCP
Inflammatory Bowel Disease Association	• No	• Yes
Increased Risk for Cholangiocarcinoma	• No	• Yes
Treatment	• Ursodeoxycholic acid • Liver transplant if end-stage	• ERCP to relieve biliary obstruction • Liver transplant if end-stage

PBC = primary biliary cirrhosis; PSC = primary sclerosing cholangitis.

Table 4-27
Overview of Cirrhosis

ETIOLOGY	DISEASE	PRESENTATION	DIAGNOSIS	TREATMENT

Viral	• Hepatitis B
	• Hepatitis C
		• May be asymptomatic
		• Physical exam findings
		  - Spider angioma
		  - Gynecomastia
		  - Dupreyten contracture
		  - Splenomegaly
		  - Testicular atrophy
		• If decompensated may present with variceal bleeding or encephalopathy
		• Ascites frequent but not specific
			• Gold standard is liver biopsy
			• Laboratory abnormalities:
			  - Increased amino-transferases
			  - Hyperbilirubinemia, hypoalbuminemia
			  - Thrombocytopenia
			  - Increased prothrombin time
				• Management of decompensated cirrhosis (below)
				• Screen for hepato-cellular carcinoma
				• Screen for varices with upper endoscopy
				• Consider nonselec-tive beta-blockers as prophylactic for varices
				• Liver transplant is the only definitive treatment

Toxin	• Alcohol			
Autoimmune	• Autoimmune hepatitis			
Metabolic	• Hemochromatosis • Wilson disease			
Biliary disease	• Primary biliary cirrhosis • Primary scleros-ing cholangitis			
Hepatic outflow obstruction	• Budd-Chiari syndrome • Congestive heart failure			

Table 4-28

Causes of Ascites, by Serum-Ascites Albumin Gradient (SAAG)

High SAAG (>1.1 g/dL)	Low SAAG (<1.1 g/dL)
SAAG = serum albumin level – ascites fluid albumin level	
• Chronic liver disease • Fulminant hepatic failure • Mixed (portal hypertension with another cause) • Heart failure • Budd-Chiari • Portal vein thrombosis	• Malignancy • Tuberculosis • Nephrotic syndrome • Peritoneal dialysis

Table 4-29

Management of Decompensated Cirrhosis by Complication

Complication	Clinical Presentation	Etiology	Diagnosis	Treatment/Prophylaxis
Portal hypertension	• Ascites or varices	• Caused by intra-hepatic resistance to portal blood flow and increased portal blood flow due to splanchnic vasodilation		
Variceal bleeding	• Hematemesis • Melena • Maroon stools	• Portal hypertension	• EGD screening	• EGD with band ligation, sclerotherapy • Prophylaxis with beta-blocker
Ascites	• Distended abdomen • Fluid wave • Shifting dullness • 30% of patients with cirrhosis	• Portal hypertension	• Ultrasound/CT • Diagnostic paracentesis	• Weight monitoring • Fluid restriction • Sodium restriction • Diuresis (spironolactone, furosemide) • Therapeutic paracentesis • TIPS if refractory
SBP	• New onset ascites • Abdominal pain • Fever	• Translocation of enteric bacteria into ascites fluid	• Diagnostic paracentesis: polymorpho-nuclear leukocyte count >250/µl • Cultures of ascites	• Antibiotics • Prophylaxis with antibiotics, especially if variceal bleeding

Table 4-29

Management of Decompensated Cirrhosis by Complication (continued)

COMPLICATION	CLINICAL PRESENTATION	ETIOLOGY	DIAGNOSIS	TREATMENT/PROPHYLAXIS
Hepatic Encephalopathy	• Mood changes (e.g., irritability) • Mental status changes (e.g., confusion)	Precipitating factors: • Constipation • Infections • Medications • Dehydration • Electrolyte imbalances • GI bleeding • Azotemia	• Clinical history (e.g., medication noncompliance) • Asterixis • Can check ammonia level	• Rule out predisposing factors (SBP, other infection, portal vein thrombosis) • Lactulose • Flagyl • Contraindication to TIPS

TIPS = transjugular intrahepatic portosystemic shunt; SBP = spontaneous bacterial peritonitis.

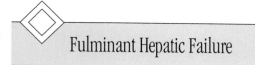

Fulminant Hepatic Failure

Definition: Development of coagulopathy and encephalopathy within 8 weeks of acute hepatocellular injury.

Etiology: The most common etiology is acetaminophen overdose. Patients need to ingest 10 g to become symptomatic unless alcoholic or malnourished. Alcohol enhances hepatic metabolism of acetaminophen to its toxic metabolite. Other etiologies include drug toxicities, viral hepatitis, autoimmune hepatitis, and Wilson disease.

Clinical Presentation: Variable. Complications include hepatic encephalopathy that progresses to coma, cerebral edema (occurs in 30–50%), acute respiratory distress syndrome (ARDS)-type pulmonary symptoms, hypoglycemia, renal failure, infections, and bleeding diathesis.

Treatment: Supportive care. *N*-acetylcysteine if acetaminophen-induced. Consider evaluation for liver transplantation.

Liver Transplantation

Indications: Viral hepatitis, alcoholic cirrhosis, and cryptogenic cirrhosis are the most common indications for transplantation, although limited hepatocellular carcinoma is also an indication.

Contraindications: Active alcohol or drug use is a contraindication to liver transplantation. Cardiac or pulmonary instability are relative contraindications.

Treatment: Immunosuppressants (steroids, cyclosporine, tacrolimus, mycophenolate mofetil, and azathioprine) reduce risk of allograft rejection.

Table 4-30

Benign, Infectious, and Malignant Hepatic Lesions

	DISEASE	CLINICAL NOTES
Benign	Hemangioma	• Most common benign tumor: occurs in 4% of population • Usually asymptomatic, but may cause pain if hemangioma bleeds or infarcts • No need for treatment unless a risk of rupture or large enough to cause mass effect
	Focal nodular hyperplasia	• Second most common benign hepatic tumor: occurs in <1% of population • Usually a solitary lesion and characterized by a stellate scar • Controversial if estrogens increase growth and increase hemorrhage rate • Usually asymptomatic • No need for treatment if no symptoms and lesions do not change
	Hepatic adenoma	• Rare tumor occurring in women of childbearing age • Associated with oral contraceptive use, pregnancy, and diabetes • Can be removed surgically • May transform into a malignant lesion
	Hepatic cysts	• Congenital lesions found in 1% of adults • Fluid accumulation usually recurs after aspiration • Further evaluation usually not needed • May have single or multiple cysts
Infectious	Hytatid cysts	• Hepatic cyst with daughter cysts and calcifications • Serologic test to rule out echinococcal disease
	Hepatic abscesses	• Amebic abscesses found in travelers returning from subtropical areas • Amebic abscesses respond well to metronidazole • Pyogenic abscesses require ultrasound guided aspiration for gram stain/culture • Pyogenic abscesses may need percutaneous drainage. Surgery rarely needed
Malignant	Metastasis from nonhepatic cancers	• Most common etiology • Resection of solitary colorectal cancer metastatic lesions may improve survival
	Hepatocellular carcinoma	• Usually occurs in cirrhotic patients • Most frequent primary liver cancer • Alpha-fetoprotein levels may be elevated, but it is a poor screening tool due to low sensitivity and fair specificity • Small lesions may be cured by curative transplant (cancer may recur in graft liver) • Large lesions have a poor prognosis. Treat with chemotherapy and/or chemoembolization
	Fibrolamellar carcinoma	• Occurs in young patients without cirrhosis
	Cholangiocarcinoma	• Increased risk in patients with primary sclerosing cholangitis

Table 4-31
Liver Diseases in Pregnancy, by Trimester

TRIMESTER	DISEASE	SYMPTOMS	LABORATORY VALUES	TREATMENT/MISCELLANEOUS
First	Hyperemesis gravidarum	• Nausea • Vomiting	• Mildly elevated transaminases	• Antiemetics • Hydration
Second or Third	Cholestasis of pregnancy	• Pruritus	• Mildly elevated alkaline phosphatase and bilirubin • Moderately elevated transaminases	• Ursodeoxycholic acid • Early delivery
Third	HELLP syndrome	• Abdominal pain • Nausea • Vomiting	• Hemolysis • Moderately elevated transaminases • Platelet <100,000	• Delivery of fetus
	Acute fatty liver of pregnancy	• Abdominal pain • Nausea	• Moderately elevated transaminases	• Delivery of fetus
	Preeclampsia/ eclampsia	• Abdominal pain • Edema • Hypertension	• Moderately elevated transaminases • Proteinuria	• Expectant delivery
Any	Viral hepatitis	• Fever • Nausea • Vomiting • Fatigue	• Severely elevated transaminases • 20% of pregnant women with hepatitis E develop fulminant hepatic failure	• Supportive care • Severity of hepatitis caused by hepatitis E, herpes zoster, or herpes simplex increased in pregnancy
	Drug-induced hepatitis	• RUQ pain • Nausea	• Mildly to severely elevated transaminases	• Remove offending agent
	Biliary tract disease	• RUQ pain • Nausea • Fever	• Elevated bilirubin and alkaline phosphatase if biliary obstruction	• Depends on exact disease
Normal Pregnancy	Serum albumin decreases throughout a normal pregnancy due to volume expansion Serum alkaline phosphatase levels increase during the third trimester			

HELLP = hemolysis, elevated liver enzymes, and low platelets; RUQ = right upper quadrant.

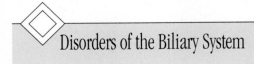

Disorders of the Biliary System

Mirizzi Syndrome

Definition: Uncommon complication when gallstone impacted in cystic duct of the neck of the gallbladder causing extrinsic compression of, or fistula formation to, the adjacent bile duct.

Clinical Presentation: Jaundice and recurrent cholangitis.

Diagnosis: Imaging shows dilation of common hepatic and intrahepatic ducts, but distal common bile duct normal.

Treatment: Endoscopic stenting of common bile duct and stone remove.

Table 4-32
Cholelithiasis and Choledocolithiasis

	CHOLELITHIASIS	CHOLEDOCHOLITHIASIS
Definition	• Solid bodies formed from bile components, with 80% made of cholesterol	• Gallstones in the common bile duct (formed de novo or migrated from gallbladder)
Risk Factors	• Obesity • Rapid weight loss • Female gender • Multiparity • Age greater than 40 years • Ethnicity (Native Americans and Chileans are at higher risk) • Use of total parental nutrition • Patients with cirrhosis also develop gallstones more frequently	• Risk factors for gallstone formation
Epidemiology	• 20.5 million people in the United States aged 20–74 have gallstones	• Most common cause of acute pancreatitis worldwide
Clinical Presentation	• Often asymptomatic • Symptoms develop at a rate of 1–2% per year • Constant right upper quadrant pain occurring an hour after a fatty meal and lasting several hours is classic (biliary colic) • Pain may be severe and associated with nausea, vomiting and diaphoresis • Biliary sludge (microlithiasis) may produce similar symptoms as cholelithiasis	• Symptoms of cholelithiasis or pancreatitis • May also causes cholangitis and secondary biliary cirrhosis
Imaging	• Ultrasound evaluation if symptomatic • Most discovered incidentally	• Dilation of the common bile duct (low sensitivity) on ultrasound • ERCP or MRI cholangrophy can show stone

Table 4-32

Cholelithiasis and Choledocolithiasis (continued)

	CHOLELITHIASIS	CHOLEDOCHOLITHIASIS
Laboratory		• Increased transaminases, alkaline phosphatase, and bilirubin

Treatment	• If asymptomatic, no need for treatment
	• Cholecystectomy indicated if symptomatic because 50% of patients will have repeat episodes
	• Complications occur when stone become impacted in the biliary tree:
	  - Cholecystitis (most common)
	  - Cholangitis (6–9%)
	  - Mirizzi syndrome (rare)
		• Requires multidisciplinary approach and depends on comorbidities. Options include surgical or ERCP approaches
		• Most patients with mild pancreatitis pass stone spontaneously

Table 4-33
Cholecystitis, Cholangitis

	ACUTE CHOLECYSTITIS	ACALCULOUS CHOLECYSTITIS	ACUTE CHOLANGITIS
Etiology	• Cystic duct obstruction from gallstone leading to distention and inflammation of the gallbladder • Most common complication of gallstone disease	• Necroinflammatory disease of the gallbladder with a multifactorial pathogenesis • Inflammation of the gallbladder without detectable stones • Acute or chronic	• Biliary obstruction and stasis secondary to benign calculi or stricture leading to subsequent suppurative infection within biliary tree
Clinical Presentation	• RUQ pain • Murphy sign (pain and interruption of deep inspiration when pressure applied to beneath the right costal arch) • 50% with acute cholecystitis have a secondary infection of the bile or gallbladder (fever and pain for >6 hours) • Mortality = 1%	• Acute: biliary colic with fever • Acute: mortality = 10–50% • Acute: often occurs in mechanically ventilated burn or trauma patients • Chronic: reduced rate of gallbladder emptying (gallbladder dyskinesia) associated with sphincter of Oddi dysfunction	• Charcot triad in 50–100%: pain, fever and RUQ pain • Reynolds pentad associated with high mortality: pain, fever, jaundice, hypotension, and mental confusion
Diagnosis	• Clinical, laboratory, radiographic	• Clinical and radiographic	• Clinical, laboratory, radiographic
Laboratory	• Leukocytosis	• Bacterial or viral causes (*Salmonella* or CMV)	• Increased transaminases, alkaline phosphatase, and bilirubin (often >2mg/dL) • Bacteremia in 20–80%, usually gram-negative bacilli and enterococci
Ultrasound	• Gallstone visualized • Thickened gallbladder wall and pericholecystic fluid • Best technique for evaluating the gallbladder	• Absence of gallstones or sludge • Thickened gallbladder wall and pericholecystic fluid	• Dilation of the common bile duct • Limited by sensitivity

Other Imaging	• Nonvisualization of the gallbladder on biliary scintigraphy	• Chronic: radionuclide scintigraphy demonstrate cholecystokinin-stimulated gallbladder ejection fraction of less than 35%	• MRCP: increased sensitivity for common bile duct stones • ERCP and endoscopic ultrasound: increased diagnostic potential
Treatment	• Hospitalization • Hydration • Antibiotics • Treatment of choice: laparoscopic cholecystectomy • Poor operative candidates: percutaneous cholecystostomy	• Antibiotics • If acute, urgent cholecystecomy • If chronic, planned cholecystectomy	• Hospitalization and hydration • Antibiotics: ureidopenicillin plus metronidazole or aminoglycoside, third-generation cephalosporin • Treatment of choice: ERCP with sphincterectomy • If a poor ERCP candidate: percutaneous drainage • AIDS cholangiopathy affects HIV patients whose CD4 is less than 200/μL

CMV = cytomegalovirus.

131

Disorders of the Pancreas

Table 4-34

Acute and Chronic Pancreatitis

	DEFINITION	CLINICAL PRESENTATION:	DIAGNOSIS	TREATMENT (GENERAL)	NOTES
Acute Pancreatitis	• Acute inflammation of the pancreas	• Abdominal pain (epigastric and radiating to the back)–steady and can last for days • Nausea • Vomiting • Signs/symptoms of cardiovascular compromise	• History and physical • Lipase elevated (more specific than amylase) • Amylase elevated (may be normal if an alcoholic) • CT: inflammation surrounding the pancreas • Initial evaluation should identify high-risk patients requiring intensive care (several scoring systems) • Interstitial pancreatitis = 80% • Necrotizing pancreatitis = 20%	• Supportive • Aggressive hydrated • If interstitial pancreatitis, mortality is less than 1% • In necrotizing pancreatitis, mortality is 10–30% • High-risk patients: cared for in intensive care • Low-risk: pain control. Keep NPO	• Amylase and lipase falsely elevated with: - Intra-abdominal inflammation - Renal insufficiency - Increased production of nonpancreatic enzymes
Chronic Pancreatitis	• Recurrent inflammation of the pancreas characterized by irreversible morphologic changes: - Strictures - Calculi - Dilation of the pancreatic duct	• Pancreatic insufficiency: - Steatorrhea - Diabetes (late) • Abdominal pain (epigastric radiating to the back, and worsened with meals)	• Plain films of the abdomen: pancreatic calcification • CT and MRI: dilation of the ducts • ERCP can aid diagnosis	• Pancreatic enzyme replacement before meals may relieve steatorrhea and pain • Analgesia can be a therapeutic challenge and often requires narcotics	

NPO = nothing per os; MRI = magnetic resonance imaging.

Table 4-35

Etiologies and Specific Treatments of Pancreatitis

TYPE OF PANCREATITIS	MECHANISM	EXAMPLE	NOTES	TREATMENT
Acute Pancreatitis	**Obstructive**	• Gallstone	• Most common cause • More likely in female patients, patients older than 40 years, and multiparous women, rapid weight loss and prolonged fasting	• Laparoscopic cholecystectomy
		• Microlithiasis	• Functional or mechanical causes of bile stasis as for gallstones	• Laparoscopic cholecystectomy
	Toxin	• Alcohol	• Second most common cause of acute pancreatitis	• Discontinue alcohol consumption
		• Medications	• Diuretics (furosemide and thiazides) • HIV medications (pentamidine) • Sulfa derivatives • Immunomodulating drugs (azathioprine)	• Discontinue offending medication
		• Scorpion venom		
	Metabolic	• Hyperlipidemia		• Treat underlying disease
	Iatrogenic	• Post-ERCP		• Supportive

(continued)

Table 4-35

Etiologies and Specific Treatments of Pancreatitis (continued)

TYPE OF PANCREATITIS	MECHANISM	EXAMPLE	NOTES	TREATMENT
Chronic Pancreatitis	**Toxin**	• Alcohol	• Causes 60% of chronic pancreatitis in Western countries • Patients often under-report use • Often occurs in men aged 35–45 who drink 150 g or more of ethanol daily for 6+ years	• Discontinue alcohol consumption
	History	• Prior severe acute pancre-atitis		• Avoid exacerbating factors such as alcohol and smoking
	Hereditary	• Genetic	• Genetic mutations found in the CFTR for acute and chronic pancreatitis	
	Autoimmune	• Autoimmune	• Occurs in Asia • Associated with hypergammaglobun-linemia and autoantibodies	
	Infectious	• Viral • Bacterial • Parasitic	• HIV, mumps, coxsackie, influenza, CMV • Ascaris infection	• Treat infection
	Trauma	• Blunt or penetrating		• Supportive • May need drain placement if pancreas lacerated

CFTR = cystic fibrosis transmembrane conductase regulator.

Table 4-36

Complications of Pancreatitis: Description and Treatment

	NOTES	TREATMENT
Organ failure	• Adult respiratory distress syndrome • Disseminated intravascular coagulation • Renal failure • Shock	• Intensive care unit monitoring • Broad spectrum antibiotics such as imipenem • May need surgical debridement, especially if infected necrosis occurs
Psuedocyst	• CT shows a collection of pancreatic fluid surrounded by fibrous wall	• If symptomatic, endoscopic or surgical drainage
Abscess	• Visualized on CT	• Surgical drainage
Hemorrhage	• Can also be diagnosed by angiography	• Surgical drainage

Table 4-37

Pancreatic Neoplasms

DISEASE	EPIDEMIOLOGY	PRESENTATION/ DIAGNOSIS	DIAGNOSIS	TREATMENT
Adenocarcinoma	• Most common pancreatic cancer • Most occur in the pancreatic head • Age group: 60–70 • Men > women • Risk factors include tobacco, family history, and chronic pancreatitis	• Jaundice • Abdominal pain • Weight loss • Poor appetite	• Usually found on imaging (CT) • Tissue diagnosis via CT-guided biopsy, endoscopic ultrasound or ERCP with brushings for cytology • Tumor markers (carcinoembryonic antigen [CEA], CA19-9, and CA125) not useful for screening, but can be useful in diagnosis and following treatment	• Whipple resection (pancreaticoduodenectomy) if localized • Adjuvant chemotherapy (5-fluorouracil and gemcitabine) and radiation may be useful after resection • ERCP with stent placement to palliate pruritis • Poor prognosis if not resectable • Chemotherapy for palliation only if metastatic
IPMT	• Uncommon • Men > women • High malignant potential	• Abdominal pain	• Dilated pancreatic duct on imaging	• Surgical resection

(continued)

Table 4-37

Pancreatic Neoplasms (continued)

DISEASE	EPIDEMIOLOGY	PRESENTATION/ DIAGNOSIS	DIAGNOSIS	TREATMENT
Neuroendocrine tumors (gastrinoma, insulinoma, glucagonoma, VIPoma)	• Uncommon	• Functional tumors: depends on hormone released by tumor	• Octreotide scan	• Surgical resection if localized • Octreotide and chemoembolization for metastatic/ symptomatic disease
Carcinoid	• Uncommon, but most common GI neuroendocrine tumor	• Carcinoid syndrome (flushing, HTN, cramping, diarrhea) after metastatic to liver	• Increased urinary 5-HIAA • Octreotide scan	• Surgical resection if localized • Octreotide and chemoembolization for metastatic disease

CEA = carcinoembryonic antigen; IPMT = intraductal papillary mucinous tumor.

Chapter 5

Nephrology

Table 5-1

Genetic Renal Disease

		CLINICAL PRESENTATION			
DISEASE	**EPIDEMIOLOGY/ETIOLOGY**	**RENAL MANIFESTATIONS**	**EXTRA-RENAL MANIFESTATIONS**	**NOTES**	
Autosomal Dominant Inheritance					
Autosomal Dominant Polycystic Kidney Disease	• Fourth leading cause of ESRD in the United States • Relatively common: 1/1000 live births	• Multiple cysts in both kidneys • Hypertension • Hematuria • Back/flank pain • Nephrolithiasis • Renal dysfunction → ESRD	• Hepatic cysts (40–60%) • Intracranial (Berry) aneurysms • Mitral valve prolapse • Diverticular disease • Abdominal hernias	• Patients present at age >30 and often have family history	
Thin Basement Membrane Disease	• Defect in type IV collagen with diffuse thinning of the GBM	• Does not cause renal failure • Persistent microscopic hematuria		• Usually presents in childhood • Also called benign familial hematuria	
X-linked Inheritance					
Alport's Syndrome	• X-linked dominant • Primary defect in type IV collagen, an important component of the GBM	Males: • Asymptomatic hematuria • Progressive renal dysfunction → ESRD by second or third decade of life Females (carriers): • Hematuria • Varying degrees of renal insufficiency	• Sensory-neural deafness • Ocular lens defects	• Thickened glomerular basement membrane on electron microscopy	

Fabry Disease	• X-linked recessive • Deficiency in the lysosomal enzyme alpha galactosidase A (glycosphingolipid metabolism) • Accumulation of glycosphingolipids in the kidneys, heart, nervous system, and skin	• Concentrating defects • Hematuria • Proteinuria • Renal insufficiency • ESRD	• Cardiomyopathy • Conduction abnormalities • Valvular disease • Acroparesthesias • Cutaneous angiokeratomas	• Variable severity of disease
Autosomal Recessive Inheritance				
Bartter Syndrome	• Abnormal chloride transporters in ascending loop of Henle	• Hypokalemia (renal potassium wasting) • Hypochloremic metabolic alkalosis • Hypercalciuria • Normotension • "Lasix effect"	• Growth and cognitive delays	• Diagnosed in childhood/adolescents
Gitelman Syndrome	• Abnormal chloride transporters in distal tubule	• Hypokalemia (renal potassium wasting) • Normotension • Hypochloremic metabolic alkalosis • Hypocalciuria • Hypomagnesemia • "Thiazide effect"		• Adolescent or adult onset

ESRD = end-stage renal disease; GBM = glomerular basement membrane.

Table 5-2

Nephrolithiasis

	Definition	**Epidemiology**	**Etiology**	**Clinical Presentation**	**Diagnosis**	**Treatment**
Kidney Stones		Affects 1–5% of the general population: • Whites greater than African Americans and Asians • Men greater than women by two to three times • White males have a 12% lifetime risk of developing a stone	• Kidney stones may be comprised of calcium, phosphate, struvite, uric, cystine, and/or oxalate • Increased excretion of these elements in the urine lead to formation of stones • Calcium stones account for about 80% of cases	• Flank pain (colicky) • Urinary urgency/ frequency • Hematuria (macro or microscopic) • May have persistent urinary tract infections	• Evaluate with non-contrast helical CT or intravenous pyelography • Abdominal plain film radiography will miss radio-lucent uric acid stones • If multiple, bilateral calcium stones, consider hyperparathyroidism, distal renal tubular acidosis (Sjogren) or medullary sponge kidney	• Hydration • Pain control • Stone may pass on own • May need surgical intervention • Recurrence up to 50% by 10 years

CT = computed tomography.

Table 5-3

Formation of Kidney Stones

CATEGORY	ETIOLOGY	MECHANISM FOR INCREASED URINARY EXCRETION	MECHANISM FOR STONE FORMATION
Hypercalciuria	• Absorptive hypercalciuria	• Enhanced intestinal uptake of calcium • Increased 1,25 vitamin D levels (unknown mechanism)	• Hyperuricosuria: uric acid crystal serves as nidus • High oxalate levels (see below) • Hypocitraturia (see below)
	• Renal hypercalciuria	• Renal tubular calcium wasting • High sodium diet increases urinary calcium excretion • Calcium is reabsorbed passively with sodium	
	• Resorptive hypercalciuria	• Occurs in setting of hyperparathyroidism (calcium resorbed from bone)	
Elevated Urinary Oxalate Levels	• Malabsorptive states (inflammatory bowel disease, ileal bypass, or small bowel resection)	• Saponified calcium is unable to bind to oxalate in the GI tract • Unbound oxalate is reabsorbed and excreted in the urine	• In the urine, oxalate binds with calcium to form insoluble calcium oxalate crystals
	• Low calcium diet	• Not enough calcium available to bind oxalate • Unbound oxalate is reabsorbed and excreted in the urine	
	• Primary hyperoxaluria	• Rare enzymatic disorder leading to overproduction of oxalate	
Hypocitraturia	• Systemic acidosis	• Citrate consumed by systemic acidosis	• In the setting of hypocitraturia, citrate unavailable to bind to calcium. Therefore, calcium is able to bind to oxalate or phosphate to form stones
	• Diets high in animal protein	• Increased acid production consumes citrate and enhances calcium release from bone	

GI = gastointestinal.

Table 5-4

Types of Kidney Stones

Type of Stone	Typical Associated Urine pH	Diagnostic Notes	Clinical and Associated Conditions	Treatment	Notes
Radiopaque Stones					

Calcium Oxalate	• Form independent of urine pH	• Microscopic Appearance:
		  - Envelope shaped
		  - Dumbbell shaped
			• GI malabsorption
			• Low urine volume
			• Hypercalciuria
			• Hypocitraturia
			• Hyperuricosuria
			• Medullary sponge kidney
				• Hydration >2 L/day
				• If hypercalciuric consider thiazide diuretics
				• If hypokalemic consider repletion
				• If hyperparathyroid consider surgery
				• Calculi <5 mm often pass spontaneously
				• Larger stones may require urologic intervention
					• Restriction of dietary calcium may worsen stone formation unless patient has absorptive hypercalciuria
					• Stone prevention diet: low animal protein, low salt, and normal calcium intake
					• Up to 20% of calcium stone formers with medullary sponge kidney

Calcium Phosphate	• Alkaline	• Microscopic Appearance: - Coffin-lid shaped	• Type I renal tube acidosis • Hyperparathyroidism • Low urine volume • Hypercalciuria • Hypocitraturia • Hyperuricosuria • Medullary sponge kidney		
Cystine	• Acidic	• Less radiopaque than calcium stones • Microscopic Appearance: - Hexagonal shape		• Hydration • Urinary alkalinization • Consider penicillamine (cystine binder) • Often need stone removal	• Rare autosmal recessive disorder of cystine transport (cystinuria) • Do not confuse with cystinosis (accumulation of intracellular cystine causing Fanconi syndrome and renal failure)

Struvite	• Alkaline	• Radiographic Appearance: - Staghorn shaped • Microscopic Appearance: - Coffin-lid shaped	• Urease producing organisms: *Proteus*, *Pseudomonas*, *Klebsiella* • If no evidence of urinary infection, unlikely to be a struvite stone	• Treat underlying infection • Antibiotics may not be able to penetrate the stone complex • Surgical intervention may be required	• Stones composed primarily of magnesium ammonium phosphate with varying degrees of calcium • Can develop quickly
Radiolucent Stones					
Uric Acid	• Acidic	• Diagnosed via CT or intravenous pyelography • Microscopic: - Rosettes - Rhombic shapes	• Low urine volume • High uric acid production associated with: - Gout - Myeloproliferative syndromes - Dehydration - Chronic diarrhea - Ileostomy • Chronic metabolic acidosis • Chronic diarrhea	• Hydration • Urinary alkalinization with oral potassium citrate or sodium bicarbonate (to pH >6.5) can dissolve uric acid stones • Allopurinol	• More common in hot, dry climates

Renal Failure

Table 5-5

Acute Renal Failure (ARF)

CATEGORY	ETIOLOGY	CLINICAL	MANAGEMENT
Prerenal Azotemia	**• Hypovolemia** - Renal losses (diuretics, hypoadrenalism) - Extrarenal loss (burns, hemorrhage, GI losses) - Extravascular sequestration (hypoalbuminemia, pancreatitis, burns, trauma) **• Heart Failure** - MI - Valvular disease - Pericardial tamponade - Massive pulmonary embolus **• Distributive Shock** - Sepsis - Anaphylaxis - Afterload reduction **• Altered Renal Vascular Tone** - Vasoconstriction (cyclosporine, amphotericin, hypercalcemia) - Efferent arteriolar dilation causing decreased renal perfusion (e.g., ACE inhibitors)	• Most common cause of ARF • History consistent with typical etiology • Physical Exam - Orthostatic hypotension - Dry mucous membranes - Decreased skin turgor - Edema suggestive of heart or liver failure • Laboratory Results - FENa <1% (most useful test if oliguria) - Elevated BUN to creatinine ratio - Increased urinary sodium concentration • End result is acute tubular necrosis (see below)	• Remove offending agents • Treat underlying etiology (most respond well to volume replacement/increased renal perfusion) • Manage fluid balance, electrolytes and acid-base homeostasis • Avoid nephrotoxic agents (especially nonsteroidal anti-inflammatory drugs and intravenous contrast) • Renal recovery may or may not occur spontaneously over a period of 1–3 weeks • If patient taking an ACE inhibitor, screen for solitary kidney or renal vascular disease • Renal replacement therapy (continuous renal replacement or hemodialysis) indicated if uncontrolled sequelae of ARF: - Hyperkalemia - Acidosis - Volume overload - Uremic symptoms - Seizures - Pericarditis - Bleeding

Intrinsic Renal Failure			

• **Renovascular Obstruction**
  - Arterial (aortic dissection, vasculitis, embolism)
  - Atheroembolic disease
  - Venous compression or thrombosis
• **Glomerular or Microvascular Disease**
  - Glomerulonephritis
  - Vasculitis
  - Thrombotic microangiopathy
	• Arterial (atrial fibrillation, MI, aortic disease)
	• Possibly proteinuria
	• Mild hematuria
	• Atheroemboli
	• Aortic procedure followed by:
	  - Eosinophiluria
	  - Livedo reticularis
	  - Low complement levels
	  - Renal vein thrombosis
	• Proteinuria nephrotic syndrome
	• Glomerulonephritis
	• Thrombotic microangiopathy
	  - Schistocytes on smear
		• Correct underlying cause
		• Manage electrolyte and fluid balances
		• Avoid nephrotoxic agents (especially NSAIDs and intravenous contrast)
		• ARF increases mortality rate of hospitalized patients
		• Renal replacement therapy meets indications above
		• Risk of drug nephrotoxicity increases with increased number of nephrotoxic agents, age, volume depletion and new renal insufficiency	

• **Acute Tubular Necrosis/Acute Kidney Injury**
  - Ischemia (shock)
  - Exogenous toxins (intravenous contrast, aminoglycosides, cisplatin, acetaminophen)
  - Endogenous toxins
    ○ Myoglobin (rhabdomyolysis)
    ○ Hemoglobin (massive hemolysis)
    ○ Uric acid
    ○ Oxalate
• Most common cause of intrinsic renal failure in hospitalized patients
	• Muddy brown casts in urine
	• FENa >1%
	• Myoglobinuria: heme positive on dipstick with few RBCs
	• Oliguric phase (may be so brief not noticed) followed by diuresis		

(continued)

145

Table 5-5

Acute Renal Failure (continued)

CATEGORY	ETIOLOGY	CLINICAL	MANAGEMENT
Intrinsic Renal Failure (Cont.)	• Interstitial Nephritis - Allergic (penicillins, NSAIDs, sulfonamides, rifampin) - Infectious (pyelonephritis, leptospirosis, candidiasis) - Infiltrative (sarcoidosis, leukemia, lymphoma)	• Pyuria • Leukocyte casts • Eosinophilia	• See above
	• Tubular obstruction (myeloma with Bence Jones proteins, uric acid, oxalate, acyclovir, methotrexate, indinavir)	• Urine protein electrophoresis • History of chemotherapy • Urate, oxalate or medication crystals may be see in urine	
Postrenal Azotemia	• Obstructed urine flow from both kidneys at any anatomic level from the renal pelvis to the urethra • Most common cause is prostatic hypertrophy or neurogenic bladder	• May or may not have flank pain • Urinalysis frequently normal • Renal ultrasound may show hydronephrosis (may require surgical intervention)	• Usually resolves with relief of the obstruction • Management of electrolyte and fluid balance are most important • Surgical intervention often yields excellent renal recovery

Data from: Harrison's Principles of Internal Medicine. 16th ed., Table 260-1; Classification and major causes of Acute Renal Failure. 2005. Page 1645. McGraw-Hill, Inc.

ACE = angiotensin converting enzyme; ANCA = antinuclear cytoplasmic antibody; ARF = acute renal failure; BUN = blood urea nitrogen; FENa = fractional excretion of sodium; MI = myocardial infarction; NSAIDs = nonsteroidal anti-inflammatory drugs; RBC = red blood cells.

Table 5-6

Management of Chronic Kidney Disease

CATEGORY	DETAILS	TREATMENT NOTES	GENERAL NOTES

Slow Progression of Kidney Disease	• Progression of underlying acute or chronic diseases can exacerbate kidney disease	• Treat underlying etiology: diabetes, hypertension, glomerulonephritis
		• Avoid nephrotoxins
		• Reduce proteinuria
		• Angiotensin converting enzyme inhibitors and angiotensin-receptor blockers are protective
			• The National Kidney Foundation estimates that approximately 8 million people in the United States have chronic kidney disease, with over 300,000 on dialysis
			• Top etiologies of chronic renal disease:
			  - Diabetes mellitus (40%)
			  - Hypertension (27%)
			• Other causes:
			  - Chronic glomerulonephritis (13%)
			  - Renal cystic disease, including autosomal dominant polycystic kidney disease (4%)
			  - Interstitial nephritis (4%)

Control Blood Pressure	• Control of blood pressure slows progression of kidney disease and reduces risk of cardiovascular and cerebro-vascular events	• Target BP < 130/80 in chronic kidney disease, < 125/75 if proteinuria present	
Anemia	• Loss of renal interstitial cells that produce erythropoietin can cause anemia	• Consider treatment with recombinant erythropoietin—optimal goal hemoglobin unclear but 11–12 is reasonable • Treat other causes of anemia including iron, B_{12}, or folate deficiency	
Nutrition	• Balance healthy and adequate nutritional intake against renal dietary restrictions	• Dietary protein about 1 g/kg/day • Avoid foods high in potassium: citrus fruits, bananas, tomatoes • Reduce phosphorus intake, especially dairy products	

(continued)

Table 5-6

Management of Chronic Kidney Disease (continued)

CATEGORY	DETAILS	TREATMENT NOTES	GENERAL NOTES

Bone Disease	• Renal osteodystrophy (osteitis fibrosa cystica)
	  - Increased bone turnover secondary to hyperparathyroidism
		• Secondary hyperparathyroidism arises due to decreased phosphate clearance and reduced calcitriol (vitamin D_3) production
		• Treatment:
		  - Vitamin D (oral calcitriol) to increase serum calcium and decrease parathyroid secretion
		  - Dietary phosphorus restriction
		  - Oral phosphate binders
		  - Low phosphate diet
			• See above

	• Adynamic bone disease: - Excessive suppression of parathyroid hormone	• Judicious parathyroid hormone control may prevent adynamic bone disease	
	• Osteomalacia: - Bone turnover decreased secondary to aluminum toxicity (less common now)	• Avoid aluminum based antacids and phosphate binders	

Table 5-7

Chronic Renal Disease Progression

DISEASE SEVERITY	GFR (CC/MIN)	STRATEGIES TO SLOW PROGRESSION/TREAT
• Normal GFR but risk factors present or evidence of kidney damage • Stage I CKD	≥90	• Slow progression (see Management of Chronic Kidney Disease, Table 5-6 for details) • Reduce risk factors • Diagnose and treat underlying diseases and comorbidites • Decrease cardiovascular risk factors
• Kidney damage with mildly to moderately decreased GFR • Stage II-III CKD	Stage II: 60–89 Stage III: 30–59	• As above • Estimate rate of progression • Evaluate and treat complications (anemia, osteodystrophy, nutrition)
• Severely decreased GFR	15–29	• As above • Prepare for renal replacement therapy
• End-stage renal disease	<15 (or other need for dialysis)	• As above • Renal replacement

CKD = chronic kidney disease; GFR = glomerular filtration rate.

Table 5-8
Chronic Renal Disease Treatment: Renal Replacement

MODALITY	COMMENTS	INDICATION	CONTRAINDICATION

Hemodialysis	• The most common and available form of renal replacement therapy in the United States
	• Standard therapy is thrice weekly (3.5–4 hours)
	• Access (fistula, graft, catheter)
	  - Problems include infection and access malfunction from clotting or infiltration
	• 20% yearly mortality
	• 50% of deaths occur because of cardiovascular disease
	• 20% of death due to infectious etiologies
	• Dialysis patients with endocarditis have an estimated 50% mortality rate
		• Absolute
		  - Hyperkalemia
		  - Metabolic acidosis
		  - Volume overload
		  - Pericarditis
		• Relative
		  - GFR <10 mL/min
		  - Uremic symptoms
			• Severe dementia
			• Other debilitating chronic disease

Peritoneal Dialysis	• Less frequently used modality of dialysis • Similar mortality rates as with hemodialysis	• As an option for those unable to tolerate or perform hemodialysis	• As above
Renal Transplantation	• Significant survival benefit (cadaveric or living donor) over dialysis when match for age and renal disease • Improved quality of life and decreased medical expenses with transplant • Donor supply limited • Immunosuppression required after transplant • Higher rates of cutaneous and lymphoid neoplasia after transplant	• Early referral to nephrologists key to optimizing treatment options	• Dementia • Noncompliance with medical therapy • Severe cardiopulmonary or hepatic disease • Recent active cancer • HIV and hepatitis C are no longer absolute contraindications to transplantation

Medical Renal Disease

Table 5-9
Nephrotic and Nephritic Kidney Disease

	DEFINITION	DIAGNOSIS	CLINICAL NOTES	TREATMENT
Nephrotic Range Proteinuria	> 3.5 g/day of proteinuria			
Nephrotic Syndrome	• Nephrotic range proteinuria and: - Peripheral edema (common) - Hypoalbuminemia - Hyperlipidemia	• If diabetic, 90% of cases due to diabetes • If not diabetic, need renal biopsy to determine etiology • Urinalysis • Clinical examination	• Loss of antithrombin III in the urine may increase hypercoagulability	• Controversial and depends on specific etiology • Generally: Angiotensin-converting enzyme inhibitors or receptor blockers alone or in combination with immunosuppression • Hyperlipidemia poorly responsive to dietary changes • Consider HMG-CoA reductase inhibitor
Nephritic Kidney Disease: Acute Glomerulonephritis	• Usually nonnephrotic range proteinuria • Characterized by abrupt onset of hematuria and ARF	• Urinalysis • Clinical examination	• Oliguria • Erythrocyte casts • Hypertension	• Sometimes reversible with immunosuppression • Adequate hydration

Table 5-10

Causes of Proteinuria

Category	Type	Disease	Clinical Presentation/Treatment	Diagnosis
Glomerular Proteinuria	**Primary**	Minimal change disease	• Steroid responsive glomerular disease	• Proteinuria usually discovered on routine urinalysis • Urine dipstick detects albumin but not light chains (i.e., Bence Jones proteins in multiple myeloma) • Proteinuria should be quantified, either with a 24-hour urine collection or with a random urine protein to creatinine ratio • If diabetes and microalbuminuria present (30–300 mg of urine protein) consider angiotensin-converting enzyme inhibitor therapy • Treat underlying disease if known • Work-up for specific etiology depends on history and inspection of urine sediment
		Focal segmental glomerulosclerosis	• Most frequent cause of idiopathic nephrotic syndrome in adults • Loss of nephrons (subtotal nephrectomy, sickle cell, morbid obesity) is a predisposing risk factor	
		Membranous nephropathy	• Incidence of deep venous thrombosis higher than in other nephrotic syndromes • If idiopathic, one-third develop end-stage renal disease in 10 years, one-third stable, and one-third have spontaneous remission	
		Membranoproliferative glomerulonephritis	• Type I often have underlying hepatitis C	
		Diabetes mellitus	• Progression may be slowed by controlling glycemic level and blood pressure and by decreasing proteinuria through blockage of the renin-angiotensin system	
	Secondary	Hypertension		
		Systemic lupus erythematosus		

	HIV associated nephropathy	Focal segmental glomerular nephrosis collapsing pattern	• See above
Tubular Proteinuria			
Nephrotoxins	Medications: gold, penicillamine lithium		
	Medications: NSAIDs (acute interstitial nephritis)		
	Metals: mercury, lead		
Tubulointerstitial Disease	Infections	• Biopsy often unrevealing • Inflammation and fibrosis correlates with progression to renal insufficiency
	Crystal induced	
	Immunologic diseases	
	Analgesics	
	Obstruction (myeloma kidney)	
Overflow Proteinuria	Multiple myeloma	• Renal involvement frequent with amyloid A (AA) amyloidosis and amyloid light chain (AL) amyloidosis, but not other types
	Light chain deposition disease	
	Pigment nephropathy (myoglobinuria, hemoglobinuria)	
	Amyloidosis	
Other	Exercise	
	Fever	
	Benign positional proteinuria	

Table 5-11

Summary of Hematuria

TYPE	DEFINITION	MAJOR CAUSES	DIAGNOSIS	FALSE RESULTS
Macroscopic (gross)	• Visible blood in urine specimen • As little as 1mL in 1 L of urine can cause gross hematuria	• May originate from anywhere along the urinary tract • Most frequently associated with - Urinary tract infection - Trauma to urogenitury tract - Exercise	• A positive urine dipstick should be verified using microscopic analysis • Casts on microscopic analysis suggest glomerular source of bleeding	• False-positive dipstick caused by: - Myoglobin - Contamination with other blood • False-negative dipstick caused by: - Ascorbic acid • Other causes of "red" urine - Myoglobin - Blackberries and blueberries - Drugs (sulfonamides, nitrofurantoin, rifampin, phenytoin, levodopa, doxorubicin)
Microscopic	>3 RBCs per high-power microscopic field from a centrifuged midstream voided urine sample	• Frequently originates from the kidney • May be associated with systemic or glomerular disease		

Note: See Urology section for further details.

Disorders of Electrolyte Balance

Table 5-12
Hyponatremia (Sodium >130 mEq/L)

Total Body Sodium	Extracellular Volemic State	Mechanism	Laboratory Findings	Clinical Presentation	Treatment
Decreased	**Hypovolemia**	• Renal losses: - Renal disease, including Bartter syndrome - diuretics	• High urinary sodium excretion (>20 mEq/L) • Hyperkalemia (except in Bartter syndrome) • Low plasma osmolality • Elevated urine osmolality	• Clinical symptoms usually manifest when the hyponatremia develops acutely and/or serum sodium concentration <120 mEq/L • Common problem in hospitalized patients • Signs/symptoms: - Nausea - Vomiting - Irritability - Headache - Decreased urine output if hypovolemic - Muscle cramps - Ataxia - Seizures - Coma	• Treatment depends on volume status - Hypovolemic: volume expansion with normal saline - Hypervolemic: treat underlying disorder and restrict free water/salt intake. Loop diuretic may be helpful as favor excretion of water over sodium - Euvolemic: treat underlying disorder • If chronic asymptomatic hyponatremia, consider slow correction with water restriction • Consider hypertonic saline if severe symptoms (delirium, seizure, coma) and/or serum sodium is less than 120 mEq/L • Correction of hyponatremia faster than 8–12 mEq/L in the first 12 hours or overcorrection can result in central pontine myelinolysis

(continued)

Table 5-12

Hyponatremia (Sodium >130 mEq/L) (continued)

TOTAL BODY SODIUM	EXTRACELLULAR VOLEMIC STATE	MECHANISM	LABORATORY FINDINGS	CLINICAL PRESENTATION	TREATMENT
Decreased (cont.)	**Hypovolemia (cont.)**	• Extrarenal losses: - GI loss (diarrhea, vomiting) - Sweat - Pancreatitis - Burns - Effusions	• Low urinary sodium (<20 mEq/L) • Hypokalemia • Low plasma osmolality	• See above	
Increased	**Hypervolemia**	• Congestive heart failure • Nephrotic syndrome • Cirrhosis	• Low urinary sodium (<20 mEq/L) • Low plasma osmolality		
Normal	**Euvolemia**	• SIADH • Pain, nausea • Adrenal dysfunction (Addison disease, CAH, adrenal hemorrhage) • Acute renal failure with severe oliguria • Hypothyroidism	• Low serum BUN and uric acid • Inappropriately elevated urine osmolality • Low plasma osmolality		
Pseudohyponatremia		• Increased nonaqueous phase of serum (hyperlipidemia or hyperproteinemia) • Hypertonic hyponatremia (hypertonic mannitol or severe hyperglycemia)	• Normal or high plasma osmolality • Osmolal gap (10 mOsm/kg between measured and calculated osmolality: $Posm = 2 [Na]$ • Other causes of osmolal gap are ethanol (most common), methanol, and ethylene glycol		

ADH = antidiuretic hormone; CAH = congenital adrenal hyperplasia; SIADH = syndrome of inappropriate anti-diuretic hormone.

Table 5-13

Syndrome of Inappropriate Anti-Diuresis

Definition	Etiology	Clinical Presentation	Diagnosis	Treatment

ADH secreted in the absence of intravascular depletion or increased serum osmolarity	• Increased hypothalamic production of ADH
	  - Drugs (haloperidol, fluoxetine, cyclophosphamide)
	  - Pulmonary disease
	  - Nausea
	  - Surgery
	  - CNS infections/malignancies
	  - Psychosis
	• Ectopic production of ADH
	  - Carcinoma (small-cell lung, bronchogenic, neuroblastoma)
	• Potentiation of ADH effect on the kidney
	  - Medications (tolbutamide, chlorpropamide)
		• Severity of symptoms depends on both the serum sodium level and the rate of fluctuation
		• Symptoms usually develop when serum sodium levels are below <120 mEq/L
			• Hyponatremia (<125 mEq/L)
			• Decreased BUN, serum uric acid and serum hypoosmolality
			• Elevated urine sodium (>20mEq/L), urine osmolality, and urine specific gravity
				• Fluid restriction
				• Sodium replacement
				• Treat underlying cause
				• Consider hypertonic saline and diuretic if seizures or profound changes in mental status
				• May need to consider vasopressin-2 antagonists (conivaptan)

CNS = central nervous system.

Table 5-14

Hypernatremia (Sodium > 145 mEq/L)

TOTAL BODY SODIUM	EXTRACELLULAR VOLUME STATUS	MECHANISM	CLINICAL PRESENTATION	DIAGNOSIS/ LABORATORY FINDINGS	TREATMENT

Decreased	**Hypovolemia**	• GI losses
		  - Diarrhea
		  - Vomiting/
		    Nasogastric suction
		  - Laxative abuse
		• Renal losses
		  - Osmotic diuresis
		  - Postobstructive
		    diuresis
		  - Diabetes insipidus
		• Skin losses
		  - Burns
		  - Fever
			• Mental status changes
			• Weakness/lethargy
			• Coma
			• Convulsion
			• All etiologies must include an impaired access to or desire for water:
			  - May be due to dementia, delirium, reduced thirst from hypothalamic dysfunction, or physical/medical restraints
				• Serum sodium concentration >145 mEq/L
				• Urinary sodium is <20 mEq/L
				• Urine sodium may be higher if etiology is renal loss
					• Administer free water enterally or parentally
					• Cerebral edema can result if free water deficit is corrected faster than 0.5–1 mEq/hour

Increased	**Hypervolemia**	• Iatrogenic - Hypertonic infusions • Hyperaldosteronism			
Normal	**Euvolemia**	• Central diabetes insipidus • Nephrogenic diabetes insipidus • Patients will become hypovolemic without water support			

Free water deficit (L) $= 0.6$(weight in kg)$(Na_{observed} - Na_{expected})/Na_{expected}$.

Table 5-15

Hypernatremia, Urine Osmolality, and Serum ADH

CAUSE OF HYPERNATREMIA	APPROPRIATELY CONCENTRATED URINE? (URINE OSMOLALITY)	SERUM ADH LEVEL
Decreased Water Intake	Yes (>500 mOsm/kg)	• High (appropriately)
Central Diabetes Insipidus	No (<300 mOsm/kg)	• Low or zero
Nephrogenic Diabetes Insipidus	No (<300 mOsm/kg)	• Normal or increased

Table 5-16

Disorders of Water Balance

	POLYURIA	CENTRAL DIABETES INSIPIDUS (DI)	NEPHROGENIC DIABETES INSIPIDUS
Description	• Increased frequency and/or volume of urination in a patient who is not drinking excessive amounts of fluid	• ADH deficiency	• ADH resistance

Etiology	• Nephrogenic DI
	• Central DI
	• Diabetes (high serum glucose)
	• Partial urinary tract obstruction
	• Hypercalcemia
	• Diuretic treatment
	• Patients with psychogenic polydipsia have polyuria because of excessive intake of fluid
		• Head trauma
		• Hypoxic brain injury
		• Infiltrative diseases (TB, sarcoid)
		• Neoplasm
		• Meningitis
			• Inherited
			  - Vasopressin V2 receptor mutation (x-linked)
			  - Aquaporin mutation (autosomal recessive)
			• Acquired
			  - Sickle cell disease/trait
			  - Amyloidosis
			  - Obstructive uropathy
			  - Electrolyte imbalance (hypercalcemia, hypokalemia)
			  - Medications (lithium and foscarnet)

Clinical Presentation	• Depends on etiology	• Polydipsia • Polyuria • Nocturia • Dehydration • Headaches	

(*continued*)

Table 5-16

Disorders of Water Balance (continued)

	POLYURIA	CENTRAL DIABETES INSIPIDUS (DI)	NEPHROGENIC DIABETES INSIPIDUS
Diagnosis	• Pathology unlikely if urine S.G. ≥1.020 • Psychogenic polydipsia: normal serum sodium and osmolarity with low urine osmolarity	• Elevated serum osmolarity • Low urine osmolarity (S.G. <1.010) • Hypernatremia • Distinguish from nephrogenic DI with intravenous vasopressin (dDAVP) challenge	• Elevated vasopressin levels • Elevated serum osmolarity • Low urine osmolarity (S.G. <1.010) • Hypernatremia • Distinguish from nephrogenic DI with intravenous vasopressin (dDAVP) challenge
Corrects with dDAVP?		• Yes	• No
Treatment	• Treat underlying cause	• Arginine vasopressin, titrated to clinical effect	• Low sodium diet • Close monitoring of hydration status • Diuretics, specifically hydrochlorothiazide
Notes	• Psychogenic polydipsia is often confused with DI	• Normally, ADH acts at the level of the renal tubule collecting ducts to increase water resorption, resulting in concentrated urine. DI occurs when the renal tubule is unable to concentrate the urine, resulting in excessive free water loss and subsequent hypernatremia	

DI = diabetes insipidus; S.G. = specific gravity; TB = tuberculosis.

Table 5-17

Hypokalemia (Potassium Level <4.0 mEq/L)

	Urinary Potassium Level	Extrarenal Losses	Urinary Losses	Intracellular Shift
Etiology	**High**	• N/A	• Diuretics (common) • Primary aldosteronism • Proximal and distal RTA • Medications (amphotericin B, trimethoprim, pentamidine) • Bartter syndrome (urinary chloride >10 mEq/L)	
	Low	• Gastrointestinal loss (common) - Protracted vomiting - Diarrhea • Laxative abuse • Hyperhidrosis (excessive sweating)	• N/A	• Insulin • Alkalemia • Familial periodic hypokalemic paralysis
Clinical Presentation	• Electrocardiographic changes; **T** wave flattening, **U** waves • Cardiac arrhythmias • Muscle cramps • Ileus • Rhabdomyolysis			
Treatment	• Oral or parenteral potassium supplementation • Treat underlying causes • Evaluate for hyponagnesemia because often lose both intracellular ions together			

RTA: renal tubular acidosis.

Table 5-18

Hyperkalemia (Potassium >5.5 mEq/L)

Etiology	Impaired Renal Excretion	• Renal failure • Type IV RTA • Hyporeninemic hypoaldosteronism (decreased aldosterone secretion due to intra-adrenal defect and decreased angiotensin II production secondary to decreased renin function) (common cause)
	Pharmacologic	• Distal nephron K^+ secretion inhibited (e.g., amiloride, triamterene, spironolactone, trimethoprim, pentamidine) • Aldosterone production decreased (e.g., ACE inhibitors, ARBs, NSAIDs, heparin) • Cellular transport blocked (e.g., digoxin, beta-blockers, octreotide, succinylcholine)
	Extracellular Shift	• Acidemia • Insulin deficiency • Massive cellular death (e.g., rhabdomyolysis, tumor lysis) • Familial hyperkalemic periodic paralysis
Clinical Presentation		• Muscle weakness • Cardiac arrhythmias • ECG changes: peaked T waves, flattened P waves, widened QRS, and ventricular arrhythmias

Treatment	Shift Potassium to Intracellular Space	• Temporary shift of potassium from the extracellular to the intracellular space
		  - Insulin administration (with concurrent glucose support)
		  - Aerosolized beta-agonist administration

	Potassium Removal	• Loop diuretics (if normal renal function) • Cation exchange resins • Dialysis
	Cardiac Protection	• Calcium gluconate is potentially cardioprotective but does not affect serum potassium level
	Chronic	• Restrict dietary potassium • Potassium wasting diuretics (furosemide, hydrochlorothiazide) • Mineralocorticoid administration is sometimes necessary
Notes		• More than 98% of potassium is intracellular

ARB = angiotensin II receptor blockers; ECG = electrocardiogram; RTA = renal tubular acidosis.

Table 5-19

Hypophosphatemia and Hypomagnesemia

	ETIOLOGY	TREATMENT	NOTES

Hypophosphatemia	• Decreased GI absorption
	  - Use of aluminum- or magnesium-containing antacids
	• Increased urinary excretion
	  - Vitamin D deficiency
	  - Fanconi syndrome/proximal tubular dysfunction
	  - Hyperparathyroidism
	• Shift of phosphorous into intracellular space
	  - Respiratory alkalosis
	  - Increased insulin secretion (often seen during refeeding)
	  - Hungry bone syndrome (after parathyroidectomy for hyperparathyroidism)
		• Treat underlying cause
		• Oral phosphorous supplements
			• Alcoholics are prone to severe hypophosphatemia after admission to the hospital because of acute shifts of phosphate into the intracellular compartment

Hypomagnesemia	• GI loss
	  - Diarrhea
	  - Intestinal bypass
	• Renal loss
	  - Loop or thiazide diuretics
	  - Amphotericin B
	  - Aminoglycoside antibiotics
	  - Cyclosporine
	  - Gitelman syndrome
		• Treat underlying cause
		• Oral magnesium supplements
		• Intravenous supplementation if plasma magnesium level <1.0 mg/dL
			• Hypomagnesimia decreases parathyroid hormone release and efficacy
			• Uncorrected hypomagnesemia may prevent correction of hypocalcemia
			• Often associated with hypokalemia because of renal potassium wasting

Table 5-20

Summary of Renal Tubular Acidosis

RTA TYPE	MECHANISM	URINE pH	CLINICAL PRESENTATION	TREATMENT
RTA Type 1 (Distal Tubule)	• Decreased hydrogen ion (acid) excretion into the urine	• >5.5	• Hyperchloremic metabolic acidosis • Calcium kidney stones	• Daily sodium bicarbonate
RTA Type 2 (Proximal Tubule)	• Decreased absorption of sodium bicarbonate by renal tubules	• <5.5	• Hyperchloremic metabolic acidosis • Urinary potassium wasting → hypokalemia	• Hypokalemia worsened with exogenous sodium bicarbonate

Table 5-21

Approach to Acid Base Disorders

STEP	NOTES
1. Measure extracellular pH	• Indicates whether the primary disturbance has lead to acidemia or alkalemia
2. Assess serum bicarbonate and arterial Pco₂ levels	• Classifies the primary disturbance as respiratory or metabolic
3. Calculate anion gap	• Indicates if anion gap metabolic acidosis also present
4. Compare observed versus expected compensation	• A significant difference in observed versus expected compensation indicates: - Presence of a mixed acid-base disorder - Measurement of venous rather than arterial blood

Table 5-22

Compensated Acid-Base Disorders

PRIMARY DISORDER	pH	PROCESS	COMPENSATION	ADAPTIVE RESPONSE DETAILS	EXAMPLE
Metabolic Alkalosis	↑	↑ HCO_3	↑ P_{CO_2}	• 0.7 mm Hg increase in P_{CO_2} for every 1 mEq/L rise in $[HCO_3]$	• Diuretics • Vomiting
Metabolic Acidosis	↓	↓ HCO_3	↓ P_{CO_2}	• 1.2 mm Hg decrease in P_{CO_2} for every 1 mEq/L fall in $[HCO_3]$	• Sepsis • DKA • Toxins
Respiratory Alkalosis	↑	↓ P_{CO_2}	↓ HCO_3	• Acute: 1 mEq/L increase in $[HCO_3]$ for every 10 mm Hg rise in P_{CO_2} • Chronic: 3.5 mEq/L increase in $[HCO_3]$ for every 10 mm Hg rise in P_{CO_2}	• Asthma exacerbation (early) • Aspirin toxicity (early) • Pain • Fever
Respiratory Acidosis	↓	↑ P_{CO_2}	↑ HCO_3	• Acute: 1 mEq/L increase in $[HCO_3]$ for every 10 mm Hg rise in P_{CO_2} • Chronic: 3.5 mEq/L increase in $[HCO_3]$ for every 10 mm Hg rise in P_{CO_2}	• CNS injury • Respiratory failure • Obstructive sleep apnea • Barbiturate toxicity • Chronic lung disease

Table 5-23

High Anion Gap Metabolic Acidosis

CATEGORY	EXAMPLE	UNMEASURED ANION CAUSING HIGH GAP

Lactic Acidosis	• Severe mitochondrial dysfunction secondary to:
	  - Tissue hypoperfusion
	  - Drugs (metformin and nucleoside reverse transcriptase inhibitors)
		• Lactate

Ketoacidosis (Diabetic, Alcoholic)	• Hepatic production of ketones from free fatty acids
	  - Insulin deficiency in diabetes
	  - Severe starvation
	  - Prolonged alcoholic binges
		• Beta-hydroxybutyrate
		• Acetoacetate

Uremia	• Renal dysfunction inhibits clearance of organic acids	• Sulfates • Phosphate • Urate • Hippurate
Ingested Anions	• Methanol • Ethylene glycol • Paraldehyde • Salicylate	• Formate • Glycolate, oxalate • Organic anions • Ketones • Salicylate

Table 5-24

Normal Anion Gap (Hyperchloremic) Metabolic Acidosis

CATEGORY	EXAMPLE	DETAILS
GI Loss	• Diarrhea	
Reduced Renal H⁺ Secretion	• Distal (type I) RTA	• Secondary to hypercalciuria, Sjögren syndrome, amphotericin B
	• Hypoaldosteronism (type IV RTA)	• Secondary to diabetes mellitus, NSAIDs, Addison disease, long-term heparin therapy
	• Some cases of renal failure	
Renal Bicarbonate Loss	• Proximal (type II) RTA	• Includes Fanconi syndrome
	• Tubular dysfunction	• Secondary to ifosfamide, multiple myeloma, cystinosis, Wilson disease, acetazolamide

(continued)

Table 5-24

Normal Anion Gap (Hyperchloremic) Metabolic Acidosis (continued)

CATEGORY	EXAMPLE	DETAILS
Miscellaneous	• Ammonium chloride ingestion	
	• Hyperalimentation	
	• Aggressive administration of NS	• pH of NS is 7.0
	• Recovery phase of respiratory alkalosis	

NS = normal saline.

Note: No increase in anion gap because chloride replaces the lost bicarbonate.

Metabolic Alkalosis

Table 5-25

Causes of Metabolic Alkalosis

MECHANISM	ETIOLOGY	EXAMPLE	NOTES.
Loss of Protons	GI tract proton loss	• Vomiting/nasogastric suction • Chloride rich diarrhea (Villous adenoma or factitious diarrhea)	• Vomitting and diuretics are common causes of metabolic alkalosis • One milliequivalent of hydrogen lost generates one milliequivalent of bicarbonate • Renal mechanism: increased distal hydrogen excretion • Citrate in blood product causes metabolic alkalosis
	Kidney proton loss	• Loop or thiazide diuretics • Primary mineralocorticoid excess • Bartter and Gitelman syndromes	
	H^+ shift into cells	• Hypokalemia (K–H^+ exchange)	
HCO_3^- Administration/ Retention	Excess bicarbonate	• Massive blood transfusion • Milk-alkali syndrome	

Table 5-25

Causes of Metabolic Alkalosis (continued)

MECHANISM	ETIOLOGY	EXAMPLE	NOTES
Contraction Alkalosis	• Loss of relatively large volumes of bicarbonate-free fluid leaves a relatively constant quantity of extracellular bicarbonate (alkalosis) but a "contraction" of extracellular volume	• Loop or thiazide diuretics • Sweat loss in cystic fibrosis	

Table 5-26

Maintenance of Metabolic Alkalosis

PATHOPHYSIOLOGY	MECHANISM	EXAMPLE	NOTES
• Normally, the kidney can excrete enough bicarbonate to prevent significant alkalosis. Therefore, an impairment bicarbonate secretion is necessary for sustained metabolic alkalosis	• Decreased GFR	• Decreased effective arterial volume • Renal failure	• Many causes of decreased effective arterial volume
	• Increased reabsorption of bicarbonate	• Decreased effective arterial volume • Chloride depletion • Hypokalemia • Hyperaldosteronism	• Hypokalemia and hyperaldosteronism impairs the ability of the kidney to absorb protons distally and, therefore, to excrete bicarbonate

Table 5-27

Responsiveness of Metabolic Alkalosis to Saline Treatment

TYPE	URINE CHLORIDE LEVEL	TYPICAL ETIOLOGY
Saline Responsive	**<10 mEq/L**	• Gastric fluid loss • Chloride-rich diarrhea • Sweat loss in cystic fibrosis • Diuretics (remote use)
Saline Resistant	**>20 mEq/L**	• Hyperaldosteronism • Bartter or Gitelman syndromes • Severe hypokalemia • Diuretics (recent use)

168

Chapter 5   ◆   Nephrology

Table 5-28

Respiratory Acidosis

CAUSE	EXAMPLE	CLINICAL PRESENTATION	TREATMENT
General Note -	• Any cause of decreased alveolar ventilation can cause CO_2 retention and thus respiratory acidosis	• May be acute or chronic • CNS distortions • Blurred vision • Restlessness • Anxiety • Delirium • Coma	• Treat underlying etiology • Increase minute ventilation when possible • If pH <7.2, consider administration of sodium bicarbonate
CNS—Medullary Respiratory Center Inhibition	• Sedatives, opiates, anesthetics • Cardiac arrest • O_2 administration in chronic hypercapnea		
Respiratory Muscle and Chest Wall Disorders	• Guillain-Barré • Severe hypokalemia and hypophosphatemia • ALS, poliomyelitis, multiple sclerosis and spinal cord injury (chronic respiratory acidosis) • Obesity hypoventilation		
Gas Exchange Disorders	• Pulmonary edema/ARDS • Severe asthma • Pneumothorax • COPD (acute or chronic respiratory acidosis)		
Airway Obstruction	• Laryngospasm • Obstructive sleep apnea (chronic respiratory acidosis)		
Mechanical Ventilation	• Iatrogenic hypoventilation		

ALS = amyotrophic lateral sclerosis; ARDS = acute respiratory distress syndrome; COPD = chronic obstructive pulmonary disease.

Table 5-29
Respiratory Alkalosis

CAUSE OF RESPIRATORY ALKALOSIS		CLINICAL PRESENTATION	TREATMENT
CATEGORY	EXAMPLE		
Pulmonary Disease Causing Hypoxemia	• Pneumonia • Pulmonary embolus • Pulmonary edema	• Symptoms of underlying disease • Headache • Lightheadedness • Paresthesias • Carpopedal spasm	• Treat underlying etiology • Note that rapid correction of a chronic hypocapnea can cause acidemia
Other Causes of Hypoxemia	• Hypotension • Severe anemia		
Increased Respiratory Drive	• CNS tumor • Stroke • Psychiatric (anxiety, pain) • Drugs (salicylates) • Early sepsis (cytokines) • Pregnancy (increased progesterone) • Liver failure		
Mechanical Ventilation	• Iatrogenic hyperventilation		

Table 5-30
Imaging of the Kidney

STUDY	NOTES	DIAGNOSTIC USES
Noninvasive		
Renal Ultrasound with Doppler	• Inexpensive • Nontoxic • Images obtained are operator dependent	• Hydronephrosis • Kidney size and symmetry • Renal vein flow • Renal artery flow (relatively insensitive for renal artery stenosis) • Renal cysts and tumors • Calculi
CT	• More sensitive than ultrasound for renal calculi • Expensive • Risk of contrast nephropathy	• Calculi • Hydronephrosis • Cystic disease • Tumors (more sensitive than ultrasound) • Insensitive for renal artery stenosis

(continued)

Table 5-30

Imaging of the Kidney (continued)

STUDY	NOTES	DIAGNOSTIC USES
Radionuclide Imaging	• More sensitive than ultrasound for renal artery stenosis • Nontoxic • Expensive	• Renal artery stenosis (especially when used with captopril) • Hydronephrosis • Asymmetric renal function
MRI/MRA	• Much more sensitive than ultrasound for renal artery stenosis • Expensive • Can cause claustrophobia • Gadolinium contrast is implicated as a cause of nephrogenic systemic fibrosis	• Renal artery stenosis (not sensitive enough to detect fibromuscular dysplasia) • Tumors, cysts
Invasive		
Angiography	• Gold standard to diagnose renal artery stenosis • May be used for interventions • Risk of complications: contrast nephropathy and atheroembolic embolus	• Renal artery stenosis • Embolization of bleeding vessels

MRI = magnetic resonance imaging; MRA = magnetic resonance angiography.

Chapter 6

Urology

Table 6-1

Urinary Incontinence: Definition, Etiology, and Clinical Correlates

Type	Definition	Etiology	Clinical Correlates
Stress	• Leakage of urine with increased intra-abdominal pressure caused by laughing, coughing, or lifting heavy objects	• Weakened pelvic floor • Urethral hypermobility • Bladder neck prolapse	• History of pelvic surgery • Multiparity • Cystocele or rectocele on exam • Atrophic vaginitis on exam
Urge	• Leakage of urine when an involuntary bladder contraction overcomes outlet resistance	• Neurologic disorders • Infection • Intrinsic bladder lesion • Idiopathic	• Spinal cord injury, stroke, Parkinson disease or multiple sclerosis • Urinary tract infections • Bladder stone, tumor, or foreign body
Overflow	• Leakage of urine when the bladder is unable to empty fully • A high postvoid urine volume is the diagnostic hallmark	• Bladder outlet obstruction • Detrusor muscle weakness • Autonomic neuropathy • Medication side effect (anticholinergics)	• BPH • Diabetes mellitus
Total	• Constant or periodic loss of urine in settings outside of normal voiding	• Urethral sphincter abnormality • Abnormal anatomic connections	• Vesicoenteric fistulas • Ectopic ureter (ureteral orifice in the vagina)
Functional	• Physical or cognitive impairment	• Inability or unwillingness to use a toilet	
Acute	• Acute onset of any type of incontinence	• Delirium • Medications • Restricted mobility • Infection • Fecal impaction • Inflammation • Polyuric states	• Polyuric states include diabetes mellitus or insipidus, hypercalcemia, and diuretic treatment

BPH = benign prostatic hypertrophy.

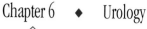
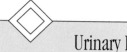

Urinary Incontinence

Definition and Etiology: There are five types of urinary incontinence: (1) stress, (2) urge, (3) overflow, (4) total, and (5) functional.

Epidemiology: Thirteen million people in the United States suffer from urinary incontinence, with a female to male ratio of 2:1. It is estimated that 35% of women and 22% of men over age 65 have some form of urinary incontinence.

Diagnosis: The evaluation of a patient with incontinence includes a detailed medical and voiding history, medications, surgeries, and parity. Physical examination should include evaluation for cystoceles and rectoceles, sphincter tone, pelvic masses. Urodynamic studies, including measurement of the postvoid residual may be valuable as well.

Treatment: See Table 6-2.

Table 6-2

Treatment (Conservative, Medical, and Surgical) of Urinary Incontinence

TYPE	CONSERVATIVE	MEDICAL	SURGICAL
Stress	• Behavioral therapy - Kegel exercises - Fluid restriction • Biofeedback • Vaginal pessaries	• Alpha-agonists to increase bladder outlet resistance • Tricyclic antidepressants • Topical estrogens may improve tissue quality and urinary control (caution if at risk for breast cancer)	• Intraurethral/bladder neck injections • Surgical approaches to strengthen/tighten pelvic floor structures
Urge	• Treat infections • Biofeedback • Timed voiding	• Anticholinergics (oxybutinin, tolterodine, hyoscyamine) • Tricyclic antidepressants	• Augmentation cystoplasty • Bladder denervation • Urinary diversion
Overflow	• Clean intermittent catheterization is preferred over an indwelling catheter • Avoid offending medication	• Alpha-blockers to decrease bladder outlet resistance (i.e., tamsulosin, doxazosin, terazosin) • Cholinergic agents to increase bladder contraction	• TURP if BPH is etiology
Total	• None	• None	• Repair of anatomic abnormality • Artificial urinary sphincter placement
Functional	• Scheduled/assisted voids • Bedside commodes or urinals	• Treat underlying illness	
Note	• Nonpharmacologic interventions are the cornerstone of treatment and should be used even when pharmacologic agents are considered		

TURP = transurethral resection of the prostate.

Table 6-3

Etiologies of Erectile Dysfunction

CATEGORY	CATEGORY	DISEASES	DETAILS
Organic	• Vascular	• Poor inflow (atherosclerosis, arterial insufficiency) • Excessive outflow (venous leak)	• Most common cause of erectile dysfunction • Mechanical obstruction → poor inflow • Ischemic injury → fibrosis → venous leak
	• Endocrine	• Hypogonadism (primary or secondary) • Hyperprolactinemia	• Consider checking LH, FSH, and prolactin
	• Neurologic	• Spinal cord injury • Diabetic neuropathy • Stroke • Parkinson disease	• Second most common cause of erectile dysfunction in older men • Often a slow onset
	• Primary disorders of the penis	• Peyronie disease • Priapism	
Iatrogenic	• Medication	• Antihypertensives → poor inflow • Anticholinergics • Medications that decrease libido	• Patients often report an acute onset • Medications that decrease libido include antidepressants, beta-blockers, and finasteride
	• Surgery	• Radical prostatectomy • Pelvic/colorectal surgery	• Surgery may disrupt penile innervation • Not responsive to sildenafil
Psychogenic	• Psychosocial	• Depression • Performance anxiety • Relationship conflict	• Patients often report an acute onset • May continue to have normal nocturnal erections
Other	• Alcohol, tobacco, illicit drugs		

LH = luteinizing hormone; FSH = follicle stimulating hormone.

Erectile Dysfunction

Definition: The inability to have or maintain an erection sufficient for penetration during sexual intercourse.

Etiology: Parasympathetic stimulation (via nitric oxide mediated cyclic guanosine monophosphate [cGMP] mechanism) relaxes the smooth muscles of the corpora cavernosa allowing increased arterial flow into the cavernosal sinusoids. As the cavernosa distends the tunica albuginea veins draining the penis are compressed, trapping blood in the penis and potentiating rigidity.

Epidemiology: Affects two-thirds of men over the age of 70 years.

Diagnosis: Evaluation includes a medical, drug, and erectile history. Physical examination includes peripheral neurovascular, genitourinary, and secondary sexual characteristics. Laboratory tests may be beneficial.

Treatment: See Table 6-4.

Table 6-4

Treatment Options for Erectile Dysfunction

TREATMENT	COMMENTS
Discontinue Offending Medication	• May not be possible to discontinue medications due to comorbid diseases
Phosphodiesterase Inhibitors (Sildenafil, Vardenafil, Tadalafil)	• Blocks phosphodiesterase type 5; prevents degradation of cGMP • Contraindicated for patients taking nitrates as the combination can lead to hypotension • Cardiac disease is not an absolute contraindication • Caution with protease inhibitors as sildenafil concentrations can rise, causing hypotension • The newer agents (vardenafil and tadalafil) do not affect color vision
Testosterone Injections/ Patches	• Consider for patients with low serum-free testosterone • Rule out central causes of low testosterone first • Rule out prostate cancer as testosterone can potentiate growth
Other	• Psychotherapy • Vasoactive intracavernous injections • Vascular surgery for small or large vessel arterial disease • Penile prosthesis for refractory cases

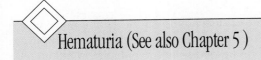

Hematuria (See also Chapter 5)

Definition: Hematuria is defined as more than three red blood cells (RBC) per high-powered field on microscopic examination of urine.

Etiology: RBC in the urine may originate directly from the epithelium of the genitourinary tract or may pass into the urinary stream due to a systemic medical problem that changes glomerular permeability.

Epidemiology: Hematuria is often intermittent, with up to 39% of adults having transient hematuria. The risk of urinary tract (kidney, ureter, or bladder) cancer as the cause of hematuria greatly increases after the age of 50.

Diagnosis: If the source of hematuria is urologic, evaluate both the upper and lower urinary tracts.

Treatment: Directed toward underlying etiology.

Table 6-5
Etiology of Hematuria

DIAGNOSIS	CLINICAL HISTORY	CLINICAL FINDINGS	DETAILS
Medical Renal Etiology	• Comorbid diseases including hypertension, diabetes, and lupus	• Proteinuria • Elevated creatinine • Anemia due to erythropoeitin deficiency	• See Chapter 5
Malignancy	• Painless hematuria	• Positive urine cytology for high grade malignancies (specific, but not sensitive)	Types of cancers: • Renal cell carcinoma • Transitional cell/bladder carcinoma • Prostate cancer • Urethral cancer
Infection	• Increased urinary frequency • Urinary urgency	• Pyuria and bacteria on urinalysis • Bacterial growth in urine culture	Types of infections: • Cystitis • Pyelonephritis • Tuberculosis (pyuria with negative urine culture)
Stones	• Colicky flank pain	• Patient often very uncomfortable	• If history of stones, work-up for stone forming state
Benign Prostatic Hypertrophy	• Hematuria tends to occurs toward the end of the urinary stream	• Enlarged prostate on digital rectal examination	• See Page 172
Urethral Atrophy	• Postmenopausal women	• Hematuria on initiation of urinary stream (anterior urethral bleeding)	• Occurs in up to 13% of postmenopausal women

Table 6-5

Etiology of Hematuria (continued)

DIAGNOSIS	CLINICAL HISTORY	CLINICAL FINDINGS	DETAILS
Trauma	• Recent surgery or trauma to the pelvis or abdomen		
Idiopathic	• No suggestive causes		
Nonhematuria Causes of Red-Tinged Urine or Positive Dipstick	• Beet ingestion • Porphyria • Myoglobinuria or hemoglobinuria	• Recent strenuous exercise or prolonged immobility • Elevated serum CPK	• Supernatant of spun urine red colored

CPK = creatine phosphokinase.

Table 6-6

RBC Morphology on Urinalysis, Associated Urinalysis Findings by Etiology of Hematuria

ETIOLOGY OF HEMATURIA	SOURCE OF RBC	RBC MORPHOLOGY	ASSOCIATED URINALYSIS FINDINGS
Medical/Systemic	• Glomerular	• Dysmorphic • Irregular shaped	• RBC casts • Proteinuria
Urologic	• Epithelial	• Regular, smooth, and rounded	• No proteinuria or casts

RBC = red blood cell.

Table 6-7

Diagnostic Tests for Evaluation of Hematuria

TEST	COMMENT
Urinalysis	• Identifies WBC and RBC casts, proteinuria, shape of RBCs, and presence of bacteria • Differentiates between glomerular versus epithelial RBCs
Urine Culture	• Pyuria with a negative urine culture raises possibility of tuberculosis
Urine Cytology	• Positive if high grade malignancy
24-hour Urine Collection for Protein	• Consider if significant proteinuria detected
CBC, Serum Electrolytes	• Consider to evaluate for anemia and renal function
Upper Tract Imaging	• See Chapter 5
Lower Tract Imaging	• Cystoscopy for thorough evaluation of the bladder • Bilateral retrograde pyelogram

WBC = white blood cell; CBC = complete blood count.

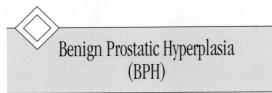

Benign Prostatic Hyperplasia (BPH)

Definition: Overgrowth of prostate tissue.

Etiology: The prostate is a walnut-sized gland located caudal to the bladder and is composed of glandular and stromal tissue. The prostate gland has three anatomical zones: the peripheral zone, the central zone, and the periurethral transition zone. BPH arises in the transition zone, while prostate cancer tends to occur in the peripheral zone. Prostatic growth is mediated by testosterone, which is converted to dihydrotestosterone (DHT) by 5-alpha-reductase. BPH can cause a mechanical compression of the urethra resulting in bladder outlet obstruction and difficulty voiding.

Epidemiology: Although up to 50% of men over the age of 50 have histological evidence of BPH, only 25–35% of men have clinical symptoms. Prevalence increases with age.

Clinical: The patient may present with a weak urinary stream, hesitancy, straining to pass urine, sensation of incomplete emptying, frequency, urgency, and occasionally, urinary retention.

Diagnosis: The digital rectal examination (DRE) evaluates the size and consistency of the prostate gland. Dullness to percussion over the lower abdomen suggests bladder distention, which may be due to bladder outlet obstruction. Measurement of prostate specific antigen (PSA) to evaluate for occult prostatic malignancy is controversial, as PSA cannot differentiate between BPH and early prostate cancer. Evaluate bladder emptying with measurement of the urine flow rate (<15 cc/s suggests obstruction) or the postvoid residual bladder volume.

Treatment: See Table 6-8.

Table 6-8

Treatment of Benign Prostatic Hypertrophy

TREATMENT	TYPE	COMMENT
Medical	Alpha1-blockers (tamsulosin, doxasozin, terazosin, alfuzosin)	• Tamsulosin is a highly selective alpha1A-blocker • Less selective alpha1-antagonists have more side effects (postural hypotension) • Symptoms tend to improve in 2–3 weeks
	5-alpha-reductase inhibitors (finasteride)	• Blocks conversion of testosterone to DHT → decrease prostate growth • Most effective in patients with large prostate glands
Surgical	TURP	• Highly effective with >90% of patients reporting symptomatic improvement • Risk of postoperative retrograde ejaculation
	TUIP	• Less invasive than TURP; can be used on smaller prostate glands

DHT = dihydrotestosterone; TUIP = transurethral incision of the prostate.

Table 6-9

Differential Diagnosis and Treatment of Scrotal Masses

	PAIN	DEFINITION	ETIOLOGY	EPIDEMIOLOGY	CLINICAL	DIAGNOSTIC ULTRASOUND FINDINGS	TREATMENT
Epididymitis	Yes	• Inflammation of the epididymis (located on the posterior aspect of the testicle)	Most frequent causes: • Age <35: sexually transmitted disease • Age > 35: urine pathogens • Less frequent causes: viral and fungal infections, sterile urine reflux, posttraumatic and amiodarone-induced chemical epididymitis	• Any age	• Most common cause of testicular pain in postpubertal men • Urinalysis: pyuria and bacteruria • Pain has gradual onset over days • Edema and erythema of the testes • Cremasteric reflex preserved • May have abdominal or flank pain, fever, urethral discharge or UTI symptoms • Resolves in 2–4 weeks	• Increased testicular blood flow	• Scrotal elevation • NSAIDs • Antibiotic therapy as indicated
Orchitis	Yes	• Inflammation of the testis	• Viruses, pyogenic bacteria, mumps, Coxsackie B, TB, syphilis and granulomatous	• Any age	• Acute onset of pain • Enlarged, indurated and tender testicle • May have high fever, nausea and vomiting • Resolves in 2–4 weeks		• Ice • Analgesics • Bed rest • Scrotal support

(continued)

Table 6-9

Differential Diagnosis and Treatment of Scrotal Masses (continued)

	PAIN	DEFINITION	ETIOLOGY	EPIDEMIOLOGY	CLINICAL	DIAGNOSTIC ULTRASOUND FINDINGS	TREATMENT
Testicular Torsion	Yes	• Twisting of the spermatic cord with strangulation of the blood supply to the affected testicle	• Bell-clapper deformity: inadequate posterior fixation of the epididymis/testis/gubernaculums to the scrotal wall	• Generally <30 years old. Peak incidence in teenage years	• Acute onset of scrotal pain, nausea, and vomiting • Absent cremasteric reflex • Scrotal edema and erythema • May have high riding, tranverse lying testicle • Salvage rate 80–100% when treated within 6 hours. At 24 hours, salvage rate is 0–20%	• Decreased testicular blood flow	• Surgical emergency
Torsion of Testicular Appendage	Yes	• Twisting of the remnant of the Muellerian duct (at upper pole of testis)	• Long, thin testicular appendage stalk	• Rare in adults. Generally occurs in 7–14 years of age	• "Blue dot" visible on scrotal skin over tender area • Paratesticular nodule • Pain has acute or subacute onset, is mild to severe and is localized in superior pole of testicle • No systemic symptoms • Usually resolves in 2 weeks	• Increased testicular blood flow. "Cold spot" indicates the appendage	• Scrotal elevation • NSAIDs • No surgery needed

Varicocele	Yes	• Tortuous dilation of the pampiniform plexus and internal spermatic vein	• Due to incompetent venous valves	• Occurs in 20–40% of males • Incidence increases with age	• Pain rare. Dull ache at the end of the day • Palpated as a "bag of worms"/painless posterior testicle mass • Can impair fertility (oligospermia, poor motility) • Occurs in up to 40% of males • If right-sided, consider IVC obstruction • If left-sided, consider renal mass	• Increased testicular blood flow/cystic mass	• No specific treatment • The most surgically correctible cause of male infertility
Testicular Cancer	Yes/ No	• Cancer arising from the cells in the testis	• 95% are germinal cell type, with 40% seminoma and 60% non-seminoma (any component of embryonal, teratoma or choriocarcinoma)	• Most common cancer in males aged 15–34 • Incidence =3.5/100,000	• Painless, hard testicular mass • Can be painful if tumor is rapidly growing and/or has area of necrosis or infarction • Does not transilluminate • *Never* biopsy, as it can spread tumor • Tumor markers: AFP/ HCG/LDH • Seminomas are sensitive to radiation • Needs prompt consultation with surgery and oncology • Can be cured if treated appropriately	• Solid mass	• Radical inguinal orchiectomy • Radiation and/or chemotherapy based on histology and extent of disease

(continued)

Table 6-9

Differential Diagnosis and Treatment of Scrotal Masses (continued)

	PAIN	DEFINITION	ETIOLOGY	EPIDEMIOLOGY	CLINICAL	DIAGNOSTIC ULTRASOUND FINDINGS	TREATMENT
Inguinal Hernia	Yes/No	• Herniation of abdominal contents into the scrotum	• Defect of abdominal wall fascia	• Incidence increases with age	• Incarceration and/or strangulation will present with pain	• Nonspecific/solid mass	• Monitor • Surgical correction (emergent if strangulated)
Hydrocele	No	• Fluid collection within the parietal and visceral layers of the tunica vaginalis	• Patent process vaginalis	• All ages	• Asymptomatic scrotal mass • Improves when lies flat • Transilluminates on physical exam	• Fluid collection/cystic mass	• Drainage if uncomfortable or disfiguring • Spontaneous resolution is frequent
Spermatocele	No	• Painless cystic mass containing spermatozoa	• Arises from testicular/epididymal tubules	• Up to 30% of men	• Pain is rare • Spermatocele is freely movable, transilluminates and is palpated superior/posterior to testes	• Cystic mass	• No surgery if concerned with fertility

AFP = alpha-fetoprotein; HCG = human chorionic gonadotropin; IVC = inferior vena cava; LDH = lactate dehydrogenase; NSAIDs = nonsteroidal anti-inflammatory drugs; TB = tuberculosis; UTI = urinary track infection.

Note: For details about urologic cancers (bladder, kidney, and testis) please refer to Oncology, Chapter 10.

Chapter 7

Infectious Diseases

Table 7-1

Common Pathogens in Bacterial Meningitis

PATHOGEN	CLINICAL PRESENTATION	PROGNOSIS	VACCINE	TREATMENT

General	• Fever
	• Headache
	• Lethargy
	• Altered mental status
	• Blurry vision
		• Complications:
		  - Seizures
		  - SIADH
		  - Hearing loss
		  - Brain abscess
		  - Death
		  - Hydrocephalus
		  - DIC
		  - Cerebrovascular events
		  - Subdural empyema
		  - Hemorrhage
				Diagnosis:
				• Lumbar puncture and CSF examination
				• CT scan recommended before lumbar puncture if:
				  - Papilledema
				  - History of CNS disease
				  - History of seizures within 1 week prior
				  - Focal neurologic abnormalities
				  - Consider if >60 years old or immunocompromised

Streptococcus pneumoniae	• Most frequent organism • There is often another foci of infection: pneumonia, mastoiditis, endocarditis	• Mortality: 20–25%	• 23-valent polysaccharide vaccine is available for adults ≥65 and those over age 2 years with chronic illness	• Initial treatment pending susceptibility results: vancomycin + third-generation cephalosporin (ceftriaxone or cefotaxime, not ceftazidime) • Adjuvant dexamethasone may reduce mortality in pneumococcal meningitis
Neisseria meningitidis	• Classic in young adults • Susceptible if complement C5–C9 deficiency • Serotype B causes up to 30% of cases in the United States	• Mortality 5–15%	• Polysaccharide conjugate vaccine for meningococcus cover serotypes A, C, Y, and W-135, but not B - Recommended for high-risk groups (military, freshman living in dorms)	• Third-generation cephalosporin • Often resistant to PCN G and ampicillin

Group B Strep	• Often occurs in those with chronic disease (diabetes, cardiac disease, cancer, alcoholism, liver/renal failure, collagen vascular disease, steroid use HIV)	• None	• Ampicillin or PCN G
Listeria monocytogenes	• >50 years old • Often occurs in those with chronic disease (see above) • Associated with contaminated milk, cheese, processed meat	• Mortality 15–30%	• None	• Ampicillin or PCN G (consider adding gentamicin)

CT = computed tomography; CNS = central nervous system; CSF = cerebrospinal fluid; DIC = disseminated intravascular coagulation; HIV = human immunodeficiency virus; PCN = penicillin; SIADH = syndrome of inappropriate antidiuretic hormone.

Table 7-2

Summary of CSF Findings in Meningitis

	BACTERIAL	**VIRAL**	**TUBERCULOUS**	**CRYPTOCOCCAL**
Opening pressure (cm H$_2$O)	200–500	≤250	180–300	>200
WBC count	1000–5000	50–1000	50–300	20–500 (low WBC is a poor prognostic sign)
WBC differential	PMNs (lymphocytic predominance possible in early infection)	Lymphocytes (PMN predominance possible in early infection)	Lymphocytes	Lymphocytes
Glucose	<40	>45	≤45	<40
Protein	100–500	<200	50–300	>45
Notes	• Gram stain positive in 60–90% of cases	• Often difficult to detect and diagnose	• AFB smear positive in <25% of cases	• Blood culture for Cryptococcal organism is sensitive • Cryptococcal antigen in CSF is sensitive

WBC = white blood cell; PMNs = polymorphonuclear leukocytes; cm = centimeters; AFB = acid-fast bacilli.

Table 7-3

Summary of Diagnostic Criteria for Infective Endocarditis

DIAGNOSIS		**NOTE**
Definitive endocarditis (as defined by Duke's criteria)	• 2 major criteria • 1 major + 3 minor • 5 minor	• Suspect if unexplained febrile or chronic illness • Always consider if evidence of: bacteremia, epidural abscess, splenic or renal infarcts, osteomyelitis, intra-abdominal abscess, and septic joints
Possible endocarditis	• 1 major + 1 minor • 3 minor	
Major Criteria		
Microbiologic data	• Typical pathogen grows in two separate blood cultures	• Any *Staphylococcus aureus* bacteremia should prompt echocardiography to rule out endocarditis

Table 7-3

Summary of Diagnostic Criteria for Infective Endocarditis (continued)

DIAGNOSIS		NOTE
Microbiologic data (cont.)	• Persistently positive blood cultures with any pathogen • 1 positive blood culture or positive serology for *Coxiella burnetii*	• Infection with *C. burnetii* is called Q fever
Endocardial involvement	• Evidence of vegetation, abscess, or new partial dehiscence of prosthetic valve on echocardiogram • New valvular regurgitation murmur on physical examination	• TEE more sensitive than TTE • HACEK organisms (gram-negative rods) often form large vegetations
Minor Criteria		
Serology or blood cultures not meeting major criteria		
Predisposing cardiac condition or injection drug user		• Endocarditis in injection drug users tends to be right sided (in contrast to left sided in noninjection drug users)
Fever >38.0°C (100.4°F)		
Vascular phenomena:	• Septic pulmonary infarcts • Mycotic aneurysm • Arterial emboli • Conjunctival hemorrhage • Intracranial hemorrhage • Janeway lesions (painless dark spots on palms/soles)	
Immunologic phenomena:	• Glomerulonephritis • Osler nodes (painful nodules on fingertips) • Roth spots (pale area surrounded by hemorrhage in fundoscopic examination) • + Rheumatoid factor	

HACEK = *Haemophilus, Actinobacillus, Cardiobacterium, Eikenella, Kingella*; TEE = transesophageal echocardiogram; TTE = transthoracic echocardiogram; C = celsius; F = fahrenheit.

Table 7-4

Summary of Infective Endocarditis Pathogens

CLINICAL SCENARIO	ETIOLOGY	TREATMENT (ANTIBIOTIC CHOICE DEPENDS ON ORGANISM AND LOCAL RESISTANCE PATTERNS)	NOTE	INDICATION FOR SURGERY
Native Valves	• *Streptococcus viridans* • *Streptococcus bovis* • Enterococci	• Antibiotics for 4–6 weeks depending on organisms • Consider a PCN, cephalosporin, or vancomycin for *Streptococcus* • Consider ampicillin/sulbactam or vancomycin + gentamicin for *Enterococcus* • Addition of gentamicin for 3–5 days may speed resolution of bacteremia	• If *S. bovis*, consider endoscopy to look for upper and lower GI malignancies	• New/worsened congestive heart failure • New conduction abnormality • Extension of infection around the valve • Recent prosthetic valve placement • Abscess on the valve • Failure of antibiotic treatment • Fungal infection • Consider if Staphylococci on a prosthetic valve • Consider if two major emboli or one major embolus + large residual vegetation
Prosthetic Valve, Early (<2 Months of Surgery)	• Coagulase negative Staphylococci	• Antibiotics • Usually requires valve replacement		

188

Prosthetic Valve, Late (>1 Year Postop)	• Similar to native valves	• Antibiotics as for native valves • If Staphylococci, consider adding rifampin (delay addition until the burden of organisms is reduced to avoid development of resistance)	• Prosthetic valves generally require longer antibiotic treatment than native valves	• As above
Injection Drug Users	• *S. aureus* (MSSA and MRSA) • Gram-negative rods	Antibiotics for 4–6 weeks: • MSSA: consider PCN, cephalosporin, or vancomycin • MRSA: consider vancomycin + gentamicin • Gram-negative rod: consider ceftriaxone or ampicillin + gentamicin		
Culture Negative		• Antibiotics for 4–6 weeks • Multiple antibiotic regimens possible such as vancomycin, gentamicin, and ciprofloxacin		

GI = gastrointestinal; MRSA = methicillin-resistant *S. aureus*; MSSA = methicillin-sensitive *S. aureus*.

Table 7-5

Community Acquired Pneumonia (CAP)

PATHOGEN	PRESENTATION	DIAGNOSIS	TREATMENT
General	• Typical signs/symptoms: - Cough - Variable sputum production - Malaise - Fevers - Dyspnea - Rigors - Pleuritic chest pain • Typical examination: - Egophony - Dullness to percussion - Tachypnea - Bronchial breath sounds - Hypoxia	• CXR • Blood cultures if hospitalized • Sputum Gram stain and culture • Specific pathogen often not recovered	Empiric therapy: • Target pneumococci and atypical pathogens using beta-lactams combined with macrolides or respiratory fluoroquinolones Outpatient therapy: • Oral respiratory fluoroquinolones OR beta-lactams combined with macrolides or fluoroquinolones
S. pneumoniae	• Most common cause of CAP • Acute onset of rigors • Rust-colored sputum classic		• Beta-lactams, less commonly fluoroquinolones
Moraxella catarrhalis, Haemophilus influenzae	• Productive cough • Typical CAP symptoms as above	• Sputum Gram stain and culture • CXR: lobar infiltrate	• Beta-lactams, azithromycin, or fluoroquinolones
S. aureus	• Productive cough • Typical CAP symptoms as above		• Beta-lactams if not MRSA • Vancomycin or linezolid if PCN allergy • Usually methicillin sensitive when community acquired. However, community-acquired MRSA becoming more common

Atypicals

Mycoplasma pneumoniae	• Typically in younger patients: "walking pneumonia"
	• Headache
	• Sore throat
	• Paroxysmal dry cough worse at night
	• Erythema multiforme
	• CNS symptoms
		• Positive cold agglutinins
		• Mycoplasma titers
		• PCR of BAL fluid or sputum
		• Throat swab
		• Hemolytic anemia
		• CXR: patchy infiltrates
			• Azithromycin or clarithromycin
			  OR
			• Fluoroquinolone
			  OR
			• Doxycycline

Chlamydia pneumoniae	• Sore throat
	• Headache
	• Cough can be long-lasting if untreated
	• Scant sputum production
		• Serum titers
		• PCR of sputum or BAL fluid
		• Sputum culture
		• CXR: circumscribed infiltrate
			• Azithromycin or clarithromycin
			  OR
			• Fluoroquinolone
			  OR
			• Doxycycline

Legionella pneumophila	• Can be most severe atypical CAP
	• Symptoms range from mild cough to respiratory failure
	• Myalgias
	• Malaise
	• Anorexia
	• Abdominal pain
	• Diarrhea
	• Pleuritic pain
	• Hemoptysis
		• DFA or PCR of sputum or BAL fluid
		• Urine *Legionella* antigen
		• Serum titers
		• Hyponatremia
		• Microscopic hematuria
		• Leukocytosis
		• Elevated LFTs
		• Hypophosphatemia
		• CXR: patchy consolidations
			• Fluoroquinolone
			  OR
			• Azithromycin or clarithromycin
			  OR
			• Doxycycline

CNS = central nervous system; PCR = polymerase chain reaction; BAL = bronchial alveolar lavage; CXR = chest x-ray; CAP = community acquired pneumonia; DFA = direct fluorescent antibody; LFTs = liver function tests.

Table 7-6

Summary of Tuberculosis (TB)

TYPE	CLINICAL PRESENTATION	DIAGNOSIS	TREATMENT*
Primary Pulmonary TB (Active)	• Cough • Fevers • Malaise See Table 7-8 for tuberculin skin testing	Imaging: • Middle/lower lung zone consolidation • Hilar lymphadenopathy • Atelectasis, miliary pattern • Three induced sputum samples obtained at least 12 hours apart for AFB smear and culture (important to confirm sensitivities)	Testing prior to treatment: • Culture/susceptibility • Baseline labs prior to treatment Common regimen: INH, ethambutol, pyrazinamide, rifampin; 8 weeks induction, then 18 weeks with INH and rifampin • Mnemonic: - 6 months total antibiotic treatment - 4 drugs × 2 months - 2 drugs × 4 months
Reactivation Pulmonary TB (Active)	• Fever • Wasting • Ill-appearing • Cough • Malaise	Imaging: • Upper lobes affected more often, but can have infiltrates in lower lobes • Cavitations • Pleural effusion • Three induced sputum samples obtained at least 12 hours apart for AFB smear and culture	• As for active primary pulmonary TB
Latent	• Asymptomatic	Imaging: • CXR can be normal or with evidence of old TB • Positive PPD and no active pulmonary disease (normal CXR or negative AFB sputum smears × 3)	• INH for 9 months • Alternative: rifampin for 4 months • No longer recommended: rifampin and pyrazinamide (hepatotoxicity)

| Extrapulmonary | • More common if immunosuppressed
• Lymphadenitis (particularly cervical) most common manifestation
• Pleural disease:
  - Cough, pleuritic chest pain, fever, dyspnea
• Osteoarticular disease:
  - Back pain from spinal disease (Pott disease), slowly progressive monoarthritis
• CNS disease:
  - Cranial nerve defects, altered mental status, seizures, headache, meningitis
• GU tract disease:
  - Dysuria, sterile pyuria, hematuria, flank pain
• Abdominal:
  - Abdominal pain, diarrhea, weight loss
  - peritonitis
• Cardiac:
  - Pericarditis | • CXR may be normal
• AFB smear and culture from appropriate tissue (CSF, gastric aspirate, urine, joint, bone, etc.)
• NAAT may be helpful for rapid identification, but sensitivity limited
• Pleural fluid: usually exudative, with lymphocyte predominance (PMN early in course); adenosine deaminase, lysozyme, and interferon-alfa may be elevated | • Four drug therapy (as for active TB above) × 2 months, then INH and rifampin × 4–10 months
• CNS: 9–12 months of therapy; adjuvant steroids
• Consider extended therapy if bone or joint involvement |

*Multidrug-resistant TB requires different regimens.

GU = genitourinary; INH = isoniazid; NAAT = nucleic acid amplification testing; PPD = purified protein derivative; TB = tuberculosis; AFB = acid-fast bacilli; CXR = chest radiograph; CNS = central nervous system; PMN = polymorphonuclear.

Table 7-7

TB Medications and Side Effects

TB DRUG	SELECT ADVERSE REACTIONS	NOTE
Pyrazinamide	• Hepatitis • Hyperuricemia • Arthralgias	• Baseline LFTs and uric acid prior to treatment
Ethambutol	• Red-green color blindness • Optic neuritis	• Assess baseline red-green color blindness prior to treatment
Rifampin	• Hepatitis • Orange discoloration of body fluids • Flu-like illness	• Baseline LFTs prior to treatment • Significant drug-drug interactions between rifampin and PIs/NNRTIs • Substitute rifabutin for HIV+ patients on HAART
INH	• Hepatitis • Anemia • GI symptoms • Peripheral neuropathy • Rash	• Baseline LFTs and CBC prior to treatment • Discontinue if LFTs > 3× upper limit of normal and symptomatic or > 5× and asymptomatic • Pyridoxine may prevent peripheral neuropathy

CBC = complete blood count; HAART = high active antiretroviral therapy; NNRTIs = nonnucleoside reverse transcriptase inhibitors; PIs = protease inhibitors; LFT = liver function test; GI = gastrointestinal; HIV = human immuno deficiency virus.

Table 7-8

Summary of Tuberculin Skin Testing

RISK CATEGORY	RISK FACTOR	MM INDURATION CONSIDERED POSITIVE
High	• HIV+ • Immunosuppressant treatment • Recent contacts with active TB patients • CXR with evidence of previous TB	>5 mm
Medium	• Healthcare workers • IV drug users • Residents of high-risk institutions (prison, nursing homes, homeless shelters, etc.) • Recent immigrants (<5 years) from endemic areas • Mycobacteriology lab personnel	>10 mm

Table 7-8

Summary of Tuberculin Skin Testing (continued)

RISK CATEGORY	RISK FACTOR	MM INDURATION CONSIDERED POSITIVE
Medium (cont.)	• Chronic disease: - Diabetes - Organ transplant recipient - Long-term corticosteroid use - Head and neck cancer - Leukemia and lymphoma - End-stage renal disease - Chronic malabsorption states - >10% below ideal body weight - Gastric bypass	
Low	• None of the above risk factors	>15 mm
BCG Recipient	• Vaccine does not prevent infection • Reduces complications, such as TB meningitis in children • Usually given in places where TB is endemic, making it difficult to discern between BCG reaction or actual exposure	• Common teaching in the United States is to ignore BCG status when interpreting PPD, particularly with a PPD result ≥15 mm • Newly developed interferon-gamma release assays using whole blood can distinguish between *Mycobacterium tuberculosis* infection and BCG vaccination. However, accurate assessments of the sensitivity of these tests for detection of latent TB are complicated by the absence of a gold standard for this diagnosis

BCG = Bacille Calmette-Guérin; IV = intravenous.

Table 7-9

Summary of Urinary Tract Infections (UTI)

Type of UTI	Definition	Risk Factors/Clinical Presentation	Diagnosis	Common Treatment
Acute Uncomplicated Cystitis	• Dysuria, frequency, and/or urgency confirmed by the presence of bacteriuria in adult non-pregnant women with normal urinary tract	• Burning/itching on urination	• Clinical history • Urine culture not needed for diagnosis	• TMP/SMX × 3 days • Consider quinolone if resistance to TMP/SMX is present in the community

Acute Complicated Cystitis	• Dysuria, frequency, and/or urgency confirmed by the presence of bacteriuria in adults with risk factors	• Risk factors:
		  - Abnormal urinary tract
		  - Indwelling catheter
		  - History of stones or obstruction, symptoms > 7 days
		  - Recent antibiotic use or hospitalization
		  - Recent instrumentation of urinary tract
		  - Age >65 years
		  - Male
		  - Pregnancy
		  - Host susceptibility: diabetes, immunocompromised, chronic kidney disease
			• Clinical history
			• UA
			• Urine culture
				• TMP/SMX (or quinolone depending on culture and sensitivities) × 7–10 days

Recurrent UTI	• >3 UTI episodes in 12 months	• Risk factors:
		  - Intercourse
		  - Spermicide
		  - Postmenopausal
		  - Indwelling catheter
		  - Repeated catheterizations
			• Clinical history
			• UA
			• Urine culture
				• Daily low-dose prophylaxis
				• Postcoital voiding and prophylaxis with TMP/SMX × 1 dose
				• Patient-initiated treatment (symptom-guided)
				• Consider estrogen cream in postmenopausal women with atrophic vaginitis

Pyelonephritis	• Infection of renal parenchyma or pelvis	Clinical presentation: • Fever • Flank pain • CVA tenderness • Nausea/vomiting	• Clinical history • UA • Urine culture	• Select, otherwise healthy patients: - Outpatient oral fluoroquinolone, amoxicillin-clavulanate, cephalosporin, or TMP/SMX - Female: 7–14 days if immunocompetent and 14–21 if immunocompromised - 14 days in men if uncomplicated - 4 weeks if acute prostatitis • If ill/elderly: - Inpatient, IV fluoroquinolone, aminoglycoside +/− ampicillin, or third-generation cephalosporin - Follow cultures for sensitivities - Patients often bacteremic - If treatment fails, consider perinephric abscess, nephrolithiasis, obstruction, and resistant organisms
Asymptomatic Bacteriuria	• Positive UA without symptoms			• Treat if: - Pregnant (use nitrofurantoin or amoxicillin) - Planned urologic surgery - Patients with urinary outlet obstruction - Neutropenic patients - Renal transplant patients

CVA = costovertebral angle; UA = urinalysis; UTI = urinary tract infection; TMP/SMX = trimethoprim/sulfamethoxazole.

Table 7-10
Summary of Infectious Diarrhea

Disease	Etiology	Clinical Presentation	Diagnosis	Treatment	Complication	Comment
Salmonella, nontyphi	*S. paratyphi* *S. enteriditis* *S. typhimurium*	• Diarrhea (may be bloody) • Cramps • Abdominal pain • Fever • More severe in presence of immunodeficiency, hemoglobinopathies, colitis, and chronic GI disease	• Stool culture	• Supportive • Consider treatment for patients considered at risk for severe disease or extraintestinal spread • Bacteremia should always be treated • Treatment choices include TMP/SMX, ceftriaxone, or fluoroquinolone • Because of high rates of resistance, antibiotic therapy should be guided by local sensitivities	• Bacteremia • Sepsis • Meningitis	• Commonly transmitted by fecal contamination of poultry, red meat, eggs, dairy, produce • Turtles, iguanas, other reptiles are reservoirs • Screen family members only if symptomatic, or if at high risk for disease • Antibiotics usually do not change course of illness • Risk factors for extraintestinal spread: age >50 years old, prosthesis, valvular heart disease, severe atherosclerosis, immunosuppressed hosts, AIDS, lymphoproliferative disease, and uremia

Disease	Organism	Clinical Features	Diagnosis	Treatment	Complications	Notes
Typhoid Fever	*S. typhi*	• Diarrhea (may be bloody) • Relative bradycardia (lower heart rate than expected for degree of fever) • Fever • Abdominal pain • Hepatomegaly • Splenomegaly • Rose spots on trunk • Altered mental status • Meningismus	• Stool and/or blood culture • Bone marrow/urine culture • Leukopenia/leukocytosis • Proteinuria • Transaminitis • DIC • Serology not helpful due to high false-positive and false-negative rates	• TMP/SMX, ceftriaxone, or fluoroquinolone • Contact precautions until treatment finished and three stool cultures are negative • High rates of resistance	• GI hemorrhage • GI perforation • Pneumonia • Meningitis • Abscess formation	• Humans are only reservoir • Screen family members only if symptomatic • Carriage state may occur • Vaccine available
Shigellosis	*S. sonnei* *S. flexneri*	• Sudden onset of: - Fever - Watery/bloody diarrhea - Cramps - Tenesmus - Seizures	• Stool culture • Bacteremia rare • WBC or RBCs in stool suggestive of gut invasion, but not specific	• TMP/SMX or fluoroquinolone, depending on local sensitivities	• Dehydration • Shock	• Humans are only reservoir • Low inoculum size required for disease
Campylobacter	*C. jejuni*	• Diarrhea (may be bloody, watery, with pus or bile) • Fever • Headache • Cramps • Nausea • Vomiting	• Stool culture • Dark field microscopy of stool (low specificity; can be confused with Vibrio)	• Erythromycin or azithromycin will shorten length of illness	• Guillain-Barré syndrome	• Reservoir includes wild/domestic birds, young cats, dogs, hamsters • Contaminated water and milk products • May mimic appendicitis

(continued)

Table 7-10

Summary of Infectious Diarrhea (continued)

Disease	Etiology	Clinical Presentation	Diagnosis	Treatment	Complication	Comment
Escherichia coli	Enterohemorrhagic (O157:H7)	• Bloody diarrhea • Severe abdominal pain • Fever in <1/3	• Stool culture • Serologic testing available for O157:H7 serotype	• Supportive care • Consider fluoroquinolone or TMP/SMX if severe disease • Rifaximin if luminal disease only	• Dehydration • O157:H7: Hemorrhagic colitis • HUS	• Antibiotics probably do not prevent HUS • Most common cause of traveler's diarrhea
	Enterotoxigenic	• Watery diarrhea • Abdominal cramps				
	Enteroinvasive	• Bloody diarrhea				
	Enteropathogenic	• Bloody diarrhea				
Yersinia	*Y. enterocoliticia*	• Enterocolitis: - Bloody diarrhea - Fever • May mimic acute appendicitis: - Right lower quadrant pain - Abdominal tenderness - Fever	• Stool culture • Culture of throat swabs, peritoneal fluid, blood	• If septic, or immunocompromised, consider treatment with: first-generation cephalosporin or PCN	• Hepatic, splenic abscess • Bacteremia • Postinfectious: - Erythema nodosum - Arthritis	• Reservoirs: pigs, milk products • Patients with iron overload especially susceptible

Giardia	*G. lamblia*	• Foul smelling stools • Abdominal pain • Boating • Flatulence • Anorexia • Many asymptomatic	• Stool examination for trophozoites/cysts • Antigen detection in stool • Examination of duodenal aspirate	• Metronidazole • Alternatives: nitazoxanide or albendazole	• Weight loss, Malabsorption • Anemia	• Reservoirs include humans, dogs, cats, beavers • Associated with IgA deficiency • Treatment of asymptomatic carriers not recommended
Food Poisoning	*S. aureus* enterotoxin ingestion	• Abrupt onset 0.5–12 hours after food ingestion • Vomiting • Cramps • Diarrhea • Generally lasts 24–48 hours	• May recover Staphylococci from stool or vomit • Can isolate toxin from suspected food	• Supportive	• Dehydration	• Inadequate heating or storage of foods, especially meats, dairy, mayonnaise

AIDS = acquired immunodeficiency syndrome; HUS = hemolytic-uremic syndrome; RBCs = red blood cells; DIC = disseminated intravascular coagulation; TMP/SMX = trimethoprine/sulfamethoxazole.

Table 7-11

Frequent Complication Following Splenectomy/Asplenia

RISK	COMMON ORGANISM	PRESENTATION	PREVENTION
• Acute, overwhelming bacterial sepsis	Encapsulated organisms: • *S. pneumoniae* • *H. influenzae* • *N. meningitidis*	• Days to years after splenectomy • Prodrome of fevers, chills, pharyngitis, myalgias, or diarrhea • Rapid progression to sepsis and septic shock	• Patients often given amoxicillin-clavulanate, TMP/SMX, or other antibiotics to take at home at the first sign of infection

Table 7-12

Summary of Vector-Borne Diseases

DISEASE	ORGANISM/VECTOR	PRESENTATION	DIAGNOSIS	TREATMENT	NOTES

Lyme Disease	• *Borrelia burgdorferi*
	• Vector: deer tick—*Ixodes scapularis*
		• Early (days to 1 month):
		  - EM (single or multiple)
		  - Nonspecific rash
		  - Influenza-like illness
		  - Arthritis < 2 weeks/arthralgia
		  - Carditis
		• Early neurologic disease:
		  - Radiculopathy
		  - Cranial neuropathy
		  - Meningitis
		  - Encephalomyelitis
		• Late (years)
		  - Arthritis
		  - Late neurologic disease:
		  - Encephalomyelitis
		  - Peripheral neuropathy
		  - Encephalopathy
			• ELISA, confirmed by Western blot
			• Consider PCR of joint fluid if active joint disease
			• Urine antigen not helpful
			• CSF PCR has limited sensitivity
				• EM:
				  - Doxycycline; amoxicillin; or cefuroxime × 2–3 weeks if no evidence of neurologic disease
				• Early neurologic disease:
				  - Ceftriaxone × 14–28 days
				• Cardiac disease:
				  - Ceftriaxone × 14–21 days or oral therapy as for EM
				• Late arthritis:
				  - Same as EM
				• Late neurologic disease:
				  - Ceftriaxone × 14–28 days
				• Postexposure prophylaxis:
				  - Controversial
					• Lyme disease, *Babesia*, and *Ehrlichia* are carried by the same vector tick and coinfection can occur
					• Treat with doxycycline if concern about coinfection with *Ehrlichia*
					• Consider coinfection if symptoms do not resolve with treatment

Table 7-12

Summary of Vector-Borne Diseases (continued)

DISEASE	ORGANISM/VECTOR	PRESENTATION	DIAGNOSIS	TREATMENT	NOTES
Babesiosis	• *Babesia microti* • Vector: deer tick—*I. scapularis*	• Flu-like illness • Jaundice • Hemolytic anemia • Renal failure due to hemolysis (intraerythrocytic parasite) • Asplenic patients particularly at risk for complications including ARDS	Peripheral thin and thick smear: • Intraerythrocytic or free organisms • "Maltese cross" configuration • Serologies and PCR confirm diagnosis	• Symptomatic treatment • Quinine + clindamycin; OR atovaquone + azithromycin • If ≥10% para-sitemia, con-sider exchange transfusions to reduce burden of organisms	• See notes for Lyme disease
Ehrlichiosis— Human Monocytic (south central, southeastern United States)	• *Ehrlichia chaffeensis* • Vector: *Amblyomma america-num-* lone star tick	• Variable rash: mac-ular, maculopapu-lar, or petechial • Flu-like illness • Leukopenia • Thrombocytopenia • Elevated LFTs • Neurologic symp-toms: headache, stiff neck, and altered mental status	• Morula on blood smear (intraleukocytic inclusion) • Seroconversion evident during convalescence	• Treat empirically on clinical grounds • Doxycycline; minimum of 5–7 days, until improved	• See notes for Lyme disease
Ehrlichiosis— Human Granulocytic (midwestern, northeastern United States)	• *Anaplasma phagocyto-philum*	• Rash is rare • Otherwise, similar to ehrlichiosis— human monocytic	• Seroconversion evident during convalescence		
Rocky Mountain Spotted Fever	• *Rickettsia rickettsii* • Vector: wood tick or dog tick	• Petechial rash (begins on palms and soles and peripherally, spreads to trunk, convalesces) • Flu-like illness: malaise, fever, headache, nausea, vomiting	• Clinical diag-nosis • Biopsy of skin lesions with immunofluores-cent staining • ELISA positive in convales-cence	• Doxycycline • Empiric treat-ment within first 5 days of onset decreases mor-tality	• Rash may be absent or have atypical distribution at presenta-tion

(continued)

Table 7-12

Summary of Vector-Borne Diseases (continued)

DISEASE	ORGANISM/VECTOR	PRESENTATION	DIAGNOSIS	TREATMENT	NOTES
West Nile Virus	• West Nile Virus • Vector: mosquito	• 90% asymptomatic • Typically self-limited febrile illness with headache, back pain, myalgias • Maculopapular rash in ~50% of patients • Neuroinvasive disease in <1%: - Encephalitis - Meningitis - Photophobia - Movement disorders/ parkinsonism - Confusion - Slurred speech - Acute asymmetric flaccid paralysis (rare) - May have presentation similar to Guillain-Barré syndrome	• ELISA of serum or CSF if neurologic symptoms • CSF findings: pleocytosis with lymphocytic predominance, mild protein elevation, normal glucose	• Supportive care	• High risk for neurologic disease: - Diabetic - Elderly - Immunosuppressed

ARDS = acute respiratory distress syndrome; ELISA = enzyme-linked immunosorbent assay; EM = erythema migrans.

Table 7-13

Summary of Sexually Transmitted Infections (STI)*

INFECTION	PRESENTATION	DIAGNOSIS	TREATMENT	COMPLICATIONS	NOTES

Chlamydia trachomatis	• Women:
	  - Asymptomatic OR
	  - Dysuria
	  - Change in vaginal discharge
	  - Examination:
	    ○ Urethritis
	    ○ Cervicitis
	    ○ PID
	• Men:
	  - Asymptomatic OR
	  - Dysuria
	  - Unilateral testicular pain
	  - Scrotal erythema
	  - Examination:
	    ○ Urethritis
	    ○ Epididymitis
		• UA
		  - Sterile pyuria
		  - >5 WBC/hpf
		  - Negative urine culture
		  - Culture of cervix or urethra
		  - PCR: urine, cervical, or urethral sample
			• Uncomplicated:
			  - Azithromycin 1 g × 1 dose; or doxycycline bid × 7 days
			• Pregnant:
			  - Erythromycin or amoxicillin
			• PID
			  - Oral fluoroquinolone +/− metronidazole
			  - IV options: cefotetan (or cefoxitin) + doxycycline
				• PID (acute salpingitis):
				  - Abdominal pain
				  - Fever
				  - Prolonged menses
				  - Infertility
				  - Chronic pelvic pain
				  - Increases risk of ectopic pregnancy
				• Reiter syndrome:
				  - Reactive arthritis (asymmetric, polyarthritis)
				  - Conjunctivitis
				  - Urethritis
					• Partner should also be treated
					• Test for gonorrhea as well due to high rate of coinfection
					• Rescreen women 3–4 months after treatment

(*continued*)

Table 7-13

Summary of Sexually Transmitted Infections (STI)* (continued)

Infection	Presentation	Diagnosis	Treatment	Complications	Notes
Neisseria gonorrhoeae	• Urogenital infection in women: - Asymptomatic OR - Mild vaginal discharge - Abdominal pain • Urogenital infection in men: - Usually symptomatic - Dysuria - Penile discharge - Epididymitis (occasional) • Anorectal infections: - Proctitis - Anal pruritus - Anal discharge with bowel movements - Tenesmus - Bleeding more common in MSM • Pharyngeal infections: - Mild or no symptoms	• Culture of cervix or urethra • PCR: urine (men only) • Rectal or pharyngeal infections: culture is best	• Uncomplicated: - Ceftriaxone (IM) or cefixime (PO) • Pharyngeal: - More difficult to cure - Ceftriaxone 125 mg IM × 1 • PID: - Same as for chlamydia • Disseminated: - Ceftriaxone IV - Hospitalize initially • Cephalosporin allergy: - Consider spectinomycin - Fluoroquinolones no longer recommended due to high rates of resistance	• Disseminated disease via bloodstream infection: - Women more common than men • Arthritis: - Wrists, ankles, hands, feet - Tenosynovitis - Meningitis - Skin lesions - PID	• Treat for Chlamydia as well

Trichomonas vaginalis	• Women:
	  - Asymptomatic OR
	  - Vaginal discharge
	  - Pruritus
	  - Dysuria
	  - Strawberry cervix on examination
	• Men:
	  - Asymptomatic OR
	  - Dysuria
	  - Discharge
		• Direct visualization on wet mount prep	• Oral metronidazole	• PID
				• Adverse birth outcomes
					• Emerging resistance to metronidazole

Human Papillomavirus	• Often asymptomatic • Genital warts • Condylomata acuminata • Respiratory papillomatosis (rare) • Oral lesions (rare)	• Direct visualization • Application of acetic acid • Pap smear • Liquid cytology	• Topical podophyllotoxin • Imiquimod • 5-Fluorouracil • Cryotherapy • Laser therapy	• Cervical and anal cancer associated with HPV types 16, 18	• Most common sexually transmitted disease • Vaccine active against strains 6, 11, 16, 18

*Patients who are diagnosed with any STI should be screened for others, including gonorrhea, chlamydia, syphilis, and HIV.

HPV = human papillomavirus; MSM = men who have sex with men; PID = pelvic inflammatory disease; IV = intravenous; IM = intramuscular.

Table 7-14
Summary of Syphilis

STAGE OF SYPHILIS	MANIFESTATION	DIAGNOSIS	TREATMENT	NOTE
Primary	• Chancre—painless ulcer, clean base at site of inoculation • Regional lymphadenopathy	• Darkfield microscopy	• Benzathine PCN G IM × 1 dose • If PCN allergic, doxycycline, tetracycline, or erythromycin × 2 weeks	• Jarisch-Herxheimer reaction: - Clinical exacerbation 12–24 hours after initiation of treatment (any stage) - May be due to inflammatory response of dying organisms
Secondary	• Rash (palms and soles) • Fever • Malaise • Lymphadenopathy • Condylomalata • Meningitis	• Screen: serum RPR or VDRL (nontreponemal tests) • Confirm: FTA-ABS (treponemal test)	• Same as primary	- Symptoms: fevers, headache, malaise, and worsening of syphilitic symptoms - Treatment: symptomatic only
Latent	• Asymptomatic	• Same as secondary	• Early latent (<1 year): same as primary • Late latent (>1 year or unknown): benzathine PCN G in three weekly doses OR doxycycline OR tetracycline × 4 weeks	
Tertiary	• Cardiovascular: - Aortic aneurysm - Aortic regurgitation • Neurosyphilis: - Meningitis - Cranial nerve palsies - Tabes dorsalis (insidious dementia, delusions, fatigue, ataxia, Argyll-Robertson pupils, areflexia, loss of proprioception) - Gumma—monocytic infiltrates, tissue destruction of any organ	• Same as secondary • Neurosyphilis: - No gold standard - Combination of serum serologies, CSF serologies, and CSF findings (elevated WBC, lymphocyte predominance, elevated protein)	• Nonneuro: benzathine PCN G in three weekly doses • Neurosyphilis: IV PCN q4h × 2 weeks	

FTA-ABS = fluorescent treponemal antibody-absorption; RPR = rapid plasma reagin; VDRL = Venereal Disease Research Laboratory test.

Table 7-15

Summary of Treatment Details for Viral Hepatitis

For additional details, see Gastroenterology section

HEPATITIS VIRUS	TREATMENT	POTENTIAL SIDE EFFECTS	PROGNOSIS	NOTES

Hepatitis B	• Adefovir	• Pruritic rash
		 • Nausea
			• <10% of adults progress to chronic infection	• Associated with:
				   - Membranous glomerulo-nephritis
				   - Polyarteritis nodosa
				   - Suspect HDV coinfection if acute decompensation of preexisting chronic viral hepatitis
				   - HDV makes treatment more difficult and more likely to progress to cirrhosis

	• Lamivudine	• Lipodystrophy		

Hepatitis C	• Pegylated interferon	• Flu-like illness
		 • Depression
		 • Bone marrow suppression
			• Chronic infection in 80% with 10–20% progressing to cirrhosis
			 • 1–5% develop hepato-cellular carcinoma
			 • Faster progression if HIV, elderly, alcoholic, or underlying liver disease
			 • Genotype 1 harder to treat than 2 and 3
			 • Genotype 1b + HIV coinfection: sustained virologic response in 15% (45% if HIV−)
				• Associated with:
				   - Cryoglobulinemia
				   - Membranoproliferative glomerulonephritis
				   - Treatment of acute HCV may impact long-term outcomes
				   - Begin treatment if HCV viral load detectable or liver biopsy shows portal or bridging fibrosis and moderate inflammation
				   - Liver transplantation if decompensated cirrhosis

	• Ribavirin	• Hemolytic anemia • Birth defects • Worsening of cardiac disease		

HCV = hepatitis C virus; HDV = hepatitis D virus.

Table 7-16

Summary of Frequent Skin Infections

CLINICAL SCENARIO	COMMON PATHOGEN	DIAGNOSIS	TREATMENT	NOTE
Cellulitis				
Uncomplicated Cellulitis	• Streptococci, *Staphylococcus aureus*	• Localized erythema, tenderness, warmth, induration, and swelling at site of infection • Fever • CT or MRI if suspicion	• If IV required: cefazolin or nafcillin; then oral dicloxacillin or first-generation cephalosporin, total × 10–14 days • May require vancomycin or linezolid if MRSA	Prevention: • Support stockings if edematous • Good skin hygiene • Treat tinea pedis promptly
Diabetic Foot Ulcer	• Gram-negative rods • *Pseudomonas aeruginosa* • Anaerobes • *Staphylococcus* • *Enterococcus*	• Consider underlying osteomyelitis • Consider deep venous thrombosis • Ultrasound if suspicion for abscess or fluid collection	• Common first-line: ampicillin-sulbactam • Vancomycin or linezolid (for MRSA or severe infection)	• Usually polymicrobial • May not have pain, fever, or systemic signs. May see abnormal color, foul odor of wound
Human Bites	• Oral anaerobes • *Staphylococcus aureus* • *Streptococcus viridans*		• Common first-line: amoxicillin-clavulanate	
Cat or Dog Bites	• *Pasteurella multocida* • *Staphylococcus aureus* • *Neisseria canis*		• Common first-line: amoxicillin-clavulanate; alternative: moxifloxacin + clindamycin	
Salt Water Exposure to Break in Skin	• *Vibrio vulnificus* • *Mycobacterium marinarum* (fish tanks)		• Doxycycline; cefotaxime; ciprofloxacin	• *V. vulnificus* can cause hemorrhagic bullae
Fresh Water Exposure to Break in Skin	• *Aeromonas hydrophila*		• Ciprofloxacin; carbapenems	
Hot Tubs	• *Pseudomonas aeruginosa*		• Antipseudomonal PCN (ceftazidime, cefepime)	

Other Skin Infections

Community-Acquired MRSA Skin Abscesses	• MRSA	• History of exposure • Culture of drained abscess	• TMP/SMX, doxycycline, or clindamycin if sensitive • May require vancomycin or linezolid	• Higher prevalence in certain communities such as MSM, prison inmates, injection drug users, contact sports participants • Can be spread by person-to-person contact • Community incidence increasing
Necrotizing Fasciitis	• Infection of superficial fascia, usually by Group A *Streptococcus* or mixed aerobic/anaerobic infections, particularly with *Clostridium perfringens*	• Pain disproportionate to physical findings • Bullae • Tense edema • Crepitus with clostridial/gas-forming infection • Rapid progression to gangrene and sepsis • Systemic illness • Plain films more sensitive for detecting gas in tissues	• Early surgical exploration and extensive debridement • Empiric antibiotics (include clindamycin to prevent toxin formation, the Eagle effect) +/– IVIG • Consider hyperbaric therapy • +/– IVIG	• Often starts at injection sites in drug users • Fournier's gangrene: necrotizing fasciitis of male perineum, usually seen in diabetics
Toxic Shock Syndrome (TSS)	• Complication of streptococcal or staphylococcal infections	• Fulminant onset • High fever • Erythematous rash with desquamation • Hypotension • Multiorgan system failure • Occurs postsurgery, posttrauma, or in association with tampon use	• Vancomycin or antistaph PCN (Staph TSS) or PCN (Strep TSS) + clindamycin (Eagle effect) • Fluid replacement • Supportive treatment for shock • +/– IVIG	• Early onset of shock and organ failure

IVIG = intravenous immunoglobulin; MRI = magnetic resonance imaging; TSS = toxic shock syndrome.

Table 7-17

Summary of Selected Head and Neck Infections

INFECTION	CLINICAL NOTES	PRESENTATION	DIAGNOSIS	TREATMENT
Viral Sinusitis	• Most common overall	• Sinus tenderness • Fever • Congestion	• Clinical diagnosis	• Supportive care

Acute Bacterial Sinusitis	• Most commonly caused by:
	  - *S. pneumoniae*
	  - *H. influenzae, M. catarrhalis*
	  - Complications:
	    1. Meningitis
	    2. Brain abscess
	    3. Cavernous sinus thrombosis
	    4. Subdural empyema
	    5. Orbital cellulitis
		• Purulent nasal discharge
		• Unilateral maxillary or tooth pain
		• Unilateral maxillary sinus tenderness
		• Headache worse with leaning forward
		• Persistent symptoms > 7 days
			In contrast to viral sinusitis:
			• Lasts > 7 days
			• May worsen after initial improvement
			• Clinical history
			• CT can help define predisposing anatomic abnormalities but not needed for diagnosis
				• Mild disease:
				  - Amoxicillin, TMP/SMX, macrolide, or fluoroquinolone × 10–14 days
				• Allergy to PCN
				  - TMP/SMX or doxycycline
				• Moderate disease, diabetics, or recent antibiotics:
				  - Amoxicillin-clavulanate or fluoroquinolone
				• Recurrent sinusitis:
				  - CT scan
				  - May require surgical intervention

Ludwig's Angina	• Rapidly progressive gangrenous cellulitis of neck soft tissues and floor of mouth, submandibular/sublingual spaces
	• Usually begins with dental problems
	• Predisposing factors:
	  - Diabetes
	  - Alcoholism
	  - Immunocompromised
	  - Airway involvement can be fatal
		• Drooling
		• Dyspnea
		• Fever
		• Dysphagia
		• Tender neck swelling
		• Tooth pain
		• Protruding or elevated tongue
			• CT to assess extent of infection (contiguous spread)	• Airway management key
				• Dexamethasone to reduce swelling
				• Treat likely polymicrobial infection with ampicillin-sulbactam, PCN G + metronidazole, or clindamycin (PCN-allergic)

Lemierre Disease	• Acute parapharyngeal infection with secondary septic thrombophlebitis of internal jugular vein • *Fusobacterium* most common pathogen	• Oropharyngeal infection with septicemia occurring about 1 week later • Possible seeding to other organs	• Ultrasound of internal jugular vein may show thrombus • Evaluate for other sites of infection	• Ampicillin-sulbactam, ticarcillin-clavulanate, piperacillin-tazobactam, PCN + clindamycin OR metronidazole, or carbapenem • Anticoagulation is controversial • Consider ligation of internal jugular vein
Diphtheria	• Respiratory failure can be life threatening	• Pharyngitis • "Bull neck" (swelling) • Respiratory failure	• Gray pseudomembranes over pharynx • Culture on special media	• PCN • Respiratory droplet precautions
Retropharyngeal Abscess		• Fever • Odynophagia • Ipsilateral otalgia • Trismus • Fluctuant peritonsillar fullness • Uvula deviation	• Needle aspiration vs. incision and drainage • Imaging: CT neck, lateral neck radiographs	• PCN +/− metronidazole or clindamycin

HSV = herpes simplex virus.

Table 7-18

Frequent Complications of Antibiotics

COMPLICATION	ANTIBIOTIC/DRUG	PRESENTATION	DIAGNOSIS	TREATMENT
Dermatologic				
• **Toxic Epidermal Necrolysis** • **Stevens-Johnson Syndrome** • **Erythema Multiforme** **(The above conditions are grouped together due to the clinical similarities. See Dermatology, Chapter 14, for full explanations.)**	• Sulfonamides • Anticonvulsants • NSAIDs • Allopurinol • Many others	• See Dermatology, Chapter 14	• See Dermatology, Chapter 14	• Stop offending drug • Supportive care and fluid replacement • Steroids are controversial • Care similar to burn patients
Hypersensitivity Syndrome	• Anticonvulsants • Sulfonamides • Dapsone • Minocycline • Allopurinol • Gold salts • Many others	• Severe idiosyncratic reaction • Diffuse papulopustular skin eruption • Progresses to exfoliative dermatitis • Fever • May have visceral involvement	• Clinical diagnosis • Eosinophilia in 90% • Monocytosis in 40% • Patch tests may be used to confirm culprit drug	• Stop offending drug • Systemic (for severe) or topical (for milder presentation) steroids

GI			

Clostridium difficile Colitis	• Broad-spectrum antibiotics:
	  - PCN
	  - Cephalosporins
	  - Clindamycin
		• Symptoms range from asymptomatic to diarrhea to fulminant pseudomembranous colitis, with bandemia and sepsis
		• Onset of diarrhea after starting antibiotic therapy
			• Enzyme immunoassay for toxins A and B
			• Pseudomembranes on endoscopy
			• CT may reveal colitis
			• Significant leukocytosis
			• + fecal leukocytes
			• Hypoalbuminemia (protein-losing enteropathy)
				• Discontinue drug, IV fluids, avoid antiperistaltics
				• Metronidazole × 10–14 days (IV or PO)
				• PO vancomycin × 10–14 days if pregnant or does not respond to metronidazole
				• Treat relapses (occur in 20–25%) with another course of antibiotics
				• Severe cases: IV metronidazole + PO vancomycin
				• Colectomy and ileostomy for toxic megacolon

Antibiotic-Associated Diarrhea	• Ampicillin • Amoxicillin • Clavulanate • Cefixime • Can occur with any antibiotic	• Symptoms range from mild diarrhea to colitis • Abdominal cramping • Fever • Leukocytosis • Stool leukocytes	• CT: colonic thickening	• Supportive treatment if mild • Discontinue or change drug if more severe • Rule out *Clostridium difficile*

NSAIDs = nonsteroidal anti-inflammatory drugs; PO = per os; PCN = penicillin.

Viral Infections

Table 7-19

Summary of Influenza

EPIDEMIOLOGY	POPULATION	PREVENTION APPROACH (SEE TABLE 7-20 FOR AGENTS)	TREATMENT	COMPLICATIONS
• The majority of influenza infections are caused by influenza A	• Patients in the community setting who are at high risk for complications: - Pregnant women - ≥55 years - Certain chronic medical conditions	• Vaccinate patient • If vaccinated during peak influenza activity, continue chemoprophylaxis for 2 weeks • If unvaccinated, give chemoprophylaxis during peak influenza activity in the community	• Choose agent based on strain prevalent in community • Anti-influenza agents reduce symptoms by 1–2 days • Anti-influenza agents need to be started within 48 hours of the onset of symptoms • Resistance develops quickly with current anti-influenza treatment • Consult the CDC for updated information on resistance patterns of current circulating strains	• Super infection, including pneumonia (particularly *S. aureus*) • Myositis • Myocarditis • Encephalitis • Guillain-Barré syndrome • Reye syndrome
	• Patients in a long-term care facility setting during an outbreak	• Chemoprophylaxis to all residents and all unvaccinated staff • Continue until 1 week after outbreak ends		
	• Immunocompromised patient living at home	• All family members should be vaccinated		

CDC = Centers for Disease Control.

Table 7-20
Summary of Influenza Treatment

ANTIVIRAL AGENT	TYPE OF INFLUENZA TREATED	ROLE IN PROPHYLAXIS (VACCINATION IS PRIMARY METHOD)	CLINICAL NOTES
Amantadine (M2 Inhibitor)	• Influenza A	• Influenza A	• Reduce dose with renal failure • Seizures and delirium with high levels and in elderly patients • Contraindicated in pregnancy
Rimantadine (M2 Inhibitor)	• Influenza A	• Influenza A	• Reduce if liver failure • Seizures and delirium with high levels (less neurotoxic than amantadine) • Contraindicated in pregnancy
Zanamivir (Neuraminidase Inhibitor)	• Influenza A and B		• Less resistance than amantidine or rimantadine • Inhaled powder—caution in patients with COPD or airways disease
Oseltamivir (Neuraminidase Inhibitor)	• Influenza A and B	• Influenza A and B	• Less resistance than amantidine or rimantadine • Most frequent side effect is nausea/vomiting

COPD = chronic obstructive pulmonary disease.

Table 7-21
Summary of Herpes Simplex Virus (HSV)/Varicella-Zoster Virus (VZV)

SYNDROME	TREATMENT	SUPPRESSION/PREVENTION	CLINICAL NOTES
HSV Infections			
Orolabial (Cold Sores)	• Immunocompetent: - None OR: - Topical penciclovir cream if recurrent - Oral valacyclovir also an option • Immunocompromised: - Oral or IV acyclovir up to 14 days - Topical acyclovir ointment if limited disease	• Acyclovir	• If immunocompetent, acyclovir diminishes viral shedding but not pain and duration

(*continued*)

Table 7-21

Summary of Herpes Simplex Virus (HSV)/Varicella-Zoster Virus (VZV) (continued)

SYNDROME	TREATMENT	SUPPRESSION/PREVENTION	CLINICAL NOTES
Genital	• Acyclovir, valacyclovir, or famciclovir • Longer treatment for first episode (7–10 days)	• Acyclovir • Valacyclovir • Famciclovir	• First episode often with systemic symptoms; can be severe • Treatment of first episode does not reduce recurrence • For recurrences, maximum benefit if therapy begun during prodrome
Encephalitis, Pneumonia, Hepatitis	• Acyclovir IV × 10–21 days for encephalitis (optimal duration unknown for others)	• N/A	• Mortality from encephalitis reduced with treatment • HSV pneumonia tends to occur in extremely immunocompromised hosts such as allogeneic bone marrow transplant recipients • Hepatitis can occur without overt skin lesions; prodrome with rapidly rising transaminases and thrombocytopenia; requires rapid treatment
Ocular Disease	• Trifluridine drops • Referral to ophthalmologist	• Acyclovir	
Herpetic Whitlow (HSV Infection on Fingers)	• Acyclovir	• N/A	• Local disease
VZV Infections			

Chickenpox (Primary Varicella)	• Immunocompetent:
	  - Acyclovir within 24 hours of onset
	• Immunocompromised:
	  - IV acyclovir × 7 days or longer
		• N/A	• Treatment of pregnant women controversial
			• HSV or VZV infections resistant to acyclovir may be treated with IV foscarnet

Shingles (Herpes Zoster), within 72 Hours of Onset	• Acyclovir, valacyclovir, or famciclovir × 7 days • Treatment optional if < 50 years old, and rash, pain mild • Steroids are controversial • Refer to ophthalmologist if ocular involvement	• N/A	• Unclear if postherpetic neuralgia is prevented by treatment

Table 7-21

Summary of Herpes Simplex Virus (HSV)/Varicella-Zoster Virus (VZV) (continued)

SYNDROME	TREATMENT	SUPPRESSION/PREVENTION	CLINICAL NOTES
Shingles (Herpes Zoster), Onset > 72 Hours	• If immunocompetent and no eye involvement: no treatment • Otherwise, consider treatment	• N/A	
Pneumonia, Encephalitis	• Acyclovir IV × 7days	• N/A	

N/A = not applicable; VZV = varicella-zoster virus.

Table 7-22

Summary and Treatment of Cytomegalovirus (CMV)

CMV OCCURS IN THREE MAIN CLINICAL SETTINGS	TREATMENT OPTIONS	SELECT SIDE EFFECTS	NOTES
1. Infectious mono-nucleosis, monospot negative (usually only supportive care is needed) 2. HIV+, with CD4 <50 3. Transplant patients	Ganciclovir	• CNS • Teratogenic • Neutropenia • Thrombocytopenia	• CMV retinitis: maintenance regimen needed to prevent relapse in AIDS patients • CMV esophagitis, colitis, pneumonia: usually responds to therapy • CMV pneumonia more difficult to treat in bone marrow transplant patients
	Valganciclovir	• Teratogenic • Granulocytopenia • Thrombocytopenia	• Converted to ganciclovir in intestine and liver • More bioavailable than oral ganciclovir
	Foscarnet	• Nephrotoxic • Metabolic distur-bances • CNS	• Usually works in CVM, HSV, or VZV resistant to acyclovir
	Cidofovir	• Very nephrotoxic	• Only approved for CMV retinitis, although frequently used for other indications • Aggressive hydration and coad-ministration of probenecid needed

CNS = central nervous system.

Table 7-23

Summary of Human Immunodeficiency Virus (HIV) Transmission and Testing

	DETAIL	NOTE
Transmission	• Unprotected sexual contact • Sharing contaminated needles • Maternal-fetal transmission • Transfusion/extensive contact with contaminated blood products	• Heterosexual transmission on the rise

Testing	• ELISA first
	• If positive ELISA, Western blot to confirm
	• Positive rapid HIV test results need to be confirmed with standard testing modalities
		• 20% of ELISA are indeterminate, due to:
		  - Early HIV
		  - Late stage with waning immunity
		  - Cross-reactive antibodies
		  - HIV-2 infection

Table 7-24

Summary of HIV Course

PHASE OF UNTREATED INFECTION	HIV VIRAL LOAD	CD4 COUNT	PRESENTATION
Acute Infection	• High	• Drops transiently	• Viral-like illness • Sore throat • Fever • Lymphadenopathy • Diarrhea
Recovery from Acute Infection	• Drops	• Rises back to baseline	• Convalescence from acute HIV
Latent Period (Usually Lasts Years)	• Level stabilizes (set point)—prognostic implications	• Declines over time (average 50–100 cells/year)	• Usually asymptomatic • Can have constitutional symptoms—low-grade fever, night sweats, moderate weight loss
AIDS	• Rises	• Declines (<200)	• Opportunistic infections • Wasting syndrome (rare) • Death

AIDS = acquired immunodeficiency syndrome; CD4 = cluster of differentiation 4.

Table 7-25

Evaluation of HIV+ Patient in Primary Care Setting

CATEGORY	TEST
Baseline HIV-related Tests	• CD4 • HIV viral load • HIV genotype test
Baseline Organ Function Studies	• CBC with differential, glucose, renal function • LFT, fasting lipids
Serologies	• Hepatitis A, B, and C • Annual PPD and TB exposure history • Syphilis (RPR) • Toxoplasma IgG • CMV (suggested, but rarely helpful) • Chlamydia and gonorrhea (for patients at risk)
Cancer Screening	• Cervical Pap smear at 0 and 6 months, annually thereafter if normal • Consider anal Pap • Routine age-appropriate screening
Vaccinations	• Polyvalent pneumococcal (more effective if CD4 >200) • Yearly influenza • Hepatitis B (check serologies after completion) • Hepatitis A for populations at risk
Other Screening Considerations	• Baseline eye examination (especially if CD4 <100)

RPR = rapid plasma reagin.

Table 7-26

Summary of HIV Complications

CLINICAL PICTURE	POSSIBLE PATHOGEN
Disseminated Infection	• *Coccidioides immitis* (southwestern United States) • CMV • *Histoplasma capsulatum* • *Mycobacterium avium* complex • *M. tuberculosis* • *Pneumocystis jiroveci* (formerly *carinii*)
Upper GI (Oral, Esophageal)	• Candida • HSV • CMV (ulcerative lesions) • EBV-related oral hairy leukoplakia
Lower GI (diarrhea)	• *Microsporidia* • *Isospora belli* • *Cryptosporidium* • *Cyclospora cayetanensis* • CMV (ulcerative lesions, colitis) • *M. avium* complex
Pulmonary	• *P. jiroveci* • *M. tuberculosis* • *Legionella* • Most common: community-acquired typical infections
CNS	• Cryptococcosis (meningitis) • JC virus (progressive multifocal leukoencephalopathy) • Toxoplasmosis (ring-enhancing) • HIV-associated encephalopathy • CMV (retinitis)
Vulvovaginal/Anorectal	• HPV (cervical cancer) • Candida • HSV • Lymphogranuloma venereum
Skin/Soft Tissue	• HHV-8 (Kaposi sarcoma) • VZV (shingles) • HSV
Liver	• HCV progresses more quickly, especially if CD4 counts low • Many HIV+ patients coinfected with HCV • May lose HCV seropositivity if late stage HIV • Many antiretrovirals are hepatotoxic

EBV = Epstein-Barr virus; HHV = human herpes virus.

Table 7-27

Summary of HIV Treatment

Class of Drug	Indication	Selected Major Side Effect	Note
Nucleoside Reverse Transcriptase Inhibitor (NRTI)	Indications to initiate HAART: • CD4 <200 • Symptomatic/AIDS defining illness • Pregnancy	• Entire class: lactic acidosis • Abacavir: hypersensitivity (fever, rash, nausea, vomiting, abdominal pain) usually occurring in the first 6 weeks of treatment • Didanosine: pancreatitis, peripheral neuropathy • Zidovudine: anemia, bone marrow suppression, nausea/vomiting • Stavudine: lipoatrophy, hyperlipidemia, lactic acidosis, pancreatitis, peripheral neuropathy	• Immune reconstitution inflammatory syndrome occurs as a result of successful HAART therapy - Clinical: paradoxical worsening of underlying opportunistic infections as immune system reconstitutes - Management: symptomatic. Continue HAART
Non Nucleoside Reverse Transcriptase Inhibitor (NNRTI)		• Entire class: rash, elevated LFTs • Efavirenz: vivid dreams, insomnia or somnolence, agitation, confusion • Nevirapine: fatal hypersensitivity, particularly in women with CD4 >250 or men with CD4 >400; hepatitis	
Protease Inhibitor (PI)		• Entire class: metabolic—lipodystrophy, hyperlipidemia, glucose intolerance, nausea, vomiting, diarrhea • Atazanavir: asymptomatic unconjugated hyperbilirubinemia, first-degree AV block • Indinavir: nephrolithiasis • Ritonavir is used in low doses to "boost" the levels of other PIs (interferes with their metabolism)	
Fusion Inhibitors		• Enfuvirtide: injection site reactions	

AV = atrioventricular; HAART = highly active antiretroviral therapy.

Table 7-28
Prophylaxis for Opportunistic Infections

OPPORTUNISTIC INFECTION	INITIATE PRIMARY PROPHYLAXIS IF:	DISCONTINUE TREATMENT IF:	COMMON PRIMARY PROPHYLAXIS AGENT	SECONDARY PROPHYLAXIS
Pneumocystis jiroveci (formerly known as Pneumocystic Carinii)	• CD4 <200/μL	• CD4 >200/μL for 3+ months	• Bactrim DS daily or SS daily • Alternate: dapsone daily	• Bactrim DS or SS daily
Toxoplasma gondii	• CD4 <100/μL and toxo IgG+	• CD4 >200/μL for 3+ months	• Bactrim DS daily • Alternate: atovaquone daily	• Sulfadiazine + pyrimethamine + leucovorin
Mycobacterium avium complex	• CD4 <50/μL	• CD4 >100/μL for 3+ months	• Azithromycin weekly or clarithromycin bid • Alternate: rifabutin daily	• Clarithromycin + ethambutol +/- rifabutin
Mycobacterium tuberculosis	• Positive PPD (≥5 mm) • Recent exposure to active TB and no evidence of active TB	• Usually treated for 9 months	• INH sensitive: INH + pyridoxine × 9 months • INH resistant: rifampin × 4 months	• None needed • Relapse is rare and recurrent infection usually due to reinfection

DS = double strength; SS = single strength.

Table 7-29

Summary of Candidal Infections

	CLINICAL NOTES	TREATMENT

Mucocutaneous Candidiasis	• Recurrent mucocutaneous infections associated with:
	  - Diabetes
	  - Antibiotic use
	  - Steroid use
	  - HIV
		• First line: creams, solutions, and troches of nystatin or azoles
		• If refractory: oral fluconazole
		• Oropharyngeal: 1–2 week course
		• Esophagitis: 2–3 week course

Candiduria	• Usually benign colonization
	• Treat if:
	  - Active urinary sediment
	  - Symptomatic
	  - Renal transplant patient
	  - Neutropenic
		• No need to treat colonization
		• Fluconazole

Candidemia	• If *Candida* in blood culture:
	  - Speciate to guide therapy
	  - Assess for systemic infection:
	    1. Echocardiogram (r/o endocarditis)
	    2. Ophtho examination (r/o endophthalmitis)
	    3. Consider chest and/or abdominal imaging to r/o pulmonary, hepatic, splenic involvement
	• May have rash: nontender, nonpruritic, pustular
		• Suspected localized infection:
		  - Remove all lines
		  - Treat with sensitive agent for 2 weeks from last positive culture
		• If signs of systemic infection:
		  - Treat with sensitive agent: high-dose fluconazole, amphotericin B, caspofungin
		  - Duration of therapy determined by site of infection and host's immune system

Table 7-30

Summary of Fungal Infections

Fungal Infection	High-Risk Groups	Clinical Presentation	Diagnosis	Treatment

Cryptococcosis	• AIDS: CD4 <100
	• COPD (pulmonary) cryptococcosus
	• Transplant patients
	• Chronic kidney disease
	• Cirrhosis
	• Corticosteroids
	• Heme malignancies
		• Increased ICP occurs more often in AIDS patients
		• Repeat lumbar puncture until ICP returns to normal
			• Fungal culture of CSF or BAL fluid
			• Biopsy if skin or bony disease suspected
			• Serum and/or CSF cryptococcal antigen detection
				• Non-CNS infection:
				  - Fluconazole or itraconazole × 6–12 months
				  - Amphotericin for severe cases until patient is stable
				• CNS infections:
				  - Amphotericin B + flucytosine × 2 weeks, then fluconazole × 10 weeks
				  - HIV+ patients: chronic suppression with lower-dose fluconazole until CD4 >100–200 for ≥6 months

Aspergillosis			

	• Risks for invasive disease:
	  - Neutropenia
	  - Transplant
	  - Corticosteroids
	  - Sarcoidosis
	  - Graft-versus-host disease
		• Contamination/colonization common as *Aspergillus* is ubiquitous in environment
		• Invasive disease:
		  - Hemoptysis (can be life threatening)
		  - May involve skin locally or as part of systemic infection
		  - Mortality rate up to 90% in allogeneic stem cell transplant patients
			• Chest CT:
			  - Multiple nodular lesions
			  - Halo sign occurs early (nodule with ground-glass surrounding from hemorrhage)
			  - Air-crescent sign occurs late (necrosis and cavitation)
			• Histopathologic evidence of invasion confirms diagnosis of invasive disease, but may be hard to obtain due to comorbidities
			• Positive sputum or BAL in immunocompromised host adequate to initiate treatment
			• Head imaging:
			  - Rule out CNS involvement
				• Invasive disease:
				  - First line: voriconazole or amphotericin
				  - Treat until resolved, 10–12 weeks minimum
				• Allergic bronchopulmonary disease:
				  - Corticosteroids +/– itraconazole
				• Pulmonary aspergilloma:
				  - May not require treatment
				  - If treatment required, consider surgery +/– antifungals

ICP = intracranial pressure; BAL = bronchoalveolar lavage.

Table 7-31

Summary of Endemic Mycoses

Mycosis	Geographic Region and Exposure History	Presentation	Diagnosis	Treatment
Histoplasmosis capsulatum	• Ohio, Mississippi River valleys • Exposure to bird or bat droppings • Exposure to disturbed soil	• Asymptomatic or solitary pulmonary nodule • Acute pulmonary disease: fever, headache, nonproductive cough, pleuritic chest pain; hypoxemia if severe • Chronic pulmonary disease: malaise, fever, productive cough, night sweats • Disseminated: occurs in immunocompromised	• Imaging: - Acute pulmonary disease: Normal or patches of airspace disease, adenopathy and diffuse nodules - Chronic pulmonary disease: Emphysematous, apical bullae, no adenopathy - Disseminated disease - Diffuse nodules • Diagnosis: - Culture, fungal stains, serology of affected tissue - Urine antigen can be helpful if disseminated	• Mild to moderate disease: - Itraconazole or fluconazole up to 24 months • Severe disease: - Amphotericin B until stable, then itraconazole
Blastomyces dermatitidis	• Similar to *Histoplasma* cases • Also occurs in Midwest and southeastern United States	• Asymptomatic in healthy host • Skin involvement: large papule • Pulmonary involvement: fever, cough, dyspnea, chest pain, weight loss • Disseminated disease: septicemia, meningitis; liver, spleen, kidneys	• Imaging: - Focal or diffuse infiltrates; nodules, cavities, pleural effusions • Diagnosis: - Culture, fungal stains of BAL or biopsy - Serologies usually negative	• Same as for histoplasmosis

Coccidioides immitis	• Southwestern United States, northern Mexico, Central America • Surges after dust storms	• Asymptomatic or mild respiratory disease if immunocompetent • "Valley fever": fever, sweats, anorexia, productive cough, chest pain	• Imaging: - Acute: infiltrates, pleural effusion, hilar adenopathy - Chronic: lung cavitations (thin-walled) • Diagnosis: - Serologies, culture, antigen testing - CSF: mononuclear pleocytosis, low glucose, elevated protein	• No treatment if mild disease, immunocompetent and symptoms resolve • Otherwise, same as for histoplasmosis • CNS disease: - Fluconazole or itraconazole +/– intrathecal amphotericin - Risk of hydrocephalus - If responds to azole, continue therapy for life

CSF = cerebrospinal fluid.

Table 7-32
Summary of Antifungal Medications

Antifungal	Selected Side Effects	Notes
Fluconazole	• Elevated LFTs common • Less common: drug interactions	• Treats most *Candida*, but *C. krusei* and *C. glabrata* are often resistant • Commonly used as prophylaxis for immunocompromised patients
Itraconazole	• Heart failure; hepatitis, hyperbilirubinemia, drug interactions	• Poor blood-brain barrier penetration
Voriconazole	• Hepatotoxicity, rash, photosensitivity • Transient changes in vision (wavy lines, bright spots, altered color perception) • QT prolongation • P-450 inducers decrease voriconazole levels • Voriconazole will increase levels of P-450 metabolized drugs (tacrolimus)	• Must have CrCl >50 mL/min for IV formulation • Active against *Candida*, *Cryptococcus*, and *Aspergillus* • Not active against Zygomycetes (Mucormycosis)
Posaconazole	• Liver function abnormalities • Drug-drug interactions	• Only available in oral liquid; must be taken with food (required for absorption)
Amphotericin B	• Nephrotoxicity • Hypokalemia • Hypersensitivity	• Lipid formulations less nephrotoxic and often used in high-risk patients (renal failure, transplant patients, etc.)
Caspofungin	• Few (rash and flushing) • Drug interaction with cyclosporine A	• First-generation echinocandin (blocks formation of beta-glucans in cell wall of fungi) • Active against *Candida* • Poor CNS, urinary tract, and eye penetration • Not active against *Cryptococcus* or Zygomycetes (Mucormycosis)
Terbinafine	• LFT abnormalities and rare liver failure	

CrCl = creatinine clearance.

Table 7-33

Summary of Travel Medicine/Immunizations

Disease (Mode of Transmission)	Mode of Transmission	Clinical Syndrome	Endemic Areas	Vaccine Note
Yellow Fever	• Mosquitoes	• Ranges from flu-like syndrome to hemorrhagic fever and hepatitis	• Rural areas of Africa, South America, Panama	• Live attenuated vaccine - Contraindicated if pregnant, immunosuppressed
Japanese Encephalitis	• Mosquitoes	• Viral encephalitis	• Rural areas in Asia	• Vaccine indicated if staying in highly endemic area >30 days - Avoid if pregnant
Hepatitis A	• Fecal-oral	• Diarrhea to fulminant hepatitis	• Most developing countries	• Booster dose in 6–12 months prolongs immunity

***Salmonella typhi* (Typhoid Fever)**	• Contaminated food/water
	• Contact with carrier
		• Ranges from mild diarrhea to severe febrile syndrome
		• Much less common than hepatitis A
			• Most developing countries	• Live attenuated oral
				  - 5 years protection
				  - Avoid if pregnant or immunocompromised
				• Inactivated injection
				  - 2 years protection

Neisseria meningitidis	• Droplet	• Meningitis, disseminated disease	• Sub-Saharan Africa	• Vaccines do not protect against serotype B
Rabies	• Mammal bites		• Developing countries • Increased risk depends on occupational or recreational activities	• Consider preexposure rabies vaccination if extended travel in endemic areas or high-risk occupation/recreation planned • Rabies vaccine and rabies immunoglobulin should be given after in case of exposure

Table 7-34

Summary of Malaria Prophylaxis

APPROACH	DETAILS
Prevention	• DEET-based insect repellent for skin • Permethrin-based formula for clothing • Long sleeved clothing • Mosquito netting • Dusk to dawn highest risk
Chemoprophylaxis	• Generally begin before departure and continue use after return • Specific agent depends on resistance patterns in country of travel (http://www.cdc.gov for current recommendations) • Malaria is resistant to chloroquine in many parts of the world • Other options include mefloquine, doxycycline, or atovaquone/proguanil

DEET = meta-*N,N*-diethyl toluamide.

Table 7-35

Summary of Bioterrorism Pathogens

DISEASE	CLINICAL PRESENTATION	DIAGNOSIS	TREATMENT	VACCINE/POSTEXPOSURE PROPHYLAXIS	PRECAUTIONS
Smallpox (of *Poxviridae* Family)	• Fever • Headache • Uniform, evenly distributed rash: begins as macules, progresses to papules, then crusts and sloughs • Rash: involves palms and soles • Complications include encephalitis	• Electron microscopy of vesicle fluid • Viral culture	• Supportive	• Live vaccine • Avoid vaccination unless exposed if: - Immunocompromised AIDS, transplant - Pregnant - Eczema	• Respiratory • Contact (person-to-person spread)
Anthrax (*Bacillus anthracis*)	• Cutaneous: - Papule > vesicle > ulcerated black eschar • Pulmonary: - Rapid onset - Shortness of breath - Stridor - Tachycardia - Can progress to shock and death in 24–48 hours - Hemorrhagic meningitis	Cutaneous: • Gram stain, wound/blood culture Inhaled: • Rapid ELISA CXR: • Widened mediastinum and/or bloody pleural effusions	• Ciprofloxacin, doxycycline, or IV PCN • Add clindamycin if significant symptoms • Rifampin if CNS involvement	• Acellular vaccine • Ciprofloxacin or doxycycline × 60 days if exposed	• No special precautions—no person-to-person transmission has occurred
Plague (*Yersinia pestis*)	• "Buboes"—necrotizing lymphadenitis • Septicemia • Pulmonary involvement with cavitations or hemorrhagic pleural effusions • Shock and death within 2–4 days	• Clinical • Gram stain shows "safety pin" morphology • Sputum, blood, CSF Wright's stain—safety pin appearance	• Streptomycin • Gentamicin • Ciprofloxacin • Doxycycline	• No vaccine available • Doxycycline, ciprofloxacin, or tetracycline × 7 days if exposed	• Droplet precautions × 48 hours (person-to-person spread)

(continued)

Table 7-35

Summary of Bioterrorism Pathogens (continued)

Disease	Clinical Presentation	Diagnosis	Treatment	Vaccine/Postexposure Prophylaxis	Precautions
Tularemia (*Francisella tularensis*)	• Febrile illness • Many organs can be affected • In the United States, tick-associated (dog tick) and ulceroglandular most common • Untreated: 30–60% mortality	• Sputum or blood culture • DFA • Immunohistochemistry	• Streptomycin • Gentamicin • Ciprofloxacin • Treat × 10–14 days	• Live attenuated vaccine If exposed: • Doxycycline • Tetracycline • Ciprofloxacin • Treat × 14 days	• No special precaution • Notify lab, as infection can occur from culture plate
Viral Hemorrhagic Fever (Marburg, Ebola, Lassa, Junin)	• Febrile illness • Mucosal purpura • GI/GU hemorrhages • DIC, shock, death	• ELISA/IgM antibody • PCR • Viral isolation	• Supportive • Certain viruses may be susceptible to ribavirin in first 7 days	• No vaccine available • Ribavirin if Junin/Lassa	• Person-to-person spread • Strict barrier/contact precautions • Respiratory isolation/negative pressure room
Botulism (*Clostridium botulinum*)	• GI symptoms • Cranial nerve and bulbar abnormalities • Descending flaccid paralysis • Respiratory compromise • Dysphagia and dysarthria	• Clinical • Serologies • Toxin test • CSF unremarkable	• Antitoxins available from CDC • Ventilatory support	• Toxoid vaccine for certain types • No prophylaxis	• No special precautions

DFA = direct fluorescent assay.

Table 7-36
Summary of Nosocomial Infections

NOSOCOMIAL INFECTION	PATIENTS AT RISK	SELECTED COMPLICATIONS	SPECIFIC INTERVENTION TO DECREASE INFECTION RISK	GENERAL PREVENTION STRATEGIES
UTI	• Catheterized • Elderly • Debilitated • Postpartum	• Cystitis • Prostatitis • Pyelonephritis • Bacteremia	• Minimize catheter use and remove as soon as possible • Use closed sterile drainage systems for catheters • Place urinary collection bag below the bladder	• Meticulous hand disinfection • Infection control programs • Contact, respiratory, or droplet precautions as needed for individual organisms • Proper sterile technique for all procedures
Bacteremia	• Patients with central venous catheter at highest risk (femoral or internal jugular > subclavian) • Prolonged hospitalization • TPN	• Mortality rate approximately 40%	• Remove lines as soon as possible • Use chlorhexidine for skin disinfection • Use proper precautions for insertion	
Ventilator-Associated Pneumonia	• Nasal intubation • Presence of NG tube • Supine positioning • Reintubation • Malnutrition • Large gastric volumes	• Independent predictor of mortality in ICU patients	• Minimize intubation, reintubations and time on ventilator • Keep head of bed > 30 degrees • Strict attention to oral care	

TPN = total parenteral nutrition; NG = nasogastric; ICU = intensive care unit.

Table 7-37

Occupational Exposure to Infectious Disease for Health Care Workers

Disease	Postexposure Prophylaxis	Prophylaxis Notes	Notes

Hepatitis B	• Hepatitis B immune globulin + first dose vaccine or booster, depending on vaccine status	• Indicated unless patient vaccinated, and serology indicates response to vaccine
		• If the source patient has unknown HBsAg, initiate vaccination series in the unvaccinated
		• For known nonresponders, treat as if the source were HBsAg positive
			• Blood-borne pathogens
			  - Rule of 3s for risk of transmission: 30% for hepatitis B, 3% for hepatitis C, 0.3% for HIV
			• Risk factors for transmission:
			  - Deep, penetrating injury
			  - High viral load
			  - Hollow-needle puncture

HCV	• None	• Document hepatitis C seroconversion	

HIV	• Two-drug or three-drug regimen
	• HIV Ab should be tested for at baseline, 6 weeks, 12 weeks, 6 months, and consider at 1 year
		• Low risk:
		  - Mucosal exposure, solid needle puncture, superficial injury, source asymptomatic, low viral load
		  - Prophylaxis with two-drug treatment
		• High risk:
		  - More severe injury
		  - Source with symptomatic HIV or AIDS
		  - Seroconversion with high viral load
		  - Prophylaxis with three-drug treatment
		  - Best if started within 72 hours	

Hepatitis A	• Immune globulin	• Indicated for exposure during outbreak	
Pertussis	• Erythromycin (first line) or trimethoprim/sulfamethoxazole	• Indicated for exposure to respiratory secretions (such as intubating or suctioning without a mask)	
VZV	• Immune globulin +/- acyclovir	• Indicated if negative serology for varicella in health care worker	• For transmission, need close and prolonged exposure/skin-to-skin contact with lesions • Pregnant health care workers without a history of VZV should avoid exposure to VZV
Tetanus	• Tetanus toxoid	Indicated if: • Wound is clean and last vaccine >10 years ago • Wound is dirty and last vaccine >5 years ago	• Tdap should be given in place of Td if health care worker has never received Tdap

Ab = antibody; HBsAg = surface antigen of the hepatitis B virus; Tdap = tetanus, diphtheria, and pertussis.

Chapter

8

Endocrinology

Table 8-1

Hyper- and Hypothyroid States

	DEFINITION	ETIOLOGY	EXAMPLES	CLINICAL PRESENTATION	NOTES
Hyperthyroid	• Excess concentrations of free thyroid hormones (usually T4)	• Autoimmune	• Graves disease	• Weight loss with increased appetite	• Most frequent causes:
		• Secondary to viral infection	• de Quervain Thyroiditis	• Tachycardia/palpitations	- Graves disease
				• Heat intolerance	- Beta-blockers can help symptoms
		• Other	• Early phase Hashimoto thyroiditis	• Goiter	- Older patients may have apathetic thyrotoxicosis (asymptomatic or with decreased energy)
			• Toxic adenoma	• Hyperreflexia	
			• Multinodular goiter	• Menstrual irregularities	
			• Thyroid storm	• Pretibial myxedema	
				• Thyroid storm	
Hypothyroid	• Deficient synthesis or activity of thyroid hormone	• Hashimoto thyroiditis	• (see Table 8-4)	• Weight gain with poor appetite	• Most frequent causes:
		• Iatrogenic	• Radioactive iodine	• Bradycardia	- Hashimoto thyroiditis
			• Subtotal/total thyroidectomy	• Cold intolerance	- Radioiodine-induced (treatment of Graves disease)
			• Irradiation of neck for malignancy	• Constipation	- TSH best screen for hypothyroidism
				• Fatigue/lethargy	
		• Drugs*	• Iodine contrast	• Delayed tendon relaxation	
			• Amiodarone	• Dry skin	
			• Lithium	• Hair loss	
			• Antithyroid drugs	• Menstrual irregularities	
		• Iodine deficiency		• Diastolic hypertension	
		• Infiltrative disorders	• Amyloidosis	• Peripheral edema	
			• Sarcoidosis	• Myxedema coma if severe	
			• Hemachromatosis		
		• Secondary/central	• Hypopituitarism		
			• Hypothalamic disease		

*Many medications alter thyroid hormone levels through a variety of mechanisms.

TSH = thyroid-stimulating hormone.

Table 8-2

Hyperthyroid Diseases: Graves Disease, de Quervain Thyroiditis, and Thyroid Storm

	DEFINITION	**CLINICAL PRESENTATION**	**DIAGNOSIS**	**TREATMENT**
Graves Disease	• Autoimmune disorder • Secondary to continuous stimulation of thyroid gland by anti-TSH thyroid receptor antibodies	• Signs/symptoms of hyperthyroidism • Proptosis/exopthalmos/ophthalmopathy • Lid lag and lid retraction are frequently the first symptoms of disease • Thrill and bruit over the gland due to increased vascularity and hyperdynamic circulation	• Diffuse symmetric thyroid enlargement (70% of cases) • Serum thyroid receptor antibodies (antiperoxidase and anti-TSH receptor) present • Elevated serum T3 and T4, and decreased TSH levels • Increased I_{123} thyroid uptake on radionuclide scan	• PTU • Methimazole • Beta-blockers for symptomatic relief of tachycardia, palpitations, and anxiety attacks • Radioactive ablation with I_{131} and thyroidectomy reserved for refractory cases
De Quervain Thyroiditis (Transient Subacute/Viral Thyroiditis)	• Inflammatory destruction of the gland • Secondary to viral infection (commonly mumps, coxsackie, and influenza viruses)	• Transient hyperthyroidism (early phase) followed by transient hypothyroidism and then recovery • Self-limited • Painful enlargement of thyroid gland • Low-grade fever • Earache • Neck swelling	• High ESR and a low radioiodine uptake • Decreased uptake on I_{123} radionuclide scan • No antithyroid receptor antibodies	• Supportive care • NSAIDs or aspirin • Steroids if refractory

(continued)

Table 8-2

Hyperthyroid Diseases: Graves Disease, de Quervain Thyroiditis, and Thyroid Storm (continued)

	DEFINITION	CLINICAL PRESENTATION	DIAGNOSIS	TREATMENT

Thyroid Storm	• Severe manifestation of thyrotoxicosis (elevated thyroid hormone levels)	• Hyperthermia
		• Tachycardia
		• Arrhythmias
		• Nausea, vomiting, and diarrhea
		• Resembles sepsis, malignant hyperthermia, and pheochromocytoma
		• Risk factors:
		  - Thyroid surgery
		  - Infection
		  - Trauma
			• Significantly elevated free T4 and T3 levels with undetectable TSH levels	• Supportive care:
				• Decrease hormone synthesis: PTU and methimazole
				• Inhibit thyroid release: sodium iodide, Lugol's solution
				• Decrease heart rate: esmolol, metoprolol
				• Support circulation: steroids and intravenous fluids
				• May be life-threatening

ESR = erythrocyte sedimentation rate; NSAIDS = nonsteroidal anti-inflammatory drugs; PTU = propylthiouracil.

Table 8-3

Medications for Hyperthyroidism

Drug Name	Mechanism of Action	Side Effects	Notes
Propylthiouracil (PTU)	• Reduces synthesis of thyroid hormones: - Blocks the synthesis of T4 to T3 - Blocks coupling of iodotyrosines and organic binding of iodide - Does not cross placenta and preferred during pregnancy	• Common: - Rash - Arthralgias • Serious: - Agranulocytosis - Hepatic damage	• Significantly more T4 is secreted from the thyroid than T3 • Most circulating T3 is converted from T4 outside of the thyroid • 99% of circulating thyroid hormone is protein bound
Methimazole (MMI)	• Reduces synthesis of thyroid hormones: - Blocks coupling of iodotyrosines and organic binding of iodine		

Table 8-4

Hypothyroid Diseases: Hashimoto Thyroiditis and Myxedema Coma

	Definition	Clinical/Diagnosis	Treatment
Hashimoto Thyroiditis	• Autoimmune disorder • Lymphocytic infiltration of the thyroid gland • Antithyroid, (antiperoxidase and antithyroglobulin) antibodies	• Serum antimicrosomal and antiperoxidase antibodies • A thyroid biopsy is often unnecessary • In early stages of disease, thyroid hormone levels may be normal • In later stages, thyroid hormone levels are usually decreased and TSH elevated • Signs and symptoms of hypothyroidism	• Levothyroxine • If patient is elderly or has CAD, start levothyroxine at a lower dose and titrate slowly to prevent thyrotoxicosis and cardiac symptoms such as angina and atrial fibrillation
Myxedema Coma	• Severe manifestation of hypothyroidism	• Reduced level of consciousness • Seizures • Hypothermia • Signs and symptoms of hypothyroidism	• Levothyroxine • Intravenous steroids • Supportive care • High mortality rate

Note: Many medications alter thyroid hormone levels. Levothyroxine absorption inhibited by concomitant ingestion of oral iron preparations. CAD = coronary artery disease.

Figure 8.1

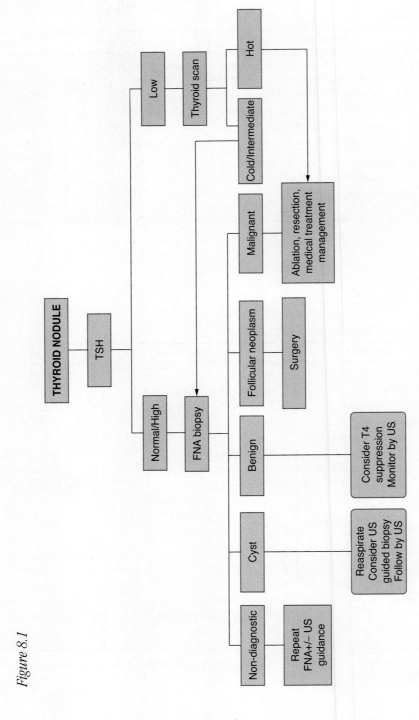

Algorithm for investigation of a thyroid nodule
US = ultrasound

Table 8-5

Thyroid Cancer

TYPE OF THYROID CANCER	ETIOLOGY/NOTE
Papillary carcinoma	• Arises from follicular cells • Most common thyroid cancer • Spreads via the lymphatics
Follicular carcinoma	• Arises from follicular cells • Spreads hematogenously • Cannot be distinguished from follicular adenoma on cytology (resection required)
Anaplastic carcinoma	• Arises from follicular cells • Highly malignant
Medullary carcinoma	• Often associated with MEN IIA and B • Arises from the C cells that produce calcitonin
Lymphoma	• Arises from lymphocytes in thyroid • Hashimoto thyroiditis is a risk factor
Clinical/Risk Factors	• History of head and neck irradiation • Age <20 or >70 • Thyroid nodule size >4 cm • Males • Family history • Iodine deficiency
Diagnosis	• On radionuclide scanning, a "hot" nodule (increased uptake) is usually benign, whereas a "cold" nodule (decreased uptake) is more worrisome for a malignant process • Cytology or pathology to distinguish type of cell
Treatment	Primary treatment options: • Surgery • Radioactive iodine therapy • Thyroxine therapy (suppresses TSH, which promotes growth of the gland and tumor)

MEN = multiple endocrine neoplasias.

Table 8-6

Calcium Regulation by Parathyroid Hormone and Vitamin D

TARGET ORGAN	ACTION	NOTES
Bone	• PTH and Vitamin D work together to stimulate osteoclasts to reabsorb calcium and phosphate from the bone	• PTH stimulates the production of 1,25-dihydroxyvitamin D (active form of vitamin D)
Kidney	• PTH increases calcium absorption and phosphate excretion	
Intestine	• Vitamin D increases the absorption of calcium and phosphate	

PTH = parathyroid hormone.

Table 8-7

Hypoparathyroidism

Definition	• Low PTH levels, usually due to destruction of parathyroid glands (acquired)		

Etiology	• Common causes:
	  - Surgery
	  - Infiltration and destruction of parathyroid glands (Wilson disease, hemochromatosis, and radiation)
	  - PTH production may be suppressed in hypomagnesemia (magnesium important for PTH homeostasis)		

Clinical Presentation	**Laboratory**	• Decreased serum PTH • Hypocalcemia • Hyperphosphatemia	• Normal 25-hydroxyvitamin D level • Decreased 1,25-dihydroxyvitamin D levels
	Symptoms (most due to hypocalcemia)	• Seizures • Constipation • Muscle cramps • Hyperreflexia • Tetany • Abdominal pain	• Lethargy • Cardiac dysrhythmia • Chvostek's sign (facial twitching when the zygomatic arch is tapped) • Trousseau's sign (forearm spasms induced by inflating BP cuff on upper arm)
Diagnosis	• Increased urine: calcium to creatinine ratio and hypophosphaturia • ECG: prolonged Q-T interval (hypocalcemia)		
Treatment	• Supplementation with calcium and 1,25-dihydroxyvitamin D • Caution with intravenous calcium administration		

BP = blood pressure; ECG = electrocardiogram.

Table 8-8

Hyperparathyroidism

Definition	• High levels of PTH levels, usually due to excessive release		
TYPE OF HPT	**ETIOLOGY/NOTE**		
Primary Hyperparathyroidism	• Parathyroid adenoma is the most common cause (85% of all hyperparathyroid cases) • Hyperplasia of the parathyroid glands • Parathyroid carcinoma (rare)		

Secondary Hyperparathyroidism	• Feedback response to hypocalcemia stimulates the parathyroid glands leading to hyperplasia and excessive PTH production
	• Causes of hypocalcemia:
	  - Renal failure is the most common cause
	  - Vitamin D deficiency
	  - Malabsorption of intestinal calcium		

Tertiary Hyperparathyroidism	• Constant stimulation of the parathyroids in secondary hyperparathyroidism causes autonomous secretion of PTH by the gland • End result is hypercalcemia because feedback response is functional • Correction of hypercalcemia associated with tertiary HPT often requires surgical resection of most of the four parathyroid glands		
Clinical Presentation	**Laboratory**	• Elevated serum PTH levels • Elevated 1,25-dihydroxyvitamin D levels	• Hypercalcemia • Hypophosphatemia
	Symptoms (most due to hypercalcemia) *"Stones, groans, and psychic moans"*	• Kidney stones • Abdominal pain • Bone pain • Depression • Nausea	• Vomiting • Weakness • Lethargy • Hypertension
Diagnosis	• Urine: decreased calcium to creatinine ratio and hyperphosphaturia • ECG: short Q-T interval (hypercalcemia)		
Treatment	• Calcium binding agents • Treat underlying etiology		

Table 8-9

Pituitary Gland Physiology

AREA OF PITUITARY GLAND	HORMONES PRODUCED	
Adenohypophysis (Anterior Pituitary Gland)	• GH—(deficiency in adults causes decreased lean body mass and bone mineral density) • Prolactin • ACTH	• Thyrotropin (TSH) • LH • FSH
Neurohypophysis (Posterior Pituitary Gland)	• Antidiuretic hormone (vasopressin) • Oxytocin	

ACTH = adrenocorticotropic hormone; FSH = follicular-stimulating hormone; GH = growth hormone; LH = luteinizing hormone.

Table 8-10

Hypopituitarism

Definition	• Deficiency of one or more of the hormones produced by the pituitary
Etiology	• Mass effect (most commonly secondary to a pituitary tumor—nonfunctioning tumors usually large and cause visual field loss) • Postpartum necrosis of pituitary (Sheehan syndrome) • Vascular infarction (diabetes or coronary artery bypass surgery) • Hemorrhagic (pituitary apoplexy) See table 18–12 • Traumatic (damaged or severed pituitary stalk) • Common after radiation therapy to pituitary area
Clinical Presentation	• Prevalence of gonadotropin deficiency at the time of diagnosis of a pituitary tumor: GH > LH/FSH > TSH > ACTH • Presentation depends on deficiency
Diagnosis	• Clinical • Serum measurements of pituitary hormones
Treatment	• See Table 8-11

Table 8-11

Pituitary Insufficiency Hormone Replacement Regimens

DEFICIENCY/DISEASE	REPLACEMENT* (COMMON DOSING OPTION)
Adrenal Insufficiency	• Hydrocortisone (20 mg in morning and 10 mg in evening)
Hypothyroidism	• Levothyroxine (1.6 µg/kg/day)
Hypogonadism (Men)	• Daily androgen replacement (patch or gel)
Hypogonadism (Women)	• Daily hormone replacement (oral contraceptive pills or hormone replacement therapy)
Diabetes Insipidus	• DDAVP (vasopressin analogue) tablets or nasal spray

*Replacement of target hormone usually more successful than pituitary trophic hormones.

Table 8-12

Pituitary Apoplexy

Definition/Etiology	• Acute infarction of a pituitary adenoma
Clinical	• Hemorrhage may cause compression of surrounding structures such as cranial nerves in the cavernous sinuses (ptosis and ocular paralysis) • Sudden severe headache with collapse • Anterior pituitary insufficiency frequent while posterior pituitary function usually preserved
Treatment	• Most recover spontaneously
Note	• Subacute forms of pituitary apoplexy are seen in patients with sickle cell disease and DM

DM = diabetes mellitus.

Table 8-13

Acromegaly

Definition/Etiology	• Overproduction of GH by a pituitary tumor • GH affects peripheral tissues by stimulating the production of IGF-1/somatomedin C in the liver and other organs	
Clinical Presentation	• Coarse features/bony enlargement of face • Enlarged hands and feet (soft tissue enlargement) • Degenerative joint disease • DM	• Hypertension • Excess sweating and skin tags • Colonic polyps
Diagnosis	• IGF-1 levels elevated • MRI to detect pituitary tumor	

Treatment	• Treatment of choice: transsphenoidal surgery
	• Medical management:
	  - Octreotide (somatostatin analogue that suppresses GH)
	  - Pegvisomant (blocks GH action at peripheral receptors, improving IGF-1 levels)
	  - Colon cancer monitoring	

IGF = insulin-like growth factor; MRI = magnetic resonance imaging.

Figure 8.2

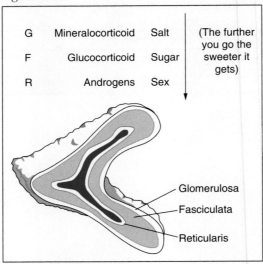

Adrenal gland. (Reproduced, with permission, from Meyer GK, DeLaMora PA. *Last Minute Pediatrics,* 1st ed. Figure 14-1. Page 274. New York: McGraw-Hill, 2004.)

Figure 8.3

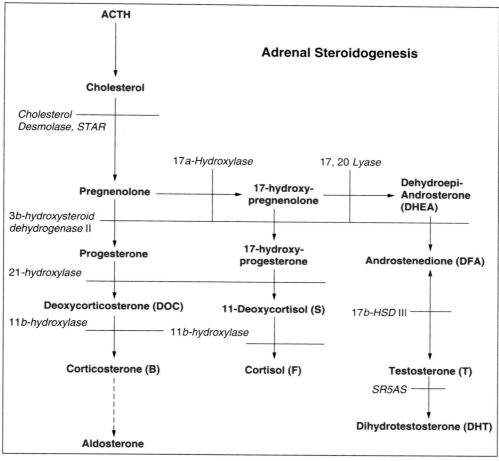

Adrenal steroidogenesis. (Reproduced, with permission, from Meyer GK, DeLaMora, PA. *Last Minute Pediatrics,* 1st ed. Figure 14-2. Page 275. New York: McGraw-Hill, 2004.)

Table 8-14

Adrenal Insufficiency

TYPE OF ADRENAL INSUFFICIENCY	ETIOLOGY/NOTES
Primary Adrenal Insufficiency (Addison Disease)	• Caused by destruction or dysfunction of the adrenal cortex • See Table 8-15
Secondary Adrenal Insufficiency	• Reduced secretion of ACTH • No hyperpigmentation or hyperkalemia
Tertiary Adrenal Insufficiency	• Usually caused by long-term use of suppressive doses of glucocorticoids, which suppresses release of CRH from the hypothalamus

CRH = corticotropin-releasing hormone.

Table 8-15
Addison Disease and Adrenal Crisis

	ETIOLOGY	CLINICAL PRESENTATION	DIAGNOSIS	TREATMENT

Addison Disease	• Primary adrenal insufficiency due to destruction of adrenal cortex
	• Glucocorticoid and mineralocorticoid function affected
	• Causes:
	  - Autoimmune destruction (most common)
	  - Infection (HIV, fungal, and tuberculosis)
	  - Hemorrhage
		• Symptoms:
		  - Weakness/fatigue
		  - Poor appetite with weight loss
		  - Salt craving
		• Examination:
		  - Hyperpigmentation (exposed skin, palmar creases, pressure areas, knuckles) due to high circulating levels of ACTH
		  - Vitiligo
		  - Muscle wasting
			• Cosyntropin test: low plasma cortisol level (<5 µg/dL) with severe stress
			• Increased ACTH level
			• Hyperkalemia
			• Hyponatremia
			• Hypoglycemia
			• Low cortisol
			• Low aldosterone
			• Elevated renin
			• Eosinophilia
				• Glucocorticoid and mineralocorticoid replacement

Adrenal Crisis	• Severe manifestation of adrenal insufficiency	• Nausea/vomiting • Diaphoresis • Orthostatic hypotension		• Stress dose of glucocorticoids during periods of stress, infection, and adrenal crisis

Table 8-16
Primary Hyperaldosteronism

Definition/ Etiology	• Excessive production of aldosterone independent of renin-angiotensin stimulation • 70% of cases are due to bilateral hyperplasia of the adrenal glands

Clinical Presentation	• Hypertension (may be severe and resistant to conventional antihypertensive treatments)
	• Most symptoms due to hypokalemia:
	  - Weakness
	  - Muscle cramps
	  - Paresthesias
	  - Headache
	  - Palpitations
	  - Polyuria and polydipsia

Diagnosis	• Ratio of morning plasma aldosterone concentration (elevated) to plasma renin activity (decreased)
Treatment	• Aldosterone antagonists (spironolactone) • Surgery if solitary adenoma

Table 8-17
Cushing Syndrome

Definition	• Elevated levels of glucocorticoids		
Etiology	**Exogenous Causes**		• Common cause: use of exogenous steroids • Most frequent cause (overall)
	Endogenous Causes		
	• ACTH dependent		• Common cause: ACTH-producing pituitary tumors • Excess ACTH stimulates increased production of cortisol
	• ACTH independent		• Common causes: adrenal adenomas and adrenal carcinomas • Inappropriately increased cortisol production by adrenal gland
Clinical Presentation	• Buffalo hump • Hirsutism • Truncal obesity • Purple striae • Easy bruising • Weight gain	• Hypertension (esp. diastolic) • Irregular menses • Impaired glucose metabolism • Osteoporosis • Proximal muscle weakness • Depression	
Diagnosis	• Screening: 24-hour urinary free cortical excretion (>250 µg/24 hours is diagnostic) • Evaluation of etiology: hormone levels and imaging		
Treatment	• Depends on the etiology		

Table 8-18
Incidental Adrenal Mass

Definition	• Adrenal mass (usually >5 mm) found incidentally, usually on radiologic study
Incidence	• Found in 1–10% of CT and MRI studies

Workup	• **Evaluation for hormonal function:**
	  - Obtain a clinical history to evaluate for Cushing disease and pheochromocytoma
	  - Measure 24-hour urine for metanephrines and catecholamines
	  - Dexamethasone suppression test
	  - Plasma aldosterone and renin levels
	  - Serum dehydroepiandrosterone sulfate (elevated with adrenocortical carcinoma)
	• **Findings on imaging that suggest malignancy include:**
	  - Irregular shape
	  - Nonhomogeneous density
	  - High unenhanced CT attenuation values (>10 Hounsfield Units)
	  - Diameter >4 cm
	  - Tumor calcification

Treatment	• Surgery: for functional masses or those >4 cm • Patients with nonfunctional masses <4 cm should be followed by repeat imaging

Table 8-19

Pheochromocytoma

Definition/Etiology	• Catecholamine-secreting tumor that arises from the chromaffin cells (neural crests derivatives) of the adrenal medulla (usually unilateral)
Epidemiology	• Men > women • Approximately 10% of cases are extra-adrenal, 10% bilateral, 10% familial, and 10% are malignant • Commonly associated with: neurofibromatosis, von Hippel-Lindau, tuberous sclerosis, Sturge-Weber, and MEN IIA, MEN IIB, especially if bilateral tumors
Clinical Presentation	• Signs and symptoms often episodic • Abdominal pain • Hypertension (uniformly present) • Palpitations • Postural hypotension • Headaches • Diaphoresis • Nausea • Pallor • Vomiting
Diagnosis	• Measurement of plasma-free metanephrines (high sensitivity and specificity) • If free metanephrines high, consider imaging studies to localize the tumor • MIBG scintigraphy is performed in the evaluation of pheochromocytoma if MRI and CT scan reveals no tumor but the diagnosis is still suspected. MIBG resembles norepinephrine and is taken up by adrenergic tissue.
Treatment	• Surgical removal of the tumor • Perioperative alpha-blockade to control hypertension • Intra-/postoperative beta-blockade to control tachycardia

MIBG = 123-I-metaiodobenzylguanidine.

Table 8-20

Hypoglycemia and Hyperinsulinemic Hypoglycemia

CONDITION	DEFINITION	ETIOLOGY	CLINICAL PRESENTATION	DIAGNOSIS
Hypoglycemia	• Whipple's triad: 　- Low plasma glucose 　　(usually <50 mg/dL) 　- Symptoms of hypoglycemia 　- Correction of 　　hypoglycemic symptoms 　　with glucose administration	• Exogenous: 　- Use of insulin and oral 　　hypoglycemic agents • Endogenous: 　- Pancreatic islet cell 　　tumor 　- Severe liver disease	Two clinical spectrums: 1. Adrenergic: 　• Diaphoresis 　• Palpitations 　• Apprehension 　• Anxiety 　• Headache 　• Weakness 2. Neuroglycopenic: 　• Confusion 　• Irritability 　• Abnormal behavior 　• Convulsions 　• Coma	• Plasma glucose • Insulin level • C-peptide level • Proinsulin levels • Oral hypoglycemic 　levels
Hyperinsulinemic Hypoglycemia	• Hypoglycemia associated 　with elevated insulin levels 　(usually in a ratio of insulin 　to glucose >0.33)	• Insulinomas (hyperplasia 　of pancreatic beta cells) • Factitious use of insulin 　or hypoglycemic agents	• Same as hypoglycemia	• See Table 8-21

254   Chapter 8   ◆   Endocrinology

Table 8-21
Frequent Causes of Hyperinsulinemic Hypoglycemia

CAUSE	INSULIN LEVEL	C-PEPTIDE LEVEL	PROINSULIN LEVEL	DRUG SCREEN
Insulinoma	↑	↑	↑	Normal
Factitious Insulin Administration	↑	↓	↓	Normal
Factitious Use of Oral Hypoglycemics	↑	↑	Normal	Positive for sulfonyl-ureas or meglitinide

Table 8-22
Diabetes Mellitus (DM)

CONDITION	INITIAL PRESENTATION	DIAGNOSIS	NOTES
DM	• Variable	• ADA* guidelines 2005: The presence of any one of the following: - Symptoms of DM plus a random glucose concentration ≥200 mg/dL - Fasting plasma glucose ≥126 mg/dL on 2 separate occasions - Two-hour postprandial glucose ≥200 mg/dL during oral glucose tolerance test (75 mg load)	• Age is not a criteria in determining the type of DM • Hb A1c not currently recommended for diagnosis
Type 1 DM	• DKA presenting complaint in over 25% of newly diagnosed type I DM patients	• Serum insulin level low • Presence of islet cell autoantibodies • GAD65 antibodies present • Random and fasting blood glucose levels elevated • See ADA guidelines above	• 20% with other organ-specific autoimmune diseases (e.g., celiac disease, Graves disease) • Elderly patients have increasing incidence of type 1 DM

Table 8-22

Diabetes Mellitus (DM)(continued)

CONDITION	INITIAL PRESENTATION	DIAGNOSIS	NOTES
Type 2 DM	• Frequently asymptomatic • Frequently progresses from prediabetes, which may not be diagnosed • Prediabetes refers to impaired glucose tolerance. It is defined as a fasting plasma glucose ≥ 100 but ≤125 mg/dL or a 2-hour serum glucose ≥ 140 but ≤199 mg/dL during oral glucose tolerance test	• Random and fasting blood glucose levels • See ADA guidelines above	• MODY is a subset of type 2 DM with a genetic disease that presents in teens/20s

*Fasting defined as no caloric intake for > 8 hours; random defined as any time of day without regard to last meal.

ADA = American Diabetes Association; DKA = diabetic ketoacidosis; Hb = hemoglobin; GAD = glutamic acid decarboxylase; MODY = maturity onset diabetes of youth.

Table 8-23

Diabetic Ketoacidosis

Etiology	• Most frequently caused by infection or poor compliance with DM medications • More frequent in type 1 DM, but may be seen in type 2 DM	

Clinical Presentation	• Clinical:
	  - Signs and symptoms of DM
	  - Abdominal pain
	  - Nausea/vomiting
	  - Kussmaul respirations
	  - Fruity breath odor (ketones)
		• Laboratory:
		  - Hyperglycemia
		  - Ketonuria
		  - Glycosuria
		  - Hyponatremia
		  - Hypophosphatemia
		  - Metabolic acidosis (elevated anion gap)

Diagnosis	• Clinical examination • Arterial blood gas	• Laboratory tests as above

Severe Complications	• Acute cerebral edema (headache, blurry vision, vomiting, lethargy)
	  - Rare, but devastating complication
	  - Monitor closely
	  - Avoid bicarbonate administration because may contribute to cerebral edema	

Table 8-24

Treatment of Diabetic Ketoacidosis

Issue	Treatment/Notes
Dehydration	• Immediate, aggressive hydration • Administer isotonic intravenous fluids (normal saline) as bolus therapy prior to administration of insulin • Evaluate severity of dehydration (usually at least 10%)
Insulin	• Following fluid resuscitation, an insulin infusion (0.05–0.1 U/kg/h) is generally necessary to resolve the ketoacidosis and to correct the serum pH • Add glucose to IVF after the serum glucose decreases to less than 250 mg/dL
Acidosis	• If pH <7.2, risk of cardiovascular dysfunction (cardiac monitoring needed) • Consider bicarbonate replacement if pH <7 • Will normalize when hydration and insulin administration clear ketones
Potassium	• Supplement potassium aggressively (insulin drives potassium intracellularly) • Hyperkalemia may be noted on serum samples secondary to concomitant acidosis, but the patient generally has a total body deficit of potassium
Sodium	• Hyponatremia is a compensatory response to the increased osmolar load imposed by profound hyperglycemia • For each 100 mg/dL increase in serum glucose over 100 mg/dL, there is an appropriate decrease in serum sodium of 1.6 meq/L • Hyponatremia may be falsely exaggerated secondary to hyperlipidemia • For each 1 g/dL increase in triglycerides, there is a false sodium decrease of 2 meq/L
Monitoring	• Close monitoring of vital signs and hydration status (urine output) • Frequent monitoring of serum glucose, electrolytes, pH, and ketones

Serum Ketones	• Three ketone bodies are produced in DKA: two ketoacids (beta-hydroxybutyric acid and acetoacetic acid), and one neutral ketone (acetone)
	  - The reagents used to detect ketones contain nitroprusside, which reacts with acetoacetate and acetone, but not with beta-hydroxybutyrate
	  - In the initial stages of DKA, there is more beta-hydroxybutyrate than other ketones so that the initial measure of ketones may be falsely negative, although severe acidosis is present
	  - Continuous monitoring of ketones during DKA is controversial as it may increase even with successful treatment of DKA as beta-hydroxybutyrate is converted to the other ketones

Table 8-25

Nonketotic Hyperglycemic Hyperosmolar Coma

Definition	• Marked diabetic stupor with hyperglycemia and hyperosmolarity, without ketosis
Clinical Features	• Altered mental status • Visual hallucinations • Dysphagia • Seizures • Nystagmus • Hemiparesis • Bilateral or unilateral hypo- or hyperreflexia • Hemianopsia
Diagnosis	• Marked hyperglycemia (usually serum glucose >600 mg/dL) • Hyperosmolarity (serum >320 mg/dL) • Arterial pH >7.3 • Cause should be determined (e.g., workup for myocardial infarction, infection, pancreatitis, stroke or GI bleed)
Treatment	• Essentially the same treatment as DKA (see Table 8-24) • Fluid resuscitation • Replacement of electrolytes, especially potassium

GI = gastrointestinal.

Table 8-26

Risk Factors for Type 2 DM

CATEGORY	EXAMPLES
Endocrine	• Cushing syndrome • Hyperthyroidism
Pancreas	• Cystic fibrosis • Pancreatitis • Pancreatic cancer • Hemochromatosis • Abdominal trauma
Medication	• Beta-agonists • Glucocorticoids
Infection	• Congenital rubella • Cytomegalovirus mumps
Genetic Syndromes	• Down • Turner • Klinefelter

(continued)

Table 8-26

Risk Factors for Type 2 DM (continued)

CATEGORY	EXAMPLES
Consider Screening for DM if Two or More of Following Conditions Met:	
Personal Characteristics	• Age >45 • Obesity (causes insulin resistance) • Sedentary lifestyle • Member of high-risk ethnic group: Hispanics, African Americans, and Native Americans
Family History	• Family history of DM

Medical History	• Personal history of:
	  - Gestational diabetes
	  - Polycystic ovarian syndrome
	  - Dyslipidemia
	  - Hypertension
	  - Vascular disease

Table 8-27

Metabolic Syndrome

Definition	• The presence of three or more of the following:
	  - Increased waist circumference (>40 in. in men and >35 in. in women)
	  - Plasma triglycerides ≥150 mg/dL
	  - Plasma HDL <40 mg/dL in men or <50 mg/dL in women
	  - BP ≥130/85 mm Hg
	  - Fasting plasma glucose ≥100 mg/dL

Implication	• Metabolic syndrome increases oxidative stress, endothelial dysfunction, and inflammation of the vasculature causing atherosclerosis • Increased mortality due to CAD and cerebrovascular disease

Intervention	• Treat each component of the metabolic syndrome:
	  - Prevent diabetes in patients with impaired glucose tolerance (prediabetes) with lifestyle modification and pharmacologic therapy, e.g., metformin
	  - Treat dyslipidemia
	  - BP control
	  - Lifestyle modification: weight loss and exercise

HDL = high-density lipoprotein; BP = blood pressure.

Table 8-28

Complications of Diabetes Mellitus

ORGAN	COMPLICATIONS	ETIOLOGY/CLINICAL	PREVENTION/SCREENING/TREATMENT	NOTES
Eyes	• Retinopathy	Three stages: • Background retinopathy: dilated retinal venules, microaneurysms, and capillary leakage. Loss of visual acuity can occur if these changes are near the macula • Preproliferative retinopathy: retinal microinfarcts and "cotton wool" or "soft exudates" • Proliferative retinopathy: - (most severe form): retinal ischemia, proliferation of new retinal blood vessels, further hemorrhage, scarring resulting from contraction of fibrovascular proliferation, and retinal detachment	• Prevention: - Tight glycemic control and antihypertensive therapy • Screening: - DM1: initially done within 3–5 years after diagnosis - DM2: at time of diagnosis and subsequently every 1–2 years • Treatment: - Photocoagulation and intravitreal steroids for macular edema	
Kidney	• Nephropathy • Renal failure		• Screening: - Microalbuminuria: urinary albumin:creatinine ratio >30 mg/g • Primary prevention: - ACE-I should be used for BP control in diabetics without microalbuminuria • Treatment: - ACE-I or angiotensin receptor blockers are used in patients with microalbuminuria and proteinuria	• DM most common cause of ESRD in the United States

(*continued*)

Table 8-28

Complications of Diabetes Mellitus (continued)

ORGAN	COMPLICATIONS	ETIOLOGY/CLINICAL	PREVENTION/SCREENING/TREATMENT	NOTES
Nervous System	• Peripheral neuropathy	• Dysesthesias (pain, abnormal sensations) begin distally and symmetrically "stocking and glove"	• Difficult to treat • Glucose control may improve symptoms • Frequent and good foot care is important to prevent infections from unnoticed minor traumas	
Cardiovascular	• Atherosclerosis	• Diabetes is considered a CAD equivalent • CAD in diabetics is typically diffuse and involves multivessels • Diabetics tend to have blunting of ischemic pain and often have atypical angina symptoms, silent ischemia, or infarction	Prevention: • Protection against CAD with strict glycemic control has not been established in type 2 diabetes	• Most frequent cause of death in type 2
	• Autonomic neuropathy	• Orthostatic hypotension		• Can cause sudden death
GI	• Autonomic neuropathy	• Gastroparesis and diarrhea		

ACE-I = angiotensin-converting enzyme inhibitors; ESRD = end-stage renal disease; GI = gastrointestinal; CAD = coronary artery disease.

Table 8-29

Treatment of Diabetes Mellitus

CONDITION	TREATMENT OPTIONS	NOTES
Prediabetes	• Lifestyle modification: diet and exercise • Pharmacologic therapy: metformin	• Tight glycemic control is the best predictor of overall morbidity and mortality • Hb A1c for monitoring "average" glucose control over past several months (goal <7%)
Type 1	• SQ insulin: usually requires multiple daily injections of short- and long-acting insulin • Continuous SQ delivery mechanisms available • New routes of insulin administration (inhaled and oral) emerging	• Target fasting glucose of 70–130 mg/dL • Target postprandial glucose (90–120 minutes after a meal) <180 mg/dL **Combination therapy:** • Initial drug of choice is metformin unless contraindicated (renal or hepatic failure) • Addition of second agent (sulfonylurea or thiazolidinedione) if Hb A1c is >7 after 2–3 months of metformin
Type 2	• Weight loss (nutrition and/or lifestyle changes) may improve insulin resistance • Combination therapy often preferred • Frequently requires adjunctive insulin therapy when Hb A1c > 7% even with two oral agents and lifestyle changes	• Three oral agents can be used if Hb A1c is not far from goal • Addition of insulin is advised if Hb A1c is > 8.5 (or patient has hyperglycemic symptoms) despite titration of metformin

SQ = subcutaneous.

Table 8-30

Summary of Medications for Type 2 Diabetes Mellitus

MEDICATION CLASS	EXAMPLE OF AGENT	MECHANISM OF ACTION	NOTES
Oral Hypoglycemic Agent			
Sulfonylurea	• Glyburide • Glipizide	• Enhances the secretion of endogenous insulin from the pancreas	• Requires functioning beta-islet cells • Long acting • Increased risk for hypoglycemia
Meglitinide	• Nagletinide	• Enhances the secretion of endogenous insulin from the pancreas	• Requires functioning of beta-islet cells • Fast onset and short acting (must be given with each meal)
Biguanide	• Metformin	• Decreases hepatic gluconeogenesis and increases peripheral insulin sensitivity	• Less likely to cause weight gain than other agents • Renal metabolism: contraindicated if renal insufficiency • Stop if dye contrast will be used for imaging studies
Thiazolidinedione	• Rosiglitazone	• Increases insulin sensitivity by enhancing insulin action in the fat and muscle cells	• Time to maximal effect may be 4–12 weeks • Check liver function tests as can cause hepatic failure
Incretin mimetic	• Exenatide	• Improves insulin secretion and decreases absorption of glucose from the gut	• Exenatide is not currently approved for use with insulin therapy • The most common side effect is nausea
Non Oral Agent			
Insulin		• Exogenous administration of insulin	• Time to onset of action, duration of action, and routes of administration vary with formulations:

INSULIN TYPE	ONSET OF ACTION	TIME OF PEAK EFFECT	DURATION OF ACTION
Regular	About 30 minutes	2–4 hours	5–8 hours
NPH	About 2 hours	6–10 hours	18–28 hours
Insulin Glargine	About 2 hours	No peak	20 to >24 hours

Chapter 9

Hematology

Anemia

Definition: Decreased number of circulating red blood cells (RBCs). Although the hemoglobin (HGB) and hematocrit (HCT) levels defining anemia are debated, generally accepted levels are: HGB < 13.5 g/dL or a HCT < 41.0% for men and < 12.0 g/dL or < 36.0% for women. There are three classifications: normocytic, microcytic, and macrocytic.

Clinical presentation: Symptoms are based on the severity of the anemia and subsequent decreased oxygen delivery. Symptoms include fatigue, pallor, dyspnea, bounding pulses, claudication, palpitations, headache, and "roaring in the ears." Severe anemia can lead to confusion, congestive failure, angina, arrhythmia, and/or myocardial infarction.

Diagnosis: Review of the patient history, physical examination, complete blood count (CBC), and peripheral blood smear. The classification of anemia is typically based on the erythrocyte size (mean corpuscular volume [MCV]).

Treatment: Depends on etiology. See specific sections.

Table 9-1

Anemia

CATEGORY		MICROCYTIC	NORMOCYTIC	MACROCYTIC
MCV		<80 fl	80–100 fl	>100 fl
Etiology	**Nutritional deficiencies**	• Iron deficiency • Copper deficiency	• Early iron deficiency	• B_{12} deficiency • Folate deficiency
	Primarily hematologic disorders	• Thalassemia • Hereditary spherocytosis • Hereditary sideroblastic anemia • Hemoglobin E	• Sickle cell anemia • Erythroid hypoplasia/ aplastic anemia	• Myelodysplasia • Reticulocytosis
	Others	• Lead poisoning • Infection or inflammation	• Anemia of chronic disease/anemia of inflammatory block • Renal failure • Hypopituitarism • Hypothyroidism	• Liver disease

Table 9-2

Laboratory Findings for Common Anemias

Type of Anemia	Iron Deficiency	Inflammatory Block	Beta-Thalassemia Minor	Alpha-Thalassemia Minor	Folic Acid Deficiency	B12 Deficiency
HCT	↓	↓	↓ (>30%)	nl or ↓	↓	↓
MCV	↓	nl or ↓	↓↓ (<75 fl)	↓	↑	↑
RDW	↑	nl	nl	nl	nl	nl
Reticulocyte Count	↓	↓	↓	↓	↓	↓
Serum Ferritin	↓ (<15 ng/mL)	↑ (>35 ng/mL)	nl	nl		
TIBC	↑	↓				
Serum Iron	↓	↓				
Stainable Iron in Bone Marrow	No	Yes				
Red Cell Folate					↓	nl
Serum B$_{12}$					nl	<100 pg/mL
MMA					nl	↑
Homocysteine					↑	↑

MMA = methylmalonic acid; RDW = red cell distribution width; TIBC = total iron binding capacity.

Table 9-3

Iron-Deficiency Anemia

DEFINITION	EPIDEMIOLOGY	DIAGNOSIS	ETIOLOGY	EXAMPLE
• Anemia caused by inadequate iron stores • Iron is necessary for hemoglobin synthesis	• Most common cause of anemia worldwide • Occurs in 1–2% of adults • Iron deficiency without anemia occurs in 11% of women (most often premenopausal) and 4% of men • In developing countries, hookworm infection is a major cause of iron deficiency	• CBC with a serum iron level and saturation • History and physical to determine etiology	**Blood Loss (major cause)**	• GI blood loss • Occult malignancy (relative risk of GI malignancy diagnosis within 2 years of iron-deficiency anemia diagnosis is 31) • Peptic ulcer disease • Menstrual blood loss
			Increased Iron Need	• Pregnancy • Lactation
			Increased Iron Loss	• Chronic hemolytic anemia (loss of iron in urine) • Paroxysmal nocturnal hemoglobinuria • Fragmentation hemolytic syndromes • Chronic phlebotomy
			Inadequate Iron Intake	• Inadequate dietary intake • Small bowel disease • Malabsorption from tropical sprue
			Iron Stores Not Accessible	• Pulmonary hemosiderosis (chronic pulmonary hemorrhage in antiglomerular basement membrane antibody disease). Iron in pulmonary macrophages poorly available for utilization in RBC production

GI = gastrointestinal; CBC = complete blood count.

	IRON-DEFICIENCY ANEMIA	ANEMIA OF INFLAMMATORY BLOCK (ANEMIA OF CHRONIC DISEASE)	FOLATE DEFICIENCY	VITAMIN B₁₂ DEFICIENCY
Type of Anemia	• Microcytosis	• Normocytosis or mild microcytosis	• Macrocytosis	
Etiology of Anemia	• Iron required for hemoglobin synthesis	• Due to inflammatory cytokine action (tumor necrosis factor, IL-1, and interferon-gamma) • Reticuloendothelial iron stores not accessable	• Arrest of erythro-cyte maturation	• Arrest of methionine formation
Etiology of Deficiency	• See Table 9-3	• Any inflammatory disorder (autoimmune diseases, diabetes) • Renal disease (decreased epogen production) • Infectious diseases • Malignancy • Up to 40% of cases may occur in the absence of chronic disease	• Malnutrition • Inflammatory bowel disease • Increased require-ment during lactation and pregnancy • Methotrexate use • Anticonvulsant use	• Pernicious anemia • Gastritis • Small bowel disease • Pancreatitis • Crohn disease • Infection with fish tapeworm (*Diphyllobotbrium latum*) • Medications that block absorp-tion: proton pump inhibitors and metformin (reversed with oral calcium) • Strict vegans
Onset of Symptoms	• Depends on initial iron stores and bal-ance between iron loss and gain	• Depends on severity and course of underlying disease	• Months after intake diminished	• Years after intake diminished

(continued)

267

Table 9-4

Iron-Deficiency, Vitamin B$_{12}$ Deficiency, and Folate-Deficiency Anemia (continued)

	Iron-Deficiency Anemia	**Anemia of Inflammatory Block (Anemia of Chronic Disease)**	**Folate Deficiency**	**Vitamin B$_{12}$ Deficiency**
At-Risk Populations	• Pregnant and lactating women • Menstruating women • Malnourished	• Patients with chronic diseases	• Elderly • Alcoholics • Malnourished • Conditions listed under etiology	
Clinical Presentation	• Symptoms of anemia • Atrophic gastritis • Craving substances not considered food, such as clay and ice (pica) • Chelosis • Esophageal webs	• Symptoms of anemia • Symptoms of underlying disease	• Symptoms of anemia • Glossitis • Megaloblastic anemia	• Symptoms of anemia • Subacute combined demyelination of the dorsal (posterior) and lateral spinal columns • Neuropathy is symmetrical and affects the legs first • Paresthesias • Ataxia • Loss of vibration sense and proprioception • Can progress to severe weakness, spasticity, clonus, paraplegia • Memory loss, dementia, and depression
Diagnosis	• Laboratory: see Table 9-2 • Peripheral smear	• Laboratory: see Table 9-2 • Low serum epogen level • Peripheral smear	• Laboratory: See Table 9-2 • Peripheral smear	• Laboratory: see Table 9-2 • Schilling test differentiates nutritional deficiency from IF deficiency (rarely used now)
Peripheral Smear	• Teardrops • Pencil forms • Anicytosis (heterogeneous RBC shape) → increased RDW • Thrombocytopenia • Hypochromia	• Hypochromia	• Hypersegmented neutrophils on peripheral blood smear	• Hypersegmented neutrophils on peripheral blood smear

Treatment			
• Oral supplemental iron should increase the hemoglobin level 2 g/dL over 3–4 weeks • Liquid iron may be better tolerated than tablets • Intravenous iron dextran if cannot tolerate oral supplementation • An increase in reticulocyte count is maximally apparent 7–10 days after therapy • Pica responds quickly to iron supplementation	• Treat underlying disease • Recombinant erythropoietin injections • Iron supplements not likely to help unless also iron deficient or concurrent use of recombinant erythropoietin	• Folate supplementation	• Parenteral B_{12} supplementation: B_{12} IM daily for 1 week, then weekly for 4 weeks, and then monthly • For compliant patients, 1000–2000 μg orally each day equivalent to 1000 μg IM
Note			
• It is unlikely that iron deficiency is present if ferritin > 100 μg/L • Iron absorption promoted by: vitamin C, gastric acid, and amino acids • Iron absorption inhibited by: tea and vegetable fiber		• Must rule out vitamin B_{12} deficiency because folic acid replacement may raise the hemoglobin level but will not address the neurologic complications associated with vitamin B_{12} deficiency	• Not all patients with neurologic complications from B_{12} deficiency have anemia • Check serum MMA if B_{12} level borderline

IF = intrinsic factor; IL = interleukin; IM = intramuscular; MMA = methylmalonic acid.

Table 9-5

Etiologies of Iron Overload

ETIOLOGY	DEFECT/NOTE	GENETICS	POPULATION AT RISK
Common			
Hereditary Hemochromatosis	• Cys282Tyr mutation in HFE gene, on chromosome 6p • Most common cause of iron overload in the United States • Screen by measuring transferrin saturation. If >50% (women) or >60% (men), confirm with genetic testing	• Autosomal recessive	• White
Thalassemias	• Ineffective erythropoiesis secondary to decreased beta- or alpha-globin gene synthesis associated with increased iron absorption	• Autosomal recessive	• Asian • Middle Eastern • Mediterranean
Chronic Transfusion	• Can occur after 100 units of blood if given in setting without blood loss • 1 unit has one-fifth amount of total body iron stores		
Uncommon			
Hereditary Aceruloplasminemia	• Absent ceruloplasmin	• Autosomal recessive	• Japanese
Friedreich's Ataxia	• Frataxin gene, located on chromosome 9	• Autosomal recessive	

Table 9-6

Iron Overload: Complications and Treatment

ORGAN	COMPLICATION	NOTE	TREATMENT
Liver	• Elevated liver enzymes • Cirrhosis • Hepatocellular carcinoma	• Higher risk for hepatocellular carcinoma if cirrhosis present, even if iron levels optimally controlled • Iron overload potentiates development of alcoholic liver disease	• Chronic phlebotomy to keep serum ferritin less than 50 ng/mL • If anemic, avoid phlebotomy and treat with iron chelation therapy (parenteral deferoxamine) • Goal is to treat before complications occur • Most complications improve when iron levels are lowered
Heart	• Dilated cardiomyopathy • Heart failure • Conductive abnormalities		
Musculoskeletal	• Arthropathies	• Does not generally respond to iron removal	
Endocrine	• Diabetes mellitus • Hypogonadism	• Endocrine complications occur in 50% of patients with hereditary hemochromatosis • Diabetes due to iron accumulation in the pancreas • Hypogonadism due to iron deposition in the pituitary	
Immune	• Susceptible to infections	• *Listeria* and *Yersinia enterocolitica* (siderophoric) • Iron overload may inhibit macrophage function	
Skin	• Hyperpigmentation		
Brain	• Friedreich's ataxia defect causes mitochondrial accumulation of iron → cerebellar ataxia	• Friedreich's ataxia also causes cardiomyopathy and diabetes	

Table 9-7

Classification of Hemolytic Anemia

- Intracellular (intrinsic) defects refer to abnormalities of the erythrocyte membrane, hemoglobin, or enzymes that lead to red cell destruction
- Extracellular (extrinsic) defects refer to disorders in the interaction of red cells with their environment
- Hemolysis can occur in the intravascular or the extravascular space
- Elevated serum LDH and a reduced haptoglobin is highly specific for diagnosing hemolysis. Normal serum LDH and haptoglobin is highly sensitive for ruling out hemolysis

Extravascular Hemolysis

Inherited Intracellular Defects	• Membrane abnormalities	• Hereditary spherocytosis is the most common membrane defect
	• Enzyme abnormalities	• G6PD deficiency • PK deficiency
	• Hemoglobinopathies	• Congenital disorders of globin gene expression caused either by alteration of globin gene expression (i.e. thalassemia) or by changes in the physical properties of the globins (i.e. SCD)
Extracellular Defects	• Immune hemolytic anemias	• Autoimmune (cold or warm) • Drug induced
	• Infection	• Malaria • Babesia • Bartonella
	• Microangiopathic	• DIC • HUS/TTP
	• Other	• Liver disease • Hypersplenism

Intravascular Hemolysis (plasma hemoglobin elevated; hemoglobinuria; urine hemosiderin positive >7 days after start of hemolysis)

Intracellular Defects	• Acquired	• Paroxysmal nocturnal hemoglobinuria
Extracellular Defects	• Microangiopathic	• Aortic stenosis • Prosthetic valve
	• Infection	• Clostridial sepsis • Severe malaria
	• Transfusion reaction	
	• Snake bite	

DIC = disseminated intravascular coagulation; G6PD = glucose-6-phosphate dehydrogenase; HUS = hemolytic-uremic syndrome; LDH = lactate dehydrogenase; PK = pyruvate kinase; SCD = sickle cell disease; TTP = thrombotic thrombocytopenic purpura.

Table 9-8
Hemolytic Anemias

	HEREDITARY SPHEROCYTOSIS	**G6PD DEFICIENCY**	**PYRUVATE KINASE (PK) DEFICIENCY**
Definition	• Structural RBC membrane disorder resulting in hemolytic anemia and splenic sequestration	• Low average G6PD levels due to abnormally short half-life of G6PD	• PK deficiency
Genetics	• Autosomal dominant in 75% of cases	• X-linked inheritance	• Autosomal recessive
Mechanism	• An intracorpuscular membrane defect in spectrin or ankryn results in osmotic damage to the RBC membrane, resulting in intravascular hemolysis • The damaged RBCs are sequestered and removed by the spleen	• G6PD is critical for regenerating glutathione and protecting erythrocytes from oxidative damage by free radicals and peroxides • Deficiency of G6PD leads to hemolysis	• PK deficiency leads to reduced ATP production, and increased erythrocyte permeability
Epidemiology	• Most common hemolytic anemia in Northern Europeans, with a reported prevalence of 1/5000	• Most common enzymatic disorder of RBCs	• The most common deficiency in the glycolytic pathway
Clinical Presentation	• Clinical course highly variable • Generally present in childhood, but mild cases may not be brought to medical attention until adulthood • Hemolytic anemia due to increased red cell osmotic fragility • Normocytic anemia • Spherocytosis • Splenomegaly • Abdominal pain • Biliary tract symptoms/cholelithiasis • May have family history of splenectomy	• Hemolytic anemia of varying degrees may occur in settings of stress (i.e. infections) or exposure to certain medications or foods (sulfa agents, primaquine, dapsone, fava beans) • Jaundice • Pallor • Abdominal pain • Back pain	• Heterozygous: no symptoms • Homozygous: ranges from non-immune hydropsfetalis to mild, fully compensated hemolysis

(continued)

Table 9-8

Hemolytic Anemias (continued)

	HEREDITARY SPHEROCYTOSIS	G6PD DEFICIENCY	PYRUVATE KINASE (PK) DEFICIENCY
Diagnosis	• Increased red cell osmotic fragility (osmotic fragility test measures the ability of the RBC membrane to withstand lysis in varying degrees of hypotonic solution) • Peripheral smear: spherocytes • MCHC elevated	• G6PD level measured on a fresh blood sample • G6PD level may be falsely normal during a hemolysis episode because younger erythrocytes may still have "normal" levels of G6PD • If false normal level suspected, consider testing family members if acute diagnosis needed or test patient 2–3 months after episode	• Enzyme assay
Disease Course	• Ranges from hyperbilirubinemia at birth to a mild disease diagnosed incidentally in adulthood • Episodes of aplastic crisis due to parvovirus infection may occur	• Ranges from hemolytic anemia only under chemical or physical stress to profound impairment with nonspherocytic hemolytic anemia	
Treatment	• Splenectomy is the treatment of choice for moderate to severe disease and may improve quality of life • Supportive transfusions during aplastic crisis • Folic acid supplementation because of high RBC production • Vaccination for encapsulated organisms	• Avoid triggers • Supportive care (hydration and blood product transfusion) during acute hemolysis episode	• Treatment with supportive transfusions and splenectomy

ATP = adenosine triphosphate; MCHC = mean corpuscular hemoglobin concentration; G6PD = glucose-to-phosphate dehydrogenase.

Table 9-9

Autoimmune Hemolytic Anemia (AIHA)

	WARM AIHA		COLD AIHA		PAROXYSMAL COLD HEMOGLOBINURIA
	PRIMARY WARM AIHA	SECONDARY WARM AIHA	PRIMARY COLD AGGLUTININ DISEASE	SECONDARY COLD AGGLUTININ DISEASE	
Etiology	• Idiopathic • 50% of patients with AIHA	• Collagen vascular disease (i.e. SLE) • Lymphoproliferative disorders (Hodgkin disease, CLL) • Viral infections • Drugs (wide range including many antibiotics. See Table 9-10)	• Idiopathic	• Mycoplasma infection • Mononucleosis • Lymphoproliferative disorder	• Acute hemolysis after viral infections • Classically described with syphilis
Epidemiology	• Most common form of AIHA				
Mechanism	• Antibody functions at 37°C • IgG autoantibodies to blood cell antigens		• Antibody functions at 4°C • IgM autoantibodies to blood cell antigens		
Clinical Characteristic	• Depends on rapidity of hemolysis • Anemia • Jaundice • Splenomegaly		• Anemia (often mild) • Dark, purple to gray discoloration of the skin on the most acral parts relieved by warming (no hyperemia as with Raynaud's) • Jaundice • Splenomegaly		
Diagnosis	• Anemia • DAT or Coombs' test positive • Decreased haptoglobin • Elevated reticulocyte count • Elevated LDH • Smear: spherocytes, erythrophagocytosis, nucleated RBCs		• Anemia • Direct Coombs' test positive for complement (especially C3d) • High titers of a cold agglutinin • Smear: RBC agglutination		
Treatment	• Usually responds within 1–2 days of starting prednisone • Splenectomy if refractory		• Preventive measures: warm clothing; cold avoidance • Warm intravenous fluids and transfusions • Low-dose alkylating agents or rituximab • Steroids and splenectomy only in select patients • Consider plasmapheresis if severe symptoms		

CLL = chronic lymphocytic leukemia; DAT = direct antiglobulin test; C = celsius; LDH = lactate dehydrogenase; SLE = septemic lupus erythematosis.

Table 9-10
Drug-Induced Immune Hemolytic Anemia

	COMMON DRUG	MECHANISM	CLINICAL
Alteration of Antigen	• Alpha-methyldopa • Procainamide	• Drug alters antigens on the RBC, inducing production of autoantibodies (IgG and C3d) that cross-react with the unaltered antigen	• Presence of drug is NOT required for hemolysis • Hemolysis gradually ceases over 3–4 months (one red cell life span) once the altered epitope is no longer being produced
Hapten Mechanism	• Penicillin	• Drug binds with antigens on the RBC membrane • An IgG antibody forms to the drug-RBC complex	• Most common mechanism • Hemolysis ceases with drug removal • Indirect Coombs test positive

Table 9-11
Classification of Hemoglobin

HEMOGLOBIN TYPE	CHARACTERISTIC
A	• Predominant type of adult hemoglobin • Made up of four polypeptide chains, two α and two β chains
A_2	• Minor component of adult hemoglobin (~3%) • Made up of two α and two δ chains
C	• More common in African Americans • Made up of two α and two abnormal β chains • May be homozygous (CC), combined with normal hemoglobin (HbC), or combined with sickle hemoglobin (Hb SC disease.)
E	• More common in persons from Southeast Asia • Made up of two α chains and two abnormal β chains
F	• Fetal hemoglobin. After 6 months of age, normally constitutes <1% of total hemoglobin • Made up of two α chains as those in HbA, plus two γ chains • The γ chain only differs from HbA by a few amino acids • Oxygen affinity of HbF is ↑ due to ↑ 2–3 diphosphoglycerate • Facilitates enhanced transplacental transport of oxygen to the fetus
H	• More common in Asians • Made up of four β chains
S	• Sickle hemoglobin
Hemoglobinopathy	• A structural defect in hemoglobin production results in defective RBC formation and function

α = alpha; β = beta; δ = delta; γ = gamma; Hb = hemoglobin; RBC = red blood cell.

Thalassemia

Definition: There are normally four chains that make up adult hemoglobin, two alpha chains, and two beta chains. Thalassemia is a deficiency of one or more of these hemoglobin chains.

Incidence: Varies with ethnicity. Beta thalassemia is most common in Italian, Greek, and African patients; alpha thalassemia is most common in African and Chinese patients. In North America, 20% of Asian immigrants have alpha-thalassemia disease, and up to 6% of Mediterranean immigrants have beta thalassemia.

Etiology: Reduced or absent production of one or more hemoglobin chains.

Clinical Presentation: Disease ranges from silent (trait), to mild, intermediate or severe (major). The patient may present with microcytic anemia, pallor, jaundice, and hepatosplenomegaly. A family history of anemia is common.

Patients with untreated thalassemia major develop characteristic "chipmunk" facies and frontal bossing due to bone marrow expansion.

Patients with thalassemia major usually present in childhood after fetal hemoglobin disappears.

Diagnosis: Hemoglobin electrophoresis is the gold standard. A peripheral blood smear reveals hypochromic, microcytic RBCs. Tear drop and target cells may also be present.

Treatment: Severity of disease directs treatment. Mild disease and asymptomatic carriers may require no treatment. Those with thalassemia major may require regular, frequent transfusions to prevent the development of extramedullary hematopoiesis, coarse facial features, and hepatosplenomegaly. The cumulative effect of repetitive transfusion is iron overload and resultant hemosiderosis. Iron chelation therapy for iron overload is mandatory. Splenectomy should be considered in moderate to severe cases. Patients with thalassemia major are at an increased risk for development of postsplenectomy syndrome. This syndrome is characterized by severe infections with encapsulated organisms (*Streptococcus pneumoniae, Haemophilus influenzae, Neisseria meningitidis*). Genetic counseling should be provided for affected individuals and their partners.

Table 9-12
Classification of Thalassemia

	MECHANISM	ELECTROPHORESIS	EPIDEMIOLOGY	CLINICAL CHARACTERISTIC	TREATMENT
Beta-Thalassemia Minor	• Heterozygotes • Loss of one of the two beta-globin genes	• ↓ HbA • ↑↑ HbA2 • ↑ HbF	• Mediterranean, sub-Saharan African, Indian subcontinent, or Southeast Asian descent	• Mild hypochromic microcytic anemia • No evidence of clinical disease	• None
Beta-Thalassemia Major	• Homozygotes • Loss of both beta-globin genes	• ↓↓ HbA • ↓↓ HbA2 • ↑↑ HbF		• Severe clinical disease • Hemolytic anemia • Growth delay • Cardiac failure • Iron overload from transfusions • Premature death	• Transfusion dependent • Chelation therapy for iron overload • Bone marrow transplant may be an option
Alpha-Thalassemia Trait	• Two functioning alpha-globin genes	• Normal	• African or Southeast Asian descent	• Mild hypochromic, microcytic anemia	• None
Hemoglobin H Disease	• Only one functioning alpha-globin gene • Four beta-globin complex together as dysfunctional homo-tetramers (HbH)	• ↑ HbF • ↑ HbH		• Moderate to severe hypochromic, microcytic anemia • Hemolytic anemia	
Hydrops Fetalis	• Loss of four alpha-globin genes • Formation of excess gamma-globin chains (hemoglobin Bart)	• ↓↓ HbA • ↓↓ HbA2 • ↓↓ HbF		• The most severe form of alpha thal-assemia • Neonatal demise	

Table 9-13
Sickle Cell Disease (SCD) and Sickle Cell Trait

	DEFINITION	GENETICS	MECHANISM	CLINICAL PRESENTATION	DIAGNOSIS	TREATMENT
SCD	• Homozygous for a single nucleotide genetic mutation on the Beta (S) gene	• 1/375 African American births • Inheritance is autosomal recessive • Mutations: substitution of the amino acid valine for glutamine in the sixth position of the beta-globin chain on chromosome 11	• Hemoglobin S hetero-tetramers undergo autopoly-merization when deoxy-genated and deform erythrocytes • Deformed cells are rigid and occlude terminal vessels • Secondary cellular defects may promote adhesion of sickled erythrocytes to the endothelium and leukocytes	Sickle cell disease: • Chronic normochromic, normocytic hemolytic anemia • Impaired splenic function with eventual autoinfarction • After splenic infarction, patients are at increased risk for infection • Hematuria • Coexisting beta thalassemia results in a less severe anemia, less hemoglobin polymerization, and fewer episodes of crisis • For complications of disease see Table 9-14	• Hemoglobin electrophoresis is gold standard (HgbS ↑ and HgbF ↑) • Anemia • MCV normal or increased • Reticulocyte count increased • RBC decreased • Positive solubility test • Peripheral smear: sickled cells	• Hydroxyurea may promotes synthesis of HgbF (less likely to sickle) • Supportive care • Antibacterial pro-phylaxis with penicillin VK • Pneumococcal and yearly influenza vaccines to prevent life-threatening infections (the leading cause of death in sickle cell patients) • Folic acid supplementation • Test family members
Sickle Cell Trait (Carrier)	• Heterozygos for Beta (S) gene mutation as above			• May be asymptomatic or have mild symptoms of SCD	• Peripheral smear: Not likely to have sickled cells • Positive solubility test • Hgb Electrophoresis	• Test family members

Penicillin VK = penicillin V potassium.

Table 9-14

Complications of Sickle Cell Disease (SCD)

COMPLICATION	CLINICAL PRESENTATION	TREATMENT	COMMENT
Acute Chest Syndrome	• Dyspnea • Fever • Chest pain • Tachypnea • Hypoxemia	• Hydration • Antibiotics (including coverage for atypical pneumonias, *Mycoplasma*) • Oxygen supplementation if needed • Pain control	• The leading cause of death in SCD
Aplastic Crisis	• Severe anemia • Signs and symptoms of severe anemia	• Blood transfusions often necessary if severe	• Parvovirus B19 is the most common cause
Vaso-Occlusive Crisis	• Very painful • Can be precipitated by dehydration, stress, and alcohol	• Hydration • Analgesics • Blood transfusion if severe	• Common first presenting sign of SCD • Can last days
Osteomyelitis	• Signs and symptoms of osteomyelitis	• Antibiotics • Surgical intervention if needed	• *Salmonella* most frequent cause of osteomyelitis in SCD
Dactylitis	• Painful swelling of the hands and feet	• Hydration • Analgesics	• Often the first presenting sign of SCD
Priapism	• Unwanted, painful erection	• Hydration • Analgesics	
Stroke	• Signs and symptoms of stroke	• Hydration • Transfusion therapy reduces the incidence of recurrent stroke	
Infection with Encapsulated Organisms	• Signs and symptoms of infection	• Antibiotics	• *S. pneumoniae* • *H. influenzae* • *N. meningitidis*

Table 9-15

Idiopathic Thrombotic Microangiopathy

	EPIDEMIOLOGY	ETIOLOGY	CLINICAL PRESENTATION	DIAGNOSIS	TREATMENT
TTP-HUS	• TTP is more common than HUS • Three to four cases per 100,000	• Absence of ADAMTS13 activity (plasma protease that normally cleaves vWF) appears to be necessary but not required for the development of TTP • Increased frequency during pregnancy	• TTP and HUS may be indistinguishable. Some authorities believe they are different manifestations of the same disease process • Classic pentad of symptoms: 1) Fever 2) Microangiopathic hemolytic anemia 3) Thrombocytopenia 4) Renal failure 5) Neurologic symptoms	• Clinical presentation • ADAMTS13 deficiency (do not wait for test result to come back to treat patient) • Peripheral smear: schistocytes are pathognomonic • Reticulocytosis • Increased LDH • Increased bilirubin • Decreased/absent haptoglobin	• Mortality rate for untreated TTP-HUS nears 100% • FFP exchange replaces deficient protease • Plasma exchange of 1–1.5 plasma volumes should occur daily until neurologic symptoms resolve, LDH normalizes, and platelet counts are stable for 3 days • Other treatment options: splenectomy, glucocorticoids, IVIG, antiplatelet therapy, immunosuppressive therapy • Delivery of fetus does not help • Frequent relapses • Platelet transfusion may make TTP-HUS worse
Epidemic HUS	• More common in children	• Associated Shiga toxin-producing bacteria such as *Escherichia coli* strain O157:H7	• Infectious symptoms: - Gastroenteritis - Abdominal pain - Watery, bloody diarrhea - HUS symptoms occur within 2 days to 3 weeks: ○ Oliguria ○ Microangiopathic hemolytic anemia ○ Thrombocytopenia ○ Neurologic symptoms ○ Renal disease	• Normal coagulation studies • Increased creatinine (especially in HUS) • Direct Coombs' test negative • No evidence of DIC	• Usually self-limited • Supportive measures including temporary dialysis if necessary • Plasma exchange is not useful • Mortality rate ~5%.

FFP = fresh frozen plasma; IVIG = intravenous immunoglobulin; vWF = von Willebrand factor; TTP = thrombotic thrombocytopenic purpura; HUS = hemolytic-uremic syndrome; DIC = disseminated intravascular coagulation.

Thrombophilia

Definition: A disorder of hemostasis that predisposes individuals to develop thromboses in the venous or arterial system.

Etiology: Abnormalities of blood flow, the vascular endothelium, or the pro- or anticoagulant pathways may shift the complicated balance of hemostasis toward thrombosis. Risk factors for a hypercoagulable state can be genetically predetermined or acquired.

Clinical Presentation: Depends on location of clot, but may include extremity swelling, tenderness, warmth, erythema, positive Homan's sign (pain with flexion of foot), or cord palpated on calf. The patient may have signs and symptoms of pulmonary embolus: shortness of breath, tachycardia, electrocardiogram (ECG) changes, and chest pain.

Diagnosis: Evaluation of the patient with a blood clot requires a careful personal and family history in order to help define the extent of testing needed. Patients who may benefit from screening: (1) younger than 50 years with a first unprovoked venous thromboembolic event; (2) recurrent unexplained thrombotic episodes; (3) documented history of a first-degree family member with a venous thromboembolic event before age 50. Although a congenital predisposition to clot increases the risk of thrombosis in asymptomatic carriers, additional risk factors are often necessary for clot formation.

Treatment: Patients with thrombosis are frequently treated with anticoagulation. Asymptomatic patients with two congenital thrombophilia abnormalities may benefit from lifelong anticoagulation. For patients with a single thrombophilia abnormality, the risks and benefits of lifelong anticoagulation should be discussed. Asymptomatic family members of affected patients rarely need chronic anticoagulation.

Table 9-16A

Congenital Risk Factors for Thrombosis

Disorder	Risk of *Initial* Venous Thrombosis Compared to "Normals"	Mechanism	Falsely Low Levels If:	Test	Clinical Note
• **Factor V Leiden (activated protein C resistance)**		• Factor V Leiden mutation yields protein that is resistant to protein C inactivation		• Clotting assay OR • Genetic test	• Most prevalent inherited coagulation defect in patients with thrombosis • Factor V Leiden mutation yields protein that is resistant to protein C inactivation • Venous thrombosis • Mainly in white populations
• **Homozygous**	80 times higher				
• **Heterozygous**	7 times higher				
• **Heterozygous AND oral estrogen use**	35 times higher				
• Antithrombin III deficiency		• Gene mutation leads to functional deficiency • ATIII neutralizes procoagulants (e.g., factors II, IX, and X)	• Acute thrombosis • Heparin	• Functional assay	• Many mutations exist • Acquired ATIII deficiency is seen in nephrotic syndrome, DIC, liver disease, acute thrombosis, oral contraceptive use, heparin use, and L-asparaginase therapy • Venous thrombosis

(continued)

Table 9-16A

Congenital Risk Factors for Thrombosis (continued)

DISORDER	RISK OF *INITIAL* VENOUS THROMBOSIS COMPARED TO "NORMALS"	MECHANISM	FALSELY LOW LEVELS IF:	TEST	CLINICAL NOTE
• **Protein C deficiency** • **Protein S deficiency**		• Deficiency of or dysfunction of protein C, protein S • Acquired deficiencies occur in pregnancy, DIC, active thrombosis, and with the use of warfarin and oral contraceptives	• Acute thrombosis • Warfarin	• Functional assay	• Protein S bound to complement protein that increases in setting of acute thrombosis/inflammation • Functional assays can be confounded by activated protein C resistance (factor V Leiden) • Warfarin-induced skin necrosis is more common in patients with protein C abnormality • Venous thrombosis
• **Dysfibrinogenemia**					
• **Prothrombin (factor II) mutation 20210A***	• 2.8 times higher	• Heterozygous gene mutation • Increased factor II level		• Genetic test	• Second most common inherited cause of thrombosis in people of European descent • Arterial venous thrombosis
• **Plasminogen activator inhibitor**					

			Serum Level
• **Hyperhomo-cysteinemia***	• 2.5 times higher	• Homocysteine is toxic to endothelial cells, triggering thrombosis and atherosclerosis	• Measure fasting homocysteine • Deficiency in vitamin B_{12}, B_6, or folate disrupts methionine metabolism leading to increased homocysteine levels • Other causes include diabetes, hypothyroidism, inflammatory disorders, malignancy, phenytoin, thiazide diuretics, cyclosporine, methotrexate, hydroxyurea • Associated with venous and arterial thrombosis as well as atherosclerosis • Folate and B vitamin supplements decrease homocysteine levels but unclear if reduce risk of thrombosis • Venous thrombosis
• **MTHFR mutation**		• Homocysteine is converted to methionine by MTHFR • When MTHFR is mutated, homocysteine levels increase	• Associated with hyperhomocysteinemia • Homocysteine level more predictive of thrombotic risk
• **Plasminogen deficiency**			

*Consider screening in thrombophilic patients with first event at less than 50 years of age.

Table 9-16 B

Other Risk Factors for Thrombosis

	DISORDER	CLINICAL NOTE
Acquired Clotting Factor Abnormalities	• Nephrotic syndrome: urinary loss of antithrombin and plasminogen	
Acquired Secondary to Systemic Disorders	• Malignancy	• Thrombosis seen in 50% of cancer patients at autopsy • Up to 20% of patients with "idiopathic" venous thrombosis have an occult malignancy • Venous thrombosis
	• Pregnancy	
	• HIT	• See Table 9-17
	• Antiphospholipid antibody syndrome • Lupus anticoagulant • Anticardiolipin antibody	• Associated with recurrent pregnancy loss • Venous and arterial thrombosis • See Table 9-18
	• Myeloproliferative disorders • ET • PV	• Venous and arterial thrombosis • Associated with elevated platelet count (ET) and elevated HCT (PV)
	• Paroxysmal nocturnal hemoglobinuria	• Associated with leucopenia and thrombocytopenia • Thrombosis occurs in abdominal veins (mesenteric, hepatic, portal, splenic, and renal veins) and in cerebral venous circulation
	• Inflammatory bowel disease	
Situational	• Immobility	• Risks associated with air travel controversial
	• Surgery (especially orthopedic and abdominal/pelvic)	
	• Trauma or mechanical damage to vein	
	• Estrogen supplementation • Oral contraception use • Hormone replacement therapy	• Risk is 4 times higher than in "normals"
	• Altered blood flow (indwelling catheter or device, compression)	
	• Previous thrombosis	

ET = essential thrombocythemia; HIT = heparin-induced thrombocytopenia; MTHFR = methylenetetrahydrofolate reductase; PV = polycythemia vera.

Table 9-17

Heparin-Induced Thrombocytopenia (HIT)

	TYPE I HIT	TYPE II HIT
Onset	• Occurs within 2 days of heparin administration	• Platelet drop (and thrombosis) occurs 4–10 days after heparin exposure • Patients who have received heparin within past 3 months can have onset of HIT within hours • Occurs in 1–3% of patients receiving unfractionated heparin • Can occur with any heparin formulation; less often seen with LMWH • Delayed HIT can occur up to 3 weeks after discontinuation of heparin
Platelet Count	• Mild thrombocytopenia • Platelets generally > 100,000	• Decrease in platelets by 50% (platelets may still be in "normal" range) • Platelets generally range from 20,000 to 100,000
Mechanism	• Direct stimulation of platelet aggregation by heparin	• Antibodies directed against the complex of heparin and platelet factor 4. This complex binds to the Fc receptor, inducing platelet activation and release of platelet procoagulant factors
Clinical Presentation	• No risk of thrombosis	• Thrombosis occurs in 50% of patients within 30 days • 20% mortality rate if have thrombosis (HITT)
Diagnosis	• HIT antibody testing negative	• HIT antibody positive • Laboratory confirmation of HIT using both functional and antigenic assays • C-SRA is the gold standard • Heparin-PF4 ELISA assay sensitive, but may be falsely elevated in patients undergoing hemodialysis, hospitalized patients, and postcardiac bypass surgery with heparin exposure
Treatment	• Self-limited, even with continued heparin use	• Discontinue all heparin products immediately if clinical suspicion of HIT • Begin nonheparin anticoagulation such as lepirudin or argatroban. Goal aPTT = 1.5 − 2.5 × normal • Lepirudin is renally cleared and contraindicated in patients with renal insufficiency • Argatroban requires dose adjustment for liver disease • Do not use warfarin until HIT resolves (platelets normal). Lowering of protein C by warfarin can exacerbate hypercoagulable state and cause to venous limb gangrene

aPTT = activated partial thromboplastin time; C-SRA = C-serotonin release assay; ELISA = enzyme-linked immunosorbent assay; HITT = heparin-induced thrombocytopenia with thrombosis; LMWH = low molecular weight heparin.

Table 9-18
Antiphospholipid Syndrome

Etiology	• Idiopathic • Systemic lupus erythematosus • Cancer (lymphoma) • Infections (*Pneumocystis carinii* pneumonia) • Drugs (hydralazine, procainamide, phenothiazines, and others)
Clinical Presentation	• Recurrent fetal loss • Arterial or venous thrombosis • Thrombocytopenia • Livedo reticularis
Diagnosis	• If aPTT prolonged, test for antiphospholipid antibodies • Diagnosis requires two positive antibody tests at least 12 weeks apart
Antiphospholipid Antibodies	• IgG and/or IgM anticardiolipin antibody in moderate or high titer • IgG and/or IGM antibodies to beta$_2$-glycoprotein in high titers • Positive lupus anticoagulant: dRVVT, kaolin plasma clotting time • May have a false positive serologic test for syphilis
Treatment	• Anticoagulation. A prospective study suggests INR of 2–3 adequate • No warfarin if patient is or could become pregnant (teratogenic). Treat with aspirin and heparin

dRVVT = dilute Russell viper venom time; INR = international normalized ratio.

Table 9-19
Treatment of Deep Venous Thrombosis

	HEPARIN	LMWH	WARFARIN
General Approach	• Anticoagulation should begin with either intravenous unfractionated heparin or subcutaneous LMWH followed by transition to oral anticoagulation with warfarin • The decision to initiate anticoagulation and how long to anticoagulate should be discussed by the patient and physician with careful review of the risks (bleeding) and benefits (thrombosis prevention)		
Length of Treatment	• If first venous thrombotic event occurred in the setting of a transient triggering factor that has resolved, may treat for 3–6 months • If no triggering factor, treat for 6 months • Consider extended anticoagulation if: (1) unprovoked event and two congenital thrombophilic abnormalities, (2) life-threatening thrombosis, (3) triggering factor does not resolve (i.e., malignancy), or (4) recurrent spontaneous thrombosis • Caution if at increased risk for bleeding		

Table 9-19

Treatment of Deep Venous Thrombosis (continued)

	HEPARIN	LMWH	WARFARIN
Mechanism	• Catalyzes ATIII activity • Neutralizes thrombin • Decreases platelet activation	• Antifactor Xa activity • Too small to bind thrombin	• Inhibits vitamin-K-dependent gamma-carboxylation of coagulation factors II, VII, IX, and X • Onset of action delayed until the normal clotting factors are cleared from the circulation
Dose	• Bolus to saturate plasma binding sites and then infusion to obtain equilibrium between free heparin and bound heparin • Adjust infusion rate to achieve goal aPTT	• Weight-based	• Based on PT/INR
Route	• Intravenous	• Subcutaneous	• Oral
Pharmacokinetics	• Immediate onset, short duration of activity • Cleared by binding to endothelial cells, macrophages, and plasma proteins	• Predictable bio-availability • Dosing interval 12–24 hours	• PT prolongs at 24–48 hours but full effect may take 5–7 days
Note	• Patients who are not therapeutic within 24 hours have a five-fold risk of recurrent venous thrombosis	• Renally cleared • Major bleeding risk is the same as for unfractionated heparin • Can monitor drug activity with anti-factor Xa levels • Consider monitoring if renal disease, extreme weight, or pregnancy	• Risk of skin necrosis related to initial drop in protein C and protein S • Concurrent heparin required until INR is > target level on consecutive days • Risk of bleeding is 2–3% per year and up to 7–9% per year in the elderly
Reversal	• Stop heparin • Protamine 1 mg/100 units of heparin	• Not reversible • Supportive care with blood products and fluids	• Vitamin K (oral or subcutaneously). Caution with intravenous vitamin K • FFP every 4–6 hours

PT = prothrombin time; FFP = fresh frozen plasma; INR = international normalized ratio.

Table 9-20
Blood Product Transfusions

	PACKED RED BLOOD CELLS (PRBC)	WHOLE BLOOD	FFP	CRYOPRECIPITATE	PLATELET TRANSFUSION
Indication	• To increase oxygen carrying capacity of blood • In chronic anemia, transfusions are indicated when Hgb <7 g/dL • Patients with cardiac disease may benefit from transfusion at higher hemoglobin levels	• To simultaneously increase blood volume and oxygen carrying capacity	• To replace coagulation factors - Dilutional coagulopathy from massive transfusion - Liver disease with bleeding - Factor deficiency/warfarin reversal - DIC - Plasmapheresis replacement • NOT appropriate for: - Volume expansion - Bleeding without coagulopathy or heparin induced bleeding - Prolonged PT/PTT without bleeding or planned procedure	• To replace fibrinogen (consider if fibrinogen < 100 mg/dL)	• Prevent bleeding from thrombocytopenia or platelet dysfunction • Spontaneous bleeding more likely to occur when platelets are less than 10,000/μL • Platelets should be maintained about 40,000/uL if bleeding, especially if bleeding in lungs or brain • Platelet dysfunction can be caused by uremia or heparin use
Expected Response	• 1 g/dL rise in hemoglobin for each unit of packed red cells transfused		• 2–4 units corrects simple factor deficiencies caused by dilution from transfusion (12–15 units PRBC) or from decreased hepatic synthesis	• 10 pooled bags = 2 g fibrinogen	• A "five-pack" (pool of 4–5 concentrates) of platelets usually increases platelet count by 22,000/μL

Lack of Response to Transfusion (Refractoriness)	• Continued bleeding • Continued consumption of RBCs				• Rise in platelet level decreased if infection, fever, hypersplenism, or consumptive coagulopathy present • Refractoriness caused by alloimmunization to HLA antigens (common in leukemia patients)
Storage	• Up to 6 weeks at 4°C				• 5 days at room temperature
Modifications	• Leukocyte-depletion/reduction decreases febrile, nonhemolytic transfusion reactions • Washing decreases allergic reaction				• Single donor platelets have less leukocytes/unit and therefore lower risk of HLA alloimmunization • Washing decreases allergic reaction
Note	• Massive transfusion may result in thrombocytopenia and dilution of coagulation factors • Monitor volume status	• Accounts for fewer than 1% of transfusions in the United States	• Efficacy limited by factor with shortest half-life (factor VII) • Made by separating plasma from whole blood	• Also contains factor VIII, vWF, factor XIII, and fibronectin • Made from FFP	

HLA = human leukocyte antigen; PTT = partial thromboplastin time.

Table 9-21

Blood Product Transfusion Reactions

	ACUTE HEMOLYTIC REACTION	DELAYED HEMOLYTIC REACTION	FEBRILE NONHEMOLYTIC TRANSFUSION REACTION	ALLERGIC REACTION	TRALI
Etiology	• Incompatible ABO blood • Usually due to improper patient identification or blood product labeling	• Amnestic response of patient alloantibody to RBC alloantigens (e.g, Rh, Kidd, Duffy, Kell, and MNSs) leads to destruction of transfused cells	• Cytokines derived from donor leukocytes • Recipient antibodies directed against donor leukocyte antigens	• Patient IgE reacts to plasma constituents	• Donor antileukocyte antibodies react against the patient's leukocytes • More common with products containing a large amount of plasma
Epidemiology	• 1:25,000 transfusions	• 1:7000 transfusions	• 0.5–1% of PRBC transfusions • Up to 30% of platelet transfusions	• 1–3% of transfusions • More common with FFP and platelets	• Rare
Clinical Characteristic	• Mortality rate = 17–70% • Symptoms occur shortly after transfusion begins • Red plasma and red urine due to intravascular hemolysis • Fever, chills • Flank and abdominal pain • Nausea, vomiting • DIC • Hypotension, tachycardia • Shortness of breath • Renal failure	• Onset 5–10 days after transfusion • Extravascular hemolysis • Drop in hemoglobin • May have fever and jaundice or may be asymptomatic	• Rise in temperature more than 1°F toward the end or after transfusion • Usually transient • May have symptoms similar to acute hemolytic reaction: fever, chills, headache, nausea, vomiting, hypertension, and tachycardia	• Rash • Urticaria • If severe, wheezing and mucosal edema • True anaphylaxis rare but can occur in IgA-deficient patients	• Respiratory distress toward the end or after transfusion • May improve in 2–3 days • May be fatal if acute respiratory distress syndrome develops

	Diagnosis				
Diagnosis	• Red urine and red plasma • Positive direct antiglobulin (Coombs') test	• Unexplained drop in hemoglobin • New alloantibody • Increase in bilirubin and LDH	• Rule out acute hemolytic transfusion reaction	• Rash	• Hypoxemia
Treatment	• Stop transfusion • Supportive care • Maintain adequate urine output	• Subsequent transfusions need to be compatible/antigen-negative	• Stop transfusion • Symptomatic treatment with antipyretics and/or steroids • Leukocyte reduce future blood products	• Stop transfusion • Antihistamines and/or steroids • Premedicate with acetaminophen and diphenhydramine before transfusing future units • Consider washing future units	• Stop transfusion • Supportive care • Caution with diuretics

TRALI = transfusion-related acute lung injury.

Table 9-22
Infectious Complications of Blood Product Transfusion

INFECTION	INCIDENCE	NOTE
Bacteria	• PRBC: >1 in 1 million units • Platelets: up to 1 in 500 units	• *Yersinia* can survive refrigerated storage • Platelet bacterial contamination higher because platelets are stored at room temperature • Chagas disease and *Babesia* are rare, but emerging concerns
Hepatitis C	• Nearly 1 in 2 million units	• HCV tends to be chronic in transfusion-transmitted disease
Hepatits B	• 1 in 58,000–269,000 units	
HIV	• 1 in 2 million units	• Blood products are screened for HIV type 1 and type 2
HTLV-1	• 1 in 2 million units	• Infection can cause T-cell leukemia/lymphoma
CMV		• Increased risk of transmission in immunocompromised recipients, particularly transplant patients • Reduce risk by using CMV-negative donors if transplant patient is CMV-negative

CMV = cytomegalovirus; HCV = hepatitis C virus; HIV = human immunodeficiency virus; HTLV-1 = human T-cell lymphotropic virus.

Table 9-23
Growth Factors

DRUG	TARGET CELL	EFFECT	INDICATION
G-CSF and GM-CSF	• Myeloid cells • Enhances production and increases activity	• Increases absolute leukocyte and ANC	• Cancer patients receiving myelosuppressive chemotherapy at high risk for serious infectious complications associated with neutropenic fever • Primary prophylactic administration in cancer patients not routinely recommended
Erythropoietins	• Erythroid progenitor cells	• Increases hemoglobin level	• Anemia associated with renal failure • Chemotherapy-induced anemia
IL-11 (Oprelvkin)	• Megakaryocytes	• Increases platelet count	• Not commonly used

ANC = absolute neutrophil count; G-CSF = granulocyte colony-stimulating factor; GM-CSF = granulocyte-macrophage colony-stimulating factor.

Table 9-24
Disorders of Blood Cell Production

Disease	Definition	Etiology	Clinical Presentation	Diagnosis	Treatment
Aplastic Anemia	• Absent (or severely diminished) myeloid progenitor and stem cells in the bone marrow	• Intrinsic defect of stem cells or immune-mediated destruction of stem cells • Idiopathic (50%) • Radiation and chemotherapy drugs • Toxins (benzene, arsenic) • Drugs (chloramphenicol, NSAIDs, sulfonamides, gold) • Infections (parvovirus, seronegative hepatitis, HIV, EBV)	• Rapidly progressive • Transfusion-dependent anemia • Recurrent infections from leukopenia • Bleeding from thrombocytopenia	• Bone marrow examination • Rule out acute leukemia and myelodysplastic syndrome	• Allogeneic stem cell transplantation, especially if younger • Immunosuppression (antithymocyte globulin, cyclosporine)
Myelodysplastic Syndromes	• Clonal disorder of hematopoietic stem cells • Ineffective hematopoiesis and cytopenias	• Clonal stem cell • Chromosomal abnormalities • Previous chemotherapy	• Median age = 65 years • Cytopenia of one or all three lineages • High risk of transformation to leukemia • Symptoms and disease course range from asymptomatic and indolent (median survival 6 years) to severe anemia with infections and rapid progression (median survival 1 year)	• Bone marrow is hypercellular • The greater the number of blasts, the more aggressive the disease • WHO classification depends on clinical factors and bone marrow results • Rule out vitamin B_{12} and folate deficiency, as well as alcohol and drug-induced cytopenias	• 5-Azacytidine • Allogeneic stem cell • Supportive care with transfusion, treatment of infections, and administration of recombinant growth factors

(continued)

Table 9-24

Disorders of Blood Cell Production (continued)

DISEASE	DEFINITION	ETIOLOGY	CLINICAL PRESENTATION	DIAGNOSIS	TREATMENT
Myeloproliferative Syndromes	• Clonal disorder of hematopoietic stem cells		• Median age of diagnosis 50–60 years • Cytopenias a late development	• No cellular dysplasia • Bone marrow hypercellular	
Chronic Myelogenous Leukemia (CML)	• Unregulated hyperproliferation of myeloid elements	• Balanced translocation t(9;22), called the Philadelphia chromosome produces the BCR-ABL gene	• Age: 50–60 • Elevated white cell count • Circulating myeloid precursors • High risk of leukemia transformation • After a proliferative, chronic phase, progresses to acute leukemic phase (blast crisis), which is often fatal	• t(9;22) by PCR or FISH or karyotype	• Imatinib mesylate inhibits BCR-ABLE and can suppress or eliminate the CML clone • Hydroxurea can decrease white count, but does not eliminate CML clone
Polycythemia Vera		• JAK2V617F mutation found in most patients	• Increased red cell mass • Clinical symptoms caused by hyperviscocsity, hypervolemia, and hypermetabolism (headache, pruritis, dyspnea, blurred vision, night sweats, facial plethora, and splenomegaly)	• Increased HCT > 60% for men and 56% for women • Rule out secondary cause of erythrocytosis • Platelets and white cells may also be elevated • Epogen level decreased	• Phlebotomy • Hydroxyurea

Polycythemia Vera (cont.)		• Bleeding thromboembolic events • Risk of cardiovascular events		• Anegrelide block megakaryocyte maturation • Aspirin if no risk of bleeding
Essential Thrombocytosis	• Clonal or autonomous thrombocytosis • JAK2V617F mutation found in half of patients	• Platelet counts exceed 600,000/uL • Symptoms include erythromelalgia, acral dysesthesia, headache, vision changes, and arterial or venous thrombosis • Bleeding can occur from intrinsic platelet dysfunction	• Elevated platelet count • Bone marrow shows fibrosis and megakaryocyte clusters • Diagnosis of exclusion	
Agnogenic Myeloid Metaplasia		• Bone marrow fibrosis that cannot be attributed to another myeloid disorder		

CML = chronic myeloid leukemia; EBV = Epstein-Barr virus; NSAIDs = nonsteroidal anti-inflammatory drugs; PCR = polymerase chain reaction; WHO = World Health Organization; FISH = fluorescent in situhybridization.

Table 9-25

Bleeding Diathesis

PROLONGED PT AND PTT	PROLONGED PTT/ NORMAL PT	PROLONGED PT/NORMAL PTT	NORMAL PT AND PTT
• Deficiency of or inhibitors to prothrombin, fibrinogen factors V and X • Combined factor deficiencies • Liver disease • DIC • Supratherapeutic doses of heparin or warfarin	• Deficiencies of factors VIII, IX, XI, XII, vWF • Inhibitors of factors VIII, IX, XI, XII • Heparin • Lupus anticoagulant	• Deficiency factor VII or vitamin K • Warfarin treatment • Inhibitors of factor VII • Liver disease	• von Willebrand disease • Thrombocytopenia • Platelet dysfunction

Table 9-26

Types of Bleeding

	THROMBOCYTOPENIA OR PLATELET DYSFUNCTION	CLOTTING FACTOR DEFICIENCY
Bleeding Response to Surgery/Cuts	• Postsurgical bleeding mild and immediate • Bleeding after minor cuts	• Postsurgical bleeding delayed • Bleeding after minor cuts less common
Typical Types of Bleeding	• Epistaxis • Gingival bleeding • Bullous hemorrhages on buccal mucosa • Petechiae • Ecchymoses (small, superficial) • GI or genitourinary bleeding • Spontaneous bleeding can occur when platelets less than 10,000/uL	• Deep bleeding (tissues, muscles, and joints) • Ecchymoses (large and palpable) • Few petechiae • Delayed bleeding

Table 9-27

Acquired Bleeding Disorders

DISEASE	ETIOLOGY	FEATURES	TREATMENT
Disseminated Intravascular Coagulation (DIC)	• Infection • Trauma • Inflammation • Malignancy	• Microangiopathic hemolysis • Low fibrinogen • Elevated PT, PTT • Thrombocytopenia	• Supportive transfusion (platelets, FFP) • Treat underlying cause

Table 9-27

Acquired Bleeding Disorders (continued)

DISEASE	ETIOLOGY	FEATURES	TREATMENT
Immune Thrombocytopenic Purpura	• IgG autoantibody-coated platelets cleared more quickly • Autoantibody often recognizes more than one platelet glycoprotein • May be idiopathic • May be secondary to lupus, HIV, hepatitis B, or lymphoproliferative disorder	• Isolated thrombocytopenia • Petechiae • Conjunctival hemorrhage • Minimal splenomegaly • Megathrombocytes	• If no clinical bleeding and platelets less than 30,000: prednisone • If clinically important bleeding or refractory to steroids: consider IVIG, anti-D immune globulin (if Rh-positive) or rituximab • 50–70% respond to steroids • Splenectomy if severe • If *Helicobacter pylori* infection present, may respond to *H. pylori* treatment
Antiphospholipid Antibodies	• See Table 9-18		
TTP-HUS	• See Table 9-15		
Thrombocytopenia	• See Table 9-29		
Platelet Dysfunction	• See Table 9-30		

Table 9-28

Pregnancy-Associated Hematologic Disorders

	TRIMESTER	CLINICAL PRESENTATION	TREATMENT/NOTES
Preeclampsia	• Third	• Hypertension and proteinuria (>300 mg/24 h) are hallmarks • Occurs after 20 week of gestation • Thrombocytopenia in many cases	• Early delivery if >34 weeks or severe disease • Conservative treatment if <34 weeks • Signs and symptoms usually resolve with delivery
HELLP	• Third • Postpartum	• Microangiopathic hemolytic anemia • Thrombocytopenia with platelets < 100,000 • AST > 70 U/L	• Early delivery if >34 weeks or severe disease • Higher maternal and fetal morbidity and mortality than with preeclampsia • Signs and symptoms usually resolve with delivery

(continued)

Table 9-28

Pregnancy-Associated Hematologic Disorders (continued)

	TRIMESTER	CLINICAL PRESENTATION	TREATMENT/NOTES
AFLP	• Third	• Nausea, vomiting, malaise, RUQ pain, dyspnea, mental status changes • Cholestatic laboratory changes • Microangiopathic hemolysis is *NOT* a significant feature • Serious consumptive coagulopathy and reduced levels of antithrombin	• Supportive care and urgent delivery
Gestational Thrombocytopenia (Incidental Thrombocytopenia of Pregnancy)	• Second or • Third	• Most common cause of thrombocytopenia in pregnant women (up to 10% of pregnancies have thrombocytopenia) • Counts usually remain over 10,000	• Fetal platelet counts normal • No adverse pregnancy outcomes
Immune Thrombocytopenia Purpura	• First • Second, or • Third	• See Table 9-27	• See Table 9-27 • Fetal platelet counts are low in 10%, severely so in 5%
SLE		• May be difficult to distinguish from preeclampsia • Decreased levels of C3 and C4	
Antiphospholipid antibodies (APLA)		• Antiphospholipid antibodies are associated with preeclampsia, HELLP, TTP, and HUS • If clinical course is unchanged with delivery, consider the presence of antiphospholipid antibodies	• See Table 9-18
TTP	• Second	• See Table 9-15	• No benefit to early delivery • See Table 9-15
HUS	• Postpartum	• See Table 9-15	• No benefit to early delivery • See Table 9-15

AFLP = acute fatty liver of pregnancy; APLA = antiphospholipid antibodies; AST = aspartate transaminase; HELLP = Hemolysis, Elevated Liver enzymes, Low Platelets; RUQ = right upper quadrant.

Table 9-29
Thrombocytopenia

	ETIOLOGY	DIAGNOSIS	TREATMENT
Drug-Induced	• Common cause of thrombocytopenia in critically ill patients • Heparin • Valproic acid • Antibiotics • Platelet GP IIb/IIIA inhibitor • Others	• Clinical history • "Peripheral smear" to rule out platelet clumping (pseudothrombocytopenia and schistocytes)	• Discontinue offending drug
Infection	• Common cause of thrombocytopenia in critically ill patients • DIC (see Table 9-26) • Antiplatelet antibodies cause enhanced clearance of platelets • Direct infection of bone marrow by viruses		• Treat underlying infection • Transfuse to keep platelets greater than 15,000–20,000
ITP	• See Table 9-27		
TTP-HUS	• See Table 9-15		
Antiphospholipid Antibody	• See Table 9-18		

ITP = idiopathic thrombocytopenic purpura.

Table 9-30
Causes of Platelet Dysfunction

CATEGORY	ETIOLOGY	TREATMENT
Chronic Renal Failure (Uremia)	• Uremia	• dDAVP • Estrogen • Platelet transfusion • Aprotinin (serine protease inhibitor) reduces blood loss in cardiac bypass surgery • Stop offending agent • Treat underlying disease
Drug	• Aspirin (irreversible) • NSAIDs (reversible) • Clopidogrel • GPIIb/IIIa receptor antagonists	
Myeloproliferative Disease		

(continued)

Table 9-30

Causes of Platelet Dysfunction (continued)

CATEGORY	ETIOLOGY	TREATMENT
Alcohol	• See Table 9-31	• See above
Genetic	• Rare • Bernard-Soulier syndrome: defect in components of the GPIb/IX/V complex, associated with thrombocytopenia	

GP = glycoprotein.

Table 9-31

Hematologic Effects of Ethanol Abuse

- Anemia of chronic disease
- Macrocytic anemia
- Dysfunctional fibrinogen
- Thrombocytopenia (marrow suppression or hypersplenism)
- Leukopenia (specifically decreased neutrophils)

Table 9-32

Acute Leukemias

	ETIOLOGY	CLINICAL PRESENTATION	DIAGNOSIS	CHROMOSOMAL ABNORMALITY	TREATMENT
AML	• Incidence increases with age • Incidence increases if exposed to chemotherapy drugs (alkylating agents and topoisomerase II inhibitors) • Multiple chromosome abnormalities	• Often presents with bleeding or infection	• Bone marrow biopsy is hypercellular • Multiple chromosomalities possible • WBC can be normal, elevated or low • Platelets often low • Blasts in peripheral blood • Uric acid may be elevated	• APL subtype is associated with t(15;17) and may have severe DIC • Monosomy 5 or 7 associated with history of chemotherapy or MDS and has poor prognosis • t(8;21) associated with a good prognosis	• Chemotherapy (may need urgently) • Xanthine oxidase inhibitor (allopurinol) given to patients prior to chemotherapy to prevent urate nephropathy (a complication of tumor lysis) • Increased risk for tumor lysis syndrome if high WBC or high tumor burden • APL subtype treated with all-trans retinoic acid and chemotherapy • Allogeneic marrow transplantation if poor prognosis
ALL	• More common in children than adults • 80% of cases are B-cell • 20% of cases are T-cell	• Often present with prodrome of fever, sore throat, and lethargy for a few weeks • Lymphadenopathy and splenomegaly may be present • CNS involvement more common than in AML • B-cell ALL has worse prognosis			• Chemotherapy (may need urgently) • Allogeneic marrow transplantation if poor prognosis • May need maintenance therapy for years • Intrathecal chemotherapy with or without radiation to treat/prevent meningeal leukemia • Up to 75% of children have long-term survival

(continued)

Table 9-32

Acute Leukemias (continued)

	Etiology	Clinical Presentation	Diagnosis	Chromosomal Abnormality	Treatment
ALL (cont.)					• Up to 40% of adults have long-term survival • Xanthine oxidase inhibitor (allopurinol) given to patients prior to chemotherapy to prevent urate nephropathy (a complication of tumor lysis) • Increased risk for tumor lysis syndrome if high WBC or high tumor burden

ALL = acute lymphoid leukemia; AML = acute myeloid leukemia; APL = acute promyelocytic leukemia; CNS = central nervous system; MDS = myelodysplastic syndrome; WBC = white blood cell.

Table 9-33

Indications for Hematologic Stem Cell Transplant

TYPE OF TRANSPLANT	ALLOGENEIC STEM CELL TRANSPLANT	AUTOLOGOUS STEM CELL TRANSPLANT
Common Indications for Transplantation in Adults	• Chronic myelogenous leukemia (CML) • Acute myelogenous leukemia (AML) • Acute lymphocytic leukemia (ALL) • Aplastic anemia • MDS	• Multiple myeloma • Amyloidosis • Chemotherapy-sensitive relapsed NHL • Relapsed Hodgkin disease
Note	• High-dose chemotherapy is given to the patient to eradicate the diseased cells. However, normal hematopoietic cells are also wiped out • Stem cells from a donor are infused into the recipient after high-dose chemotherapy in order to repopulate the bone marrow • A 6/6 HLA match often found amongst relatives of patient. However, "matches" can be unrelated • Relatively high mortality rate from procedure	• Stem cells from the patient are harvested and frozen prior to the administration of high-dose chemotherapy • High-dose chemotherapy is given to the patient to eradicate the diseased cells. However, normal hematopoietic cells are also wiped out • The patient's own cells are infused back into the patient after high-dose chemotherapy in order to repopulate the bone marrow • Lower mortality rate than from allogeneic stem cell transplant

NHL = non hodgkin lymphoma.

Oncology

Table 10-1

Biologic, Epidemiologic, Clinical Trial Terms, and Considerations in Cancer Research

TERM	DESCRIPTION	EXAMPLE
Biology		
Tumor Suppressor Gene	• Inhibits the cell cycle • If mutated, normal control mechanisms no longer work and growth proceeds unchecked	• APC gene mutations seem to be an early event in the development of colon cancer
Proto-Oncogene	• Activation of mutations activate growth signals	• Ras mutations can result in a constitutively active GTP-bound protein
Epidemiology		
Relative Cancer Risk	• The risk of cancer in one group compared to the risk of cancer in another group • Calculated by dividing the incidence in exposed group by the incidence in unexposed group	• The incidence of colon cancer among nurses with high dietary fiber divided by the incidence of colon cancer among nurses with low dietary fiber
Attributable Cancer Risk	• The additional incidence of a particular cancer related to an exposure taking into account the background rate of that cancer • Calculated by subtracting the incidence of a disease in nonexposed persons from the incidence of disease in exposed persons	• Incidence of lung cancer in smokers minus the incidence of lung cancer in nonsmokers gives the attributable risk of smoking on lung cancer
Genetic Risk Factor	• Genetic anomaly that predisposes to cancer	• Breast cancer gene 1 (BRCA 1) increases the risk of breast and ovarian cancer
Environmental Risk Factor	• Environmental factor that predisposes to cancer	• Asbestos exposure increases the risk of lung cancer and mesothelioma
Modifiable Risk Factor	• Risk factor that can be changed	• Smoking
Nonmodifiable Risk Factor	• Risk factor that cannot be changed	• Gender; genetic risk factors
Strong Risk Factor	• Risk factor with a large impact on risk	• Smoking for lung cancer
Weak Risk Factor	• Risk factor with a small impact on risk	• Alcohol intake for breast cancer

(continued)

Table 10-1

Biologic, Epidemiologic, Clinical Trial Terms, and Considerations in Cancer Research (continued)

Term	Description	Example
Clinical Trial		
Selection Bias	• Patients on different arms of a clinical trial are different in some way from each other, or from patients not enrolled in a particular trial	• Patients who can travel to an academic center to participate in a trial may be healthier than those who cannot do so—if they do better on the trial, maybe they would have done better without the trial treatment
Lead-Time Bias	• Finding a cancer earlier but without an impact on survival: the patient lives with the diagnosis longer but still dies at the same age	• If a prostate cancer is discovered 2 years earlier because of a more sensitive screening test, the patient may live with the knowledge of the prostate cancer longer. However, finding it earlier may not change the patient's survival
Length Bias	• Screening detects a greater number of slow growing tumors, which may also be less aggressive	• Yearly mammography may miss a rapidly growing tumor that developed after the last mammogram, but will catch most slow-growing tumors
Adjuvant Treatment	• Treatment given after complete resection of cancer • Goal: cure	• Hormonal therapy for early stage breast cancer
Neoadjuvant Treatment	• Treatment given before resection of cancer • Goal: shrink tumor to facilitate surgery	• Chemotherapy combined with radiation prior to surgery may improve resectability of lung cancer
Palliation	• Treatment given for metastatic cancer • Goal: relief and/or prevention of symptoms	• Radiation for pain caused by metastases to the bone

APC = adenomatosis polyposis coli; GTP = guanosine triphosphate.

Table 10-2

Cancer Risk Factors, Prevention, and Screening

CANCER	RISK FACTOR	GENETIC RISK FACTOR	PROTECTIVE FACTOR	PREVENTION	SCREENING
Breast	• Increased age • Alcohol use • Increased exposure to estrogens - Menarche at <12 years - First full-term pregnancy >30 years - Exogenous estrogens (birth control or hormone replacement) • Family history (mother or sister = 2.6 increased relative risk) • History of having a breast biopsy (even if benign findings)	• Breast cancer gene 1 and 2 (BRCA 1 and 2) autosomal dominant gene mutations: 5–10% of breast cancers • Li Fraumeni (a rare autosomal dominant disorder. p53 mutation predisposes to many forms of cancer)	• Breast feeding • Increased parity • Exercise • Oophorectomy before age 35 • Body mass index <22.9	• If high risk (BRCA 1 and 2 positive): consider prophylactic mastectomy and oophorectomy vs. intensive screening vs. tamoxifen • Tamoxifen for 5 years reduces the risk of invasive breast cancer in high-risk patients	• Mammogram • Screen for BRCA 1 and 2 if a family history of breast cancer at an early age, especially if ovarian cancer in the family or Ashkenazi Jew
Cervix (Uterine)	• HPV • Smoking • HIV infection		• HIV treatment if HIV positive	• HPV vaccination	• Regular Pap smears

(continued)

Table 10-2
Cancer Risk Factors, Prevention, and Screening (continued)

CANCER	RISK FACTOR	GENETIC RISK FACTOR	PROTECTIVE FACTOR	PREVENTION	SCREENING

Colorectal	• Family history:
	  - One first-degree relative <60 years at diagnosis
	  - Two first-degree relatives of any age at diagnosis
	• Inflammatory bowel disease
	• Diabetes
	• Cholecystectomy
	• Alcohol consumption
	• Smoking, especially at an early age
	• Physical inactivity
	• Polyps: cancer risk increases with size > 1 cm, villous histology (as opposed to tubular), and increased number of polyps
		• FAP (<1% of colon cancers): autosomal dominant. APC gene
		• HNPCC (2–6% of colon cancers): autosomal dominant
		• BRCA 1 gene mutation
		• Peutz-Jeghers: rare autosomal dominant multiple hamartomatous polyps in the gastrointestinal tract and distinctive mucocutaneous pigmentations
			• Diet rich in fruit and vegetables	• Calcium may reduce risk of adenomas
				• NSAIDs reduce recurrent polyps
				• Folic acid supplementation
					• Evolving consensus: colonoscopy starting at age 50, then every 10 years if average risk
					• High risk: regular colonoscopy.
					• Consider colectomy in second or third decade for patients with FAP

Endometrium	• Increased estrogen exposure • Obesity • Tamoxifen use • Age (usually postmenopausal women)	• HNPCC	• Oral contraceptive use • Physical activity		• None routine
Esophagus	• Smoking • Alcohol consumption • Achalasia • Barrett's • Caustic injury				• High risk (Barrett's): routine endoscopy
Head and Neck— Nasopharyngeal	• EBV				• None routine

	Risk Factors	Genetics	Prevention	Screening
Head and Neck Squamous Cell	• Alcohol consumption • Smoking		• 13-cis retinoic acid increases regression of oral leukoplakia	• None routine
Hepatocellular	• Hepatitis • Cirrhosis		• If high risk: hepatitis B vaccination	• High risk (cirrhosis, some hepatitis B carriers): ultrasound and AFP screening

Lung	• Cigarette smoke, including second-hand exposure (contributes up to 87% of cases)
	• Asbestos (concomitant smoking multiplies risk)
	• Radon
	• Arsenic and nickel exposure
	• Ionizing radiation and radon
	• Halo-ethers
	• Polycyclic aromatic hydrocarbons
	• Beta-carotene
			• Smoking cessation:
			  - Most effective cancer prevention strategy available
			  - Nicotine replacement with bupropion most effective
			  - 13-cis retinoic acid does not prevent primary lung cancer
				• None standard
				• High risk (smoker): CT scanning controversial

Leukemia	• Chemotherapy • Smoking • Radiation • Benzene • Viruses: HTLV-1 • Myelodysplatic syndrome or myeloproliferative syndromes	• Down's syndrome • Fanconi anemia • Ataxia telengiectasia • 9;22 translocation in chronic myeloid leukemia (BCR to ABL) also called Philadelphia chromosome		• None routine
Lymphoma	• Pesticides • HIV/EBV infection	• t(14:18) (lymphoma) • t(8;14) c-myc (Burkitts) • Many others		• None routine

(continued)

Table 10-2

Cancer Risk Factors, Prevention, and Screening (continued)

CANCER	RISK FACTOR	GENETIC RISK FACTOR	PROTECTIVE FACTOR	PREVENTION	SCREENING
Mesothelioma	• Asbestos • Smoking • Radiation				• None routine
Ovary	• Multiple follicle ruptures: late age at menopause, nulliparity	• BRCA 1 and 2 mutation • Family history	• Oral contraceptive use • Multiple pregnancies		• High risk: controversial. Consider oophorectomy or pelvic ultrasound twice a year with serum CA-125
Pancreas	• Smoking • Diabetes • Chronic pancreatitis	• K-ras mutation (95%) • P16 mutation (90%) • Peutz-Jeghers (STK11/LKB1 mutation has a 36% lifetime risk of pancreatic cancer) • BRCA mutations			• None routine
Prostate	• Age • High fat diet • African American	• Family history • BRCA 1 mutations			• Controversial: yearly PSA screening, digital rectal examination after age 50
Skin - Nonmelanoma - Melanoma	• Sun exposure/severe sunburn history • Immunosuppression (especially squamous) • Exposure to psoralen or UVA (especially melanoma)	• Xeroderma pigmentosum • Family history • FAMMM (familial atypical mole melanoma syndrome) • CDK N2A (P16 gene) (melanoma)	• Protection from sun exposure (sunscreen is controversial as it may encourage people to stay in the sun longer)	• Protection from sun exposure	• Regular skin examination • High risk: photo documentation of moles, frequent examinations
Testicular/ Extragonadal Germ Cell Tumors	• Cryptorchid testes increase risk for testicular cancer • Klinefelter syndrome (mediastinal germ cell tumor)	• Isochromosome of the short arm of chromosome 12: i(12p)		• Correct undescended testes before the age of 2	• Testicular examinations in men aged 20–40

FAP = familial adenomatous polyposis; HNPCC = hereditary nonpolyposis colorectal cancer; HPV = human papilloma virus; NSAIDs = nonsteroidal anti-inflammatory drugs.

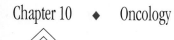

Breast Cancer

Epidemiology: Breast cancer is the most common cancer diagnosed in American females and is the second most frequent cause of cancer death in women.

Clinical Presentation: Physical examination may reveal a firm, mobile mass. Skin dimpling, skin retraction, peau d'orange skin, or bloody nipple discharge also may be seen.

Prognosis: The presence or absence of cancer in the axillary nodes is the most important prognostic factor for survival in women with early-stage breast cancer.

Table 10-3
Diagnostic Evaluation of a Breast Mass

AGE GROUP	FIRST STEP	SECOND STEP	BIOPSY	FOLLOW-UP/NOTE
Under 35 Years Old	• Ultrasound or fine needle aspiration. • Breasts may be too dense for mammogram to pick up lesion	• Send aspirated fluid for cytology	• If not clearly cystic on evaluation	• May follow for a short time if not suspicious • Always biopsy if mass persists
Over 35 Years Old	• Mammogram (misses 10–20% of palpable masses)	• Ultrasound if needed	• If not clearly cystic on evaluation	• Failure to recommend a breast biopsy increases risk for litigation

AFP = alpha-fetoprotein.

Table 10-4
Evaluation and Initial Surgical Management of a Breast Mass

Routine Workup	• Chest x-ray, liver function tests, bilateral mammogram • Bone scan and CT abdomen/pelvis to evaluate for metastatic disease if symptomatic or abnormal labs • Tumor markers are not useful for diagnosis, but may be useful to follow response to treatment
Surgical Approach	
Mastectomy	• Recommended if: - Cosmetically difficult to do lumpectomy (small breast, large tumor, multicentric disease) - Persistently positive margins after multiple surgical attempts - Prior radiation to chest

(*continued*)

Table 10-4

Evaluation and Initial Surgical Management of a Breast Mass (continued)

Breast-Conserving Surgery	• Lumpectomy and axillary node (full axillary dissection or sentinel node) followed by radiation has the same survival outcome as mastectomy
Sentinel Node	• The sentinel lymph node is established by following the drainage of the dye/radioactive tracer injected into the site of the primary breast mass • Sentinel lymph node biopsy has less morbidity (lymphedema, pain, etc.) compared to full axillary dissection • If the sentinel lymph node is negative, a full axillary dissection is avoided • If the sentinel lymph node is positive, axillary dissection should be performed

Table 10-5

Treatment for Breast Cancer—Local Disease

	ADJUVANT CHEMOTHERAPY	ADJUVANT ENDOCRINE THERAPY	RADIATION
Notes on Indication	Features that may increase the benefit of chemotherapy: • Tumor large (>1 cm) • Positive lymph nodes • "Bad" features on pathology such as lymphovascular invasion • Hormone receptor negative • Trastuzumab (monoclonal antibody) if tumor is Her2/neu positive	• Tumor should be ER and/or PR positive • Given after chemotherapy • Tamoxifen if premenopausal (5 years) • Tamoxifen and/or aromatase inhibitors if postmenoapausal (5 years)	• Given after breast-conserving surgery
Toxicities	• Cardiac (adriamycin and trastuzumab) • Neutropenia • Secondary leukemia • Premature ovarian failure/amenorrhea	• Hot flashes (can treat with venlafaxine but not hormone replacement therapy) • Vaginal dryness • Aromatase inhibitors decrease bone density • Tamoxifen increases risk of endometrial cancer (risk doubled to 1%) • DVT/pulmonary emboli	• Pneumonitis (1%) • Pericardial fibrosis • Secondary cancers (contralateral breast cancer, lung cancer, leukemia, sarcoma) • Accelerated atherosclerosis

Table 10-5

Treatment for Breast Cancer—Local Disease (continued)

	ADJUVANT CHEMOTHERAPY	ADJUVANT ENDOCRINE THERAPY	RADIATION
Prognosis	• Chemotherapy decreases absolute risk of death at 15 years by 3–10% depending on age, hormone receptor status, and lymph node status • Chemotherapy offers a larger absolute mortality benefit to younger women, to women with hormone negative tumors and women with node positive tumors • Trastuzumab (given in addition to chemotherapy) decreases risk of recurrence by up to 50% if tumor is Her2/neu positive	• 5 years of tamoxifen decreases risk of mortality by 9% at 15 years, risk of recurrence by 9–16%, and risk of contralateral breast cancer by >30% • Aromatase inhibitors are useful only in postmenopausal women	• In appropriate situations, lumpectomy plus radiation has the same survival benefit as mastectomy

DVT = deep venous thrombosis; ER = estrogen receptor; PR = progesterone receptor.

Table 10-6

Surveillance for Breast Cancer Survivors

	SCREENING	NOTES
Breast Cancer Surveillance	• Physical examination • Mammography yearly	• Scans, labs, and tumor markers are not cost-effective for routine follow-up and are not recommended unless there are specific signs or symptoms
Uterine Cancer Surveillance	• Annual gynecologic evaluation if treated with tamoxifen	• Irregular vaginal bleeding requires careful follow-up and biopsy

Table 10-7

Staging and Treatment for Advanced Breast Cancer

	Stage: Locally Advanced	**Stage: Metastatic**
Definition	• Tumor >5 cm • Extensive regional lymph node involvement • Direct involvement of skin or underlying chest wall • Inflammatory cancer (tender, firm, enlarged breast with dimpled orange peel "peau d'orange" appearance)	• Spread to distant organ
Surgical Options	• Resect if possible as potentially curable	• May be useful to palliate symptoms
Chemotherapy/ Radiation	• Give chemotherapy and radiation after surgery or before surgery (neoadjuvant) if need to shrink tumor to make resection easier	• Give chemotherapy if need a fast response, or if tumor hormone receptor negative. Multiple possible regimens
Endocrine Therapy	• Can use after chemotherapy if tumor is hormone receptor positive	• Can use if tumor less aggressive, and is hormone receptor positive
Monoclonal Antibody Treatment	• Trastuzumab if tumor is Her2/neu positive	• Can use trastuzumab if tumor is Her2/neu positive
Palliative Treatment	• N/A	• Bisphosphonates for bony metastasis • Radiation for bone/brain metastasis

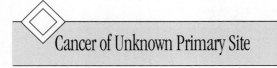

Cancer of Unknown Primary Site

Definition: Malignant cells without evidence of origin despite a full workup and a complete history. A full evaluation by histological type is suggested in Table 10-8. Although detection of the primary source is useful to guiding treatment options, the primary tumor may not be found.

Epidemiology: 3–5% of all cancer. At autopsy, the primary site is not found in 25%. The most common primary sites are lung and pancreas.

Prognosis: Generally poor.

Table 10-8

Cancer of Unknown Primary Site by Histology

BIOPSY HISTOLOGY	SITE TO EVALUATE	WORKUP	TREATMENT IF PRIMARY SITE NOT FOUND
Adenocarcinoma (70% of Unknown Primary Cancers)	• Pancreas, hepatobiliary tree, and lung account for 40–50% • Breast • Ovary • Uterus • Prostate	Depending on history and examination, consider: • CXR • Pelvic examination • Mammogram and breast examination • Hormone receptor status (estrogen/progesterone receptor) of tumor • Prostate examination and serum PSA • PSA staining of tumor • Stool for occult blood • Pattern of tumor immunohistochemistry staining for CK7 and 20 may be particularly helpful to suggest a primary site	• Depends on context: - Malignant ascites in a woman: Treat for ovarian cancer - Blastic bony disease and elevated PSA in a man: Treat for prostate cancer - Axillary nodes in a woman: Treat for breast cancer - Axillary nodes in a male smoker: Treat for lung cancer - Axillary nodes in a male nonsmoker: Treat for melanoma
Squamous Cell (5% of Unknown Primary Cancers)	• Head and neck • Lung • Esophagus • Skin • Penis • Anus • Cervix	• Skin examination • If disease is in the neck: - Chest CT - Bronchoscopy/ENT evaluation with biopsies • If disease is in the groin: - Gynecologic examination/Pap smear - Examine penis - Examine anus/anal Pap smear	• Depends on context: - Cervical nodes: Treat for head and neck cancer (even if no primary found, radical neck dissection and/or radiation can give 30–50% long-term survival) • Inguinal nodes: Treat for genital or anal cancer • Not found in cervical or inguinal nodes treat for lung cancer
Poorly differentiated (20% of Unknown Primary Cancers)	• Lymphoma (30–60%) • Carcinoma (second most common) • Extragonadal germ cell tumor • Melanoma • Sarcoma • Neuroendocrine	• Immunohistochemistry of tumor: CK7, CK29, LCA (positive in lymphoma), S-100 (positive in melanoma) and hCG/AFP (germ cell tumors)	• Aggressively rule out extragonadal germ cell tumor because these may be cured • Lymphomas often responsive to treatment

hCG = human chorionic gonadotropin; ENT = ear, nose, and throat; CK = cytokeratin; CXR = chest x-ray.

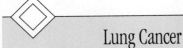

Lung Cancer

Etiology/Epidemiology: Lung cancer is the primary cause of cancer-related deaths in both men and women. Lung cancer is divided into two main types: non-small-cell lung cancer (NSCLC) (increasing in incidence) and small-cell lung cancer (SCLC) (decreasing in incidence). For histological types and relationship to smoking, see Table 10-10.

Clinical Presentation: Patients commonly present with cough, hemoptysis, and weight loss. Other common symptoms include hoarseness, anorexia, and paraneoplastic syndromes. Pleural involvement may be associated with pleuritic chest pain or shoulder/back pain.

Diagnosis: Isolated nodules on CT that double within 1 year are often usually malignant. Other suspicious radiologic features include lesions that are larger than 1 cm, have irregular borders, and lack of benign calcification patterns. Depending on tumor location and institutional expertise, tissue for pathologic diagnosis may be obtained with surgical approach, CT-guided needle biopsy, or bronchoscopy.

Table 10-9
Histology, Treatment, and Prognosis of Lung Cancer

HISTOLOGICAL TYPE	PERCENTAGE	TYPICAL PRESENTATION	TREATMENT/STAGING	PROGNOSIS	NOTES

Non-Small-Cell: Squamous	• 20–30%	• Central lesions	• Treatment: resection offers best opportunity for long-term survival:
			  - Must be fully staged
			  - Must have adequate lung capacity
			• Adjuvant chemotherapy prolongs survival after resection
			• Staging: CT chest including adrenals and bone scan if symptoms. Lymph node biopsy and mediastinoscopy may be necessary. PET scan may be useful to rule out metastatic disease
			• Stages I-III:
			  - Resect if possible
			  - Depending on pathologic stage and resectability, consider chemotherapy and/or radiation as adjuvant or definitive treatment
			• Stage IV:
			  - Metastatic disease
			  - Chemotherapy may improve survival by a few months
				• Resected stage I: 50–70% 5-year disease free survival
				• Resected stage II: 20–40% 5-year disease free survival
				• Stage III (mediastinal involvement): 2–15% 5-year survival
				• Stage IV: median survival 6–9 months
					• Bronchoalveolar subtype of adenocarcinoma (up to 20% of cases) is more common in women and non-smokers

Non-Small-Cell: Adenocarcinoma	• 30–40%	• Peripheral lesions			
Non-Small-Cell: Large Cell	• 10%				

Small Cell	• 20%	• Typically disseminated at presentation
		  - 35% with bone metastases
		  - 10% with CNS disease
			• Staging is not as important as in non-small-cell because most cases involve occult or overt metastatic disease
			• Limited stage: tumor confined to one hemithorax and fits inside radiation field
			  - Treatment combines chemotherapy and radiation
			  - Consider prophylactic brain radiation
			• Extensive stage: tumor does not fit in radiation port
			  - Chemotherapy
				• Typically responds well to chemotherapy but recurs quickly
				• Limited stage: median survival is 18–24 months
				• Extensive stage: median survival is 8–12 months
					• Most patients have a smoking history

CNS = central nervous system.

Table 10-10

Clinical Syndromes Associated with Lung Cancer

NAME	CLINICAL	CAUSE	TREATMENT
Superior Vena Cava Syndrome	• Headache • Dyspnea • Facial and upper extremity swelling and plethora • Dilated neck veins	• Obstruction of mediastinal nodes	• See Table 10-16

Pancoast Tumor	• Ipsilateral:
	  - Shoulder pain
	  - Horner syndrome
	  - Rib destruction
	  - Hand muscle atrophy from a superior sulcus tumor
		• Brachial plexus involvement by apical tumors	• Treat underlying disease, usually with radiation and chemotherapy

Horner Syndrome	• Ipsilateral:
	  - Ptosis
	  - Anhidrosis
	  - Miosis
		• Invasion of the last cervical or first thoracic segment of the sympathetic nerve trunk	

Paraneoplastic Syndrome	• Non-small-cell: adenocarcinoma:
	  - Hypertrophic pulmonary osteoarthropathy (periosteal thickening of long bones)
	  - Trousseau syndrome (hypercoagulable state)
	• Non-small-cell: squamous cell:
	  - Hypercalcemia
	• Small cell:
	  - 15% with SIADH
	  - Lambert-Eaton (proximal limb weakness and fatigue)
	  - Ectopic ACTH secretion (hypokalemia and hypertension)
		• Responsible proteins secreted by the tumor	• Severity typically parallels stage of disease, but does not necessarily imply disseminated disease
			• Symptoms typically resolve if the tumor responds to treatment

Hoarseness	• Hoarse or whispery voice	• Entrapment of recurrent laryngeal nerve (more common on left)	• Treat underlying disease
Tamponade	• Pulsus paradoxus • Low voltage on electrocardigram • Elevated jugular venous pressure • Dyspnea • Sinus tachycardia	• Direct extension of tumor to the pericardium	• Pericardiocentesis or pericardial window
Hemoptysis	• Ranges from blood-mixed sputum to life-threatening bleeding	• Tumor invades into bronchus and blood vessels	• Bronchoscopy with local treatment • Treat underlying disease

ACTH = adrenocorticotropic hormone; SIADH = syndrome of inappropriate antidiuretic hormone.

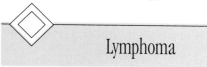

Lymphoma

Non-Hodgkin's Lymphoma

Definition: Clonal proliferations of lymphoid cells. Lymphoma can be divided into two general categories: low-grade and high-grade.

Etiology/Epidemiology: 90% of non-Hodgkin's lymphomas are derived from B-cells, 9% from T-cells, and 1% or fewer from natural killer cells or monocytes. Infectious agents such as Epstein-Barr virus (EBV), human immunodeficiency virus (HIV), and human T-lymphotropic virus (HTLV-1) can cause lymphomas (usually high-grade/aggressive). Chromosomal translocations are a common feature in all lymphomas.

Clinical Presentation: Lymphadenopathy is common, but may only be visualized on CT. Patients frequently present with night sweats, weight loss (>10% of baseline), and fever.

Diagnosis: Excisional biopsy of a lymph node is preferred over fine needle aspiration because the histological architecture is important for subtype diagnosis and treatment decisions. Bone marrow biopsy and positron emission tomography (PET) are important for staging.

Prognosis: The number of risk factors on the International Prognostic Index correlates with 5-year survival. See Table 10-13.

Table 10-11

Non-Hodgkin's Lymphoma Course, Treatment, and Prognosis

TYPE	EXAMPLE	CURABLE	URGENT TREATMENT	TREATMENT AND CLINICAL COURSE
Low Grade	• Follicular (40–45% of all lymphomas)	• No	• No	• Tend to be indolent and relapsing (i.e., slow growing, respond to chemotherapy +/– rituximab [monoclonal antibody against CD20, a B-cell marker], followed by slow return and is again responsive to treatment) • Median survival: 10 years • Can transform to aggressive disease (5–7% per year, "Richter's transformation") • MALT lymphoma found in the gastrointestinal tract and is sensitive to *Helicobacter pylori* treatment. May be cured with antibiotics if early stage
High Grade	• Diffuse large cell lymphoma (30–35% of all lymphomas)	• 40%	• Yes	• Without treatment, median survival is 6 months • Chemotherapy +/– rituximab • If relapse after initial chemotherapy response, 30% cure rate with autologous bone marrow transplant

MALT = mucosa-associated lymphoid tissue.

Hodgkin's Disease

Definition: Clonal malignancy of B-cells, typified by Reed-Sternberg cells.

Etiology/Epidemiology: Bimodal incidence: age 20–40 and >50 years.

Clinical Presentation: Commonly involves lymph nodes in the neck and/or supraclavicular area (60 to 80%). Spreads to contiguous lymph node groups.

Diagnosis: Same as for non-Hodgkin's lymphoma. Pathologic staging with exploratory laparotomy and splenectomy is rarely done now.

Treatment: Chemotherapy with or without radiation.

Prognosis: 80–85% cured; half of those not cured with initial treatment can be cured with high-dose chemotherapy and stem cell transplant. After treatment, patients have an increased rate of hematologic and solid organ cancers. Radiation to the chest increases the incidence of breast cancer, atherosclerosis, thyroid disease, pulmonary fibrosis, and pericardial stricture.

Table 10-12

Gammopathies: MGUS, Multiple Myeloma, Secondary Monoclonal Gammopathy, and Polyclonal Gammopathy

| Disease | Etiology | Diagnosis | | | | Epidemiology | Treatment | Prognosis |
		End-Organ Damage	Bone Marrow	SPEP				
MGUS	• Immunologically homogeneous protein produced by a proliferation of a single clone of plasma cells	• None	• <10% plasma cells	• IgG < 3.0 g/dL • Urine light chains = none		• Occurs in 4% of people over the age of 70 • Accounts for 2/3 of monoclonal gammopathies • 1% per year progress to multiple myeloma, macroglobulinemia, amyloidosis, or a malignant lymphoproliferative disorder	• Active surveillance with follow-up every 6–12 months	• Median survival: 2 years less than age-matched controls

(continued)

Table 10-12

Gammopathies: MGUS, Multiple Myeloma, Secondary Monoclonal Gammopathy, and Polyclonal Gammopathy (continued)

| DISEASE | ETIOLOGY | DIAGNOSIS | | | EPIDEMIOLOGY | TREATMENT | PROGNOSIS |
		END-ORGAN DAMAGE	BONE MARROW	SPEP			
Multiple Myeloma		• **Calcium** elevated • **Renal** dysfunction • **Anemia** • **Bone:** lytic lesions on skeletal survey (80% with bone pain at presentation)	• >30% plasma cells	• IgG >3.5 g/dL • IgA >2.0 g/dL • Urine light chains > 1 g/24 h	• Median age of onset is 70 years • Incidence is higher in African Americans	• High-dose chemotherapy and stem cell transplant if less than 60 years • Alkylating agent and steroids reduce myeloma burden	• Median survival is 2–2.5 years (15% die within first 3 months) • No cure even with treatment • Causes of death: sepsis, hypercalcemia, renal failure, and hemorrhage

Secondary Monoclonal Gammopathy	• Elevation of monoclonal protein secondary to systemic illnesses (rather than a proliferation of a plasma cell clone)
	• Associated with:
	  - Autoimmune disorders
	  - Malignancies (solid tumor and hematologic)
	  - Cirrhosis
	  - Parasitic diseases						

Polyclonal Gammopathy	• Elevation of immunoglobulins due to multiple plasma cell clones (broad band on SPEP)
	• Associated with:
	  - Liver disease
	  - HIV
	  - Connective tissue disorders						

MGUS = monoclonal gammopathy of unknown significance; SPEP = serum protein electrophoresis.

Prostate Cancer

Etiology/Epidemiology: Second-most frequent malignancy in men (second to nonmelanotic skin cancer.) Median age is 72 years. Most men with prostate cancer will die *with* prostate cancer rather than *from* prostate cancer. African Americans have an increased risk of disease as well as increased rates of advanced disease.

Clinical Presentation: Most cases of prostate cancer are diagnosed by prostate-specific antigen (PSA) screening and are asymptomatic. Asymmetric areas of induration or prostate nodules palpated on digital rectal examination are suggestive of prostate cancer. PSA values between 4 and 10 ng/mL may be seen with both benign prostatic hypertrophy and prostate cancer.

Biopsy is recommended for PSA >10 ng/mL and often recommended for PSA > 4 ng/mL. For PSA <4 ng/mL factors such as how fast the PSA has risen, prostate cancer risk factors, and patient preference help guide decision making. Overall, PSA screening is controversial because of the increased rate of detection without an increase in survival. In addition, there is nontrivial morbidity associated with treatment.

Diagnosis: Transrectal biopsy performed to obtain tissue for diagnosis. The Gleason score describes how aggressive the tumor cells appear under the microscope (the grade). Higher Gleason scores have a worse prognosis. Bone scan and pelvic CT for full staging if the Gleason score is greater than 6, the PSA is greater than 10, or if the patient has symptoms.

Prognosis: Generally good, unless metastatic disease is present.

Table 10-13

Prostate Cancer Treatment, Side effects, and Course by Disease Stage

STAGE	TREATMENT OPTION	SIDE EFFECTS	TREATMENT DECISION	COURSE
Localized	• Radical prostatectomy	• Up to 60% have varying degrees of incontinence • Up to 60% are impotent	• All approaches generally yield the same benefit • Choice based on patient and clinician preference, patient age/ surgical risk and side-effect profile	• 30–40% chance of biochemical relapse with any definitive local therapy • Development of metastatic disease most common in patients with biochemical relapse within 2 years, rapid PSA doubling time or poor initial prognosis
	• Radiation therapy	• Proctitis • Cystitis • Some late occurring impotence		
	• Hormone therapy	• Loss of libido/ impotence • Hot flashes • Osteoporosis		
	• Active surveillance	• Anxiety		

(continued)

Table 10-13

Prostate Cancer Treatment, Side effects, and Course by Disease Stage (continued)

STAGE	TREATMENT OPTION	SIDE EFFECTS	TREATMENT DECISION	COURSE
Advanced/ Metastatic	• Androgen deprivation therapy - LHRH agonist (stimulation lowers amount of androgen released) - Antiandrogen agent	• Loss of libido/impotence • Hot flashes • Osteoporosis	• Use hormonal treatments until proven refractory	• Palliate pain from bony metastasis with radiation
	• Chemotherapy	• Depends on treatment		

LHRH = luteinising-hormone releasing hormone.

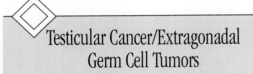

Testicular Cancer/Extragonadal Germ Cell Tumors

Definition: Malignant cells arising from the germ cells.

Etiology/Epidemiology: Most frequent malignancy in men between the ages of 20 and 35 years.

Clinical Presentation: Frequently presents as a painless, unilateral testicular mass. Many patients have a history of oligospermia or sperm abnormalities. Always consider germ cell tumors in the differential of a mediastinal mass because it is treatable.

Diagnosis: Definitive diagnosis is made by radical inguinal orchiectomy. Biopsy and/or removal of the testes through the scrotal tissue increases the risk of metastasis. Full staging consists of serum tumor markers and an abdominal CT to evaluate for retroperitoneal and para-aortic lymph nodes. It is important to distinguish between seminoma and nonseminoma (by pathology and tumor markers) because treatment differs.

Treatment: Testicular cancer is one of the most curable cancers. Even if the cancer recurs after initial treatment, most patients can be cured with chemotherapy or radiation. Therefore, careful follow-up is essential. If tumor markers are elevated, treatment should be associated with a complete decline of tumor markers to normal as predicted by their half-lives. Sperm banking should be offered to all patients. Many men recover sperm production 1–2 years after treatment and can father children.

Table 10-14

Testicular/Extragonadal Germ Cell Tumor Pathology, Cure Rates, and Treatment Issues

TUMOR TYPE	PATHOLOGY	RADIOSENSITIVE	CURE RATE	TREATMENT	RESIDUAL MASSES AFTER TREATMENT
Nonseminoma	• Contains at least one: - Embryonal carcinoma - Teratoma - Yolk-sac carcinoma - Choriocarcinoma: ○ May have a seminoma component	• No	• 70–95% depending on stage	• Stage I: orchiectomy followed by retroperitoneal dissection or active surveillance • Stage II: orchiectomy and retroperitoneal dissection with or without chemotherapy • Stage III: orchiectomy and chemotherapy	• 15% of the time • Chemotherapy-resistant teratoma may be in the residual mass • Must be removed to prevent malignant transformation
Seminoma	• Seminoma (ONLY)	• Yes	• >90% (all stages combined)	• Stage I and II: orchiectomy and retroperitoneal radiation • Stage III: orchiectomy and chemotherapy	• Often only fibrotic tissue and can be followed by serial CT

Table 10-15

Germ Cell/Testicular Tumor Markers

TUMOR MARKER	HALF-LIFE	NONSEMINOMA	PURE SEMINOMA
AFP	• 5–7 days	• Elevated	• NOT elevated
Beta-hCG	• 24–36 hours	• Elevated	• Occasionally elevated
LDH		• Elevated	• Elevated

Table 10-16
Oncologic Emergencies

EMERGENCY	SYMPTOMS/SIGN	ASSOCIATED CANCERS AND RISK FACTOR	TREATMENT
Blast Crisis	• High white count with blasts on smear • >100K blasts, or >300K myeloid cells • High percent of lymphoid cells as seen in CLL not usually a problem	• Leukemia	• Pheresis indicated if mental status changes, headache, blurry vision, chest pain, or shortness of breath • Urgent hematology/oncology consult
PE/DVT	• PE: dyspnea, pleuritic chest pain, cough • DVT: lower extremity swelling	• Any malignancy • Tamoxifen (breast cancer) • Indwelling central venous catheters	• Anticoagulation • Thrombolytic therapy if hemo-dynamically unstable (caution if platelets low)
Hypercalcemia	• Lethargy • Constipation • Nausea	• Most common in tumors with bony disease (breast cancer, prostate cancer, myeloma)	• IV hydration (if good cardiac status, urine output goal = 200 cc/h) • Furosemide AFTER hydration • Bisphosphonates • Stop thiazides and NSAIDs
Hyponatremia	• Fatigue/weakness • Nausea/vomiting/anorexia • Headache • Confusion • Coma • Seizure	• SIADH most commonly associated with SCLC	• See Table 5-12
Neutropenic Fever	• ANC <500 with a fever >101°F	• Common with many chemotherapy agents	• Empiric broad-spectrum antibiotics. Must cover gram-negative organisms • If febrile after 3 days of antibiotics without a causative agent, must reassess • May discontinue antibiotics after 3 days if no infection identified, afebrile >48 hours and ANC >500 for 2 days • May consider treating at home if very stable and very reliable

Table 10-16

Oncologic Emergencies (continued)

EMERGENCY	SYMPTOMS/SIGNS	ASSOCIATED CANCERS AND RISK FACTOR	TREATMENT

Pericardial Effusion and Tamponade	• Effusion:
	  - Dyspnea
	  - Orthopnea
	  - Chest discomfort
	• Tamponade:
	  - Pulsus paradoxus
	  - Low voltage on ECG
	  - Hypotension
	  - Sinus tachycardia
		• Lung cancer
		• Breast cancer
		• Melanoma
			• Emergent pericardiocentesis if hemodynamically unstable
			• Pericardial window if recurrent

Tumor Lysis Syndrome	• Increased creatinine, phosphorous, uric acid, and potassium levels • Decreased calcium	• Most common in hematologic malignancies with a high tumor burden	• Hydration with IV fluids • Alkalinize urine • Allopurinol • Phosphate and potassium binding resins • Loop diuretics • Insulin, glucose • May require dialysis if conservative management fails
Spinal Cord Compression	• Back pain • Sensory deficit level • Weakness • Bowel and/or bladder dysfunction • Confirm with MRI	• Breast cancer • Lung cancer • Lymphoma • Prostate	• Steroids • Radiation • Neurosurgical approaches • Outcome most dependent on neurologic condition prior to treatment

Superior Vena Cava Syndrome	• Plethora and swelling of upper extremity/face
	• Distended neck veins
	• Headache
		• Lung cancer
		• Lymphoma
		• Germ cell tumors
			• Unless impending airway obstruction, try to obtain tissue diagnosis before treating
			  - Elevate head of bed
			  - Anticoagulation controversial
			  - Steroids may mask biopsy results if lymphoma

ANC = absolute neutrophil count; CLL = chronic lymphocytic leukemia; ECG = electrocardiogram; IV = intravenous; MRI = magnetic resonance imaging; PE = pulmonary embolism; SIADH = syndrome of inappropriate anti-diuretic hormone.

Table 10-17

Late Consequences of Cancer Treatment

CHEMOTHERAPEUTIC AGENT	TYPICAL CANCER TREATED	LONG-TERM SEQUELAE OF THERAPY
Alkylating Agents and Topoisomerase II Inhibitors	• Lymphoid malignancies	• Secondary leukemia
Anthracyclines (High Doses)	• Breast cancer	• Cardiomyopathy • Risk of cardiomyathopy increases with anti-Her2/neu antibody (trastuzumab)
Bleomycin	• Testicular cancer	• Pulmonary fibrosis
Glucocorticoids	• Many, typically lymphomas	• Osteoporosis • Avascular necrosis

Radiation	• Many	• Depends on tissues lying within the radiation port
		  - Secondary solid tumor in or at border of radiation field (risk = 1% per year)
		  - Cataracts
		  - Pulmonary fibrosis (especially if a smoker)
		  - Infertility/premature menopause
		  - Neuropsychiatric and cognition difficulties

Chemotherapeutic Agents in General		• Premature menopause • Psychosocial stress

Please refer to other chapters for the following malignancies

Colon Cancer:	Tables 4-15 and 4-16
Esophageal Cancer:	Table 4-3
Gastric Cancer:	Table 4-3
Leukemia:	Tables 9-32 and 9-33
Pancreatic Cancer:	Table 4-37
Skin Cancer:	Table 14-3

Chapter 11

Rheumatology

Table 11-1

Osteoarthritis (OA)

DEFINITION/ETIOLOGY	EPIDEMIOLOGY/CLINICAL	DIAGNOSIS	TREATMENT/NOTE

• Altered cartilage physiology
• Excess weight is a risk factor for knee OA
• Acute injury (e.g., meniscal tear, cruciate ligament tear) or excessive use predispose to early OA
	• Epidemiology
	  - More common in elderly, especially postmenopausal women
	• Clinical presentation:
	  - Pain worse at the end of the day and relieved by rest
	• Pain worse with cold, damp weather
	• Clinical examination:
	  - Crepitus
	  - Decreased range of motion
	  - Joint effusions
	  - Joint instability
	  - "Locking" and "catching" are late findings
		• Clinical examination
		• Radiologic findings:
		  - Bony proliferation (osteophytes, spurs)
		  - Asymmetric joint narrowing on weight-bearing x-rays
		  - Subchondral bone sclerosis
		  - Subchondral bone cysts
		• MRI: pathologic cartilage
		• Synovial fluid: noninflammatory
			• Muscle strengthening, low impact exercises
			• Physical therapy may improve function, decrease pain, and delay need for surgical intervention
			• Acetaminophen
			• NSAIDs
			• COX-2 inhibitors
			• Glucosamine/chondroitin sulfate may decrease pain and increase mobility
			• Viscosupplementation with intra-articular hyaluronic acid
			• Intra-articular steroid injections
			• Total joint arthroplasty if failed medical therapy or function severely compromised

COX-2 = cyclooxygenase; MRI = magnetic resonance imaging; NSAIDs = nonsteroidal anti-inflammatory drugs.

Table 11-2

Rheumatoid Arthritis (RA)

DEFINITION/ETIOLOGY	EPIDEMIOLOGY/CLINICAL	DIAGNOSIS	TREATMENT/NOTE

• Systemic, inflammatory, autoimmune disease
• Proinflammatory cytokines in joint: IL-1 and TNF-alpha
• Inflammatory-proliferative synovial tissue (pannus) invades cartilage and bone
• Increased angiogenesis
	Epidemiology:
	• Prevalence: 1% of population
	• M:F ratio = 2–5/1
	• Peak occurrence: 4th–5th decade
	• Associated with ↓ life expectancy
	Clinical:
	• Symmetrical polyarticular pain and swelling
	• Affect mainly small joints of hands (wrist, MCPs, PIPs) and feet
	• Morning stiffness and fatigue
	• Complications:
	  - CAD
	  - Scleritis/episcleritis
	  - Secondary Sjögren syndrome
	  - Felty syndrome (RA+ neutropenia + splenomegaly)
	  - C-spine (C1–C2) instability → myelopathy
	  - Rheumatoid vasculitis
	  - Cricoarytenoid synovitis → dysphonia
	  - Rheumatoid nodules
	  - Baker's cyst
	  - Structural damage and disability
		• Synovial fluid: inflammatory
		• Increased ESR/CRP
		• RF+ (85%)
		• CCP
		• Anemia of chronic disease
		• X-ray: joint erosions, joint space loss, juxta-articular osteoporosis
		• Musculoskeletal ultrasound or MRI may provide earlier clues than x-ray
		• Synovial membrane biopsy
			• Early diagnosis and referral to specialist
			• NSAID therapy
			• COX-2 inhibitors (celecoxib, rofecoxib, valdecoxib)
			• Treatment of early disease with DMARDs +/− biologic agents can prevent joint destruction and long-term sequelae
			• DMARDs:
			  - Methotrexate (+ folic acid)
			  - Sulfasalazine
			  - Hydroxychloroquine
			  - Leflunomide
			  - Azathioprine
			  - Cyclosporin A
			  - Cyclophosphamide
			  - Gold
			  - Minocycline
			  - Low-dose CS
			• BRMs:
			  - TNF inhibitors (infliximab, etanercept, adalimumab)
			  - IL-1 inhibitor (anakinra)
			  - Costimulation inhibitors (abatacept)
			  - Anti-CD 20 B-cell depleting agents (rituximab)
			  - Immunoabsorbent column (Prosorba)
			• Orthopedic surgery

IL-1 = interleukin-1; TNF = tumor necrosis factor; M = male; F = female; MCP = metacarpophalangeal; PIP = proximal interphalangeal; CAD = coronary artery disease; RA = Rheumatoid Arthritis; ESR = erythrocyte sedimentation rate; CRP = C-reactive protein; RF = rheumatoid factor; CCP: cyclic citrullinated antibody; DMARDs = disease-modifying antirheumatic drugs; CS = corticosteroids; BRMs = biologic response modifiers.

Table 11-3

Crystal-Induced Arthropathies

DISEASE	DEFINITION/ETIOLOGY	CLINICAL PRESENTATION	DIAGNOSIS	TREATMENT/NOTE
Gout	• Inflammation of joint with MSU crystals in synovial fluid • Acute attacks precipitated by rapid fluctuations in serum uric acid levels, drugs, trauma, or alcohol ingestion	• Synovial fluid: MSU crystals • Typical joint affected: first MTP (podagra) • Typical presentation: sudden onset of pain, swelling, and erythema • Polyarticular disease can occur • Chronic tophaceous gout: massive urate deposition (tophi) in joints or subcutaneous tissue can cause joint erosions • Accelerated and severe course in transplant patients treated with cyclosporine • Kidney complications: urate nephropathy, uric acid nephrolithiasis Epidemiology: not common in women before menopause	• Polarized microscopy: intracellular; needle-shaped, with negative birefringence (yellow when parallel to the compensator axis) • Synovial fluid: inflammatory with PMN predominance • Hyperuricemia not always present • X-ray findings: - Acute attack: soft tissue edema - Chronic tophaceous disease: "rat bite" erosions with "overhanging" edge	• Acute attack: - NSAIDs (first line) - Colchicine - ACTH or systemic/intra-articular CS - Allopurinol **Contraindicated** during acute attack • Chronic gout: - Colchicines - Urate lowering therapy: diet, allopurinol, uricosuric agents (probenecid, sulfinpyrazone) • Reduce allopurinol dose if elevated creatinine or if concomitant azathioprine

| Pseudogout/ CPPD Deposition Disease | • Inflammation of joint with CPPD crystals in synovial fluid | • Synovial fluid: CPPD crystals
• Typical joints affected: knee, wrist, ankle
• 5–10% can have "pseudorheumatoid" symmetric polyarticular presentation
• Predisposing conditions:
  - Hyperparathyroidism
  - Hemochromatosis
  - Hypomagnesemia
  - Hypophosphatasia
• Epidemiology:
  - More common in elderly (mean age of onset is 70) | • Polarized microscopy: intracellular, rhomboid, positive birefringent (blue when parallel to the compensator axis)
• X-ray: chondrocalcinosis | • Acute attack:
• NSAIDs
• Colchicine
• Aspiration and/or systemic/ intraarticular CS |

CPPD = calcium pyrophosphate dehydrate; MSU = monosodium urate; MTP = metatarsophalangeal; PMN = polymorphonuclear; ACTH = adrenocorticotropic hormone; CS = corticosteroids.

Table 11-4

Summary of Seronegative Spondyloarthropathies

TYPE	COMMON FEATURES	EPIDEMIOLOGY/CLINICAL PRESENTATION	DIAGNOSIS	TREATMENT/NOTE
Psoriatic Arthritis	• Inflammatory back pain • Enthesitis (tendon inflammation) • Asymmetric oligoarthritis (although psoriatic can be symmetric) • High incidence of HLA-B27 positivity (though testing rarely indicated for diagnosis) • RF negative (the basis for the term "seronegative")	Epidemiology: • Family/personal history of psoriasis • Females > males Clinical: • Oligoarticular distal arthritis most specific, but polyarticular symmetric proximal arthritis (RA-like pattern) most frequent • Dactylitis ("sausage fingers") • Nail pitting • Arthritis mutilans (severe)	• Arthritis may precede skin disease in 15% of cases • Spinal involvement, especially if HLA-B27+ • X-ray: "pencil-in-cup" deformities, "fluffy" periostitis	• NSAIDs • PUVA, retinoids for skin disease • Methotrexate • Sulfasalazine • TNF-alpha inhibitors (etanercept, infliximab, adalimumab)
IBD Associated/ Enteropathic Arthritis		• Epidemiology: - 7–20% of patients with IBD develop joint symptoms. Most common extraintestinal complication of IBD • Clinical: - Pauciarticular, large joints (including sacroiliac) - Enthesitis, uveitis may be present - Peripheral arthritis waxes and wanes with bowel symptoms while axial disease independent of bowel symptoms - Arthritis may be presenting symptom of IBD	• Increased ESR, CRP • Anemia, leukocytosis, thrombocytosis • HLA-B27 may be positive in patients with sacroiliitis	• Treat underlying IBD • Physical therapy for sacroiliitis • NSAIDs (careful) • Infliximab and adalimumab may work for both IBD and arthritis

Ankylosing Spondylitis	Epidemiology: • Males > females Clinical: • Pauciarticular, large joints • Sacroiliac joint, hips, knees, heels commonly affected • Enthesopathy: inflammation of tendon insertions • Anterior uveitis common • Rare: aortic regurgitation, apical pulmonary fibrosis • Premature spinal osteoporosis • Mild trauma (e.g., fall) can cause spinal instability	• HLA-B27+ (90%) • Elevated ESR • Anemia • ANA negative • RF negative • Bilateral sacroiliitis on x-ray or CT scan • X-ray: "bamboo spine" if advanced	• NSAIDs/COX-2 inhibitors • Physical therapy • DMARDs (see Table 11-2 for details) • TNF inhibitors • Surgery
	• See above		
Reactive Arthritis	Epidemiology: • Males > females Clinical: • Oligoarticular arthritis, particularly of the lower extremities • Sterile urethritis, conjunctivitis, uveitis (rarely all three) • Enthesitis • Dactylitis ("sausage fingers") • Mucocutaneous lesions frequent ("Reiter's nails") • History of preceding infection, *Salmonella, Yersinia, Shigella, Campylobacter, Neisseria gonorrhea, Chlamydia+* • More severe in HIV+	• Stool studies if appropriate • Urethral/cervical smears • HLA-B27 • Elevated ESR • Serology for suspected pathogen if cause uncertain	• Antibiotics if active infection • Usually self-limited (3–12 months), although can see chronic or recurrent course NSAIDs • Physical therapy • DMARDs if chronic

IBD = inflammatory bowel disease; HLA = human leukocyte antigen; PUVA = ps oralen and ultraviolet A; NSAIDs = non-steroidal anti-inflammatory drugs; ANA = antinuclear antibody; CT = computed tomography; DMARDs = disease modifying anti-rheumatic drugs; HIV = human immunodeficiency virus; Nsaids.

Table 11-5
Other Arthritides

TYPE	CLINICAL PRESENTATION	DIAGNOSIS	TREATMENT/NOTE
Celiac Disease Associated Arthritis	• Polyarticular • Weight loss	• +Antiendomysial Ab • +Antigliadin Ab	• Gluten-free diet
Adult Onset Still Disease	• Females = males • Variable number joints • Daily fever spikes • Systemic signs may precede the arthritis by many years (may present as FUO) • Salmon-colored evanescent rash during fever • Hepatosplenomegaly • Lymphadenopathy • Serositis • Anemia	• Definitive diagnosis requires joint symptoms for more than 6 consecutive weeks • Leukocytosis • Increased ESR • Anemia • Thrombocytosis • Transaminitis • Chest radiograph may show pleural effusion • Echocardiogram may show pericardial effusion • RF negative • ANA negative	• Anti-inflammatories (NSAIDs) • Methotrexate • TNF-alpha inhibitors • IL-1 inhibitor (anakinra)

FUO = fever of unknown origin; Ab = antibody.

Table 11-6
Synovial Fluid Characteristics

TYPE	WBC	GLUCOSE	GRAM STAIN/CULTURE	ASSOCIATED CONDITIONS
Normal	<200 <25% PMN	Equal to serum	Negative	
Noninflammatory	<2000 <25% PMN	Equal to serum	Negative	OA, trauma
Inflammatory	>2000 >50% PMN	< serum	Negative	RA, crystal, connective tissue disease, seronegative
Septic	50,000–500,000 >75% PMN	< serum	Gram stain + Culture 25–50% +	Bacteria, mycobacteria, fungi

WBC = white blood cell.

Table 11–7

The Lupus Spectrum

TYPE	CLINICAL	DIAGNOSIS	TREATMENT/NOTE

SLE	Classification criteria:
	1. Malar rash (spares nasolabial folds)
	2. Discoid rash
	3. Photosensitivity
	4. Arthritis
	5. Oral ulcers
	6. Serositis
	7. Renal disease
	8. Neurologic:
	  - Seizures
	  - Psychosis
	9. Hematologic:
	  - Anemia (hemolytic)
	  - Lymphopenia, leukopenia
	  - Thrombocytopenia
	10. ANA+
	11. Immunologic:
	  - anti-dsDNA
	  - anti-Sm
	  - positive APLA
		• 4 of 11 criteria, serially or simultaneously
		• ANA > 95% sensitive but not specific
		• dsDNA and anti-Sm less sensitive but much more specific
		• C3 and C4 decrease and ↑ a-dsDNA correlate with disease flares, and are useful markers of disease course
		• Anti-Ro, La, and RNP antibodies may also be present, but are not specific for SLE
			• NSAIDs
			• Steroids
			• Antimalarials
			• Immunosuppressives (cyclophosphamide, azathioprine, mycophenolate mofetil)
			• Pulse cyclophosphamide plus methylprednisolone are gold standard for proliferative lupus nephritis
			• Newer data with mycophenolate mofetil have been very promising
			• Actively manage CV risk factors
			• At increased risk for:
			  - Infections (especially if on high prednisone dose)
			  - Renal failure
			  - Premature CAD

Drug-Induced Lupus	• Lupus-like syndrome
	• CNS and renal involvement uncommon
	• Common drugs:
	  - Procainamide
	  - Quinidine
	  - Hydralazine
	  - Sulfonamides
	  - INH
	  - Phenytoin
	  - Oral contraceptives
		• +/− Antihistone antibody
		• Immune complexes
			• Resolves after discontinuation of offending agent

Discoid Lupus	• Scaly rash in sun-exposed areas • No systemic signs	• Anti-Ro+	• Avoid sunlight • Anti-malarials

(*continued*)

Table 11–7

The Lupus Spectrum (continued)

Type	Clinical	Diagnosis	Treatment/Note

APLA Syndrome	• Recurrent fetal loss
	• Unexplained venous and arterial thrombosis
	• Strokes
	• Pulmonary embolus
	• Avascular bone necrosis
	• Myocardial infarcts (young age)
	• Menorrhagia
	• Cutaneous signs:
	  - Livedo reticularis
	  - Splinter hemorrhages
	  - Superficial thrombophlebitis
	  - Leg ulcers
		• Clinical event (thrombosis or fetal loss) AND positive lab test on two occasions
		• ACA +/− LA +/− anti-β2GPI Ab
		• Thrombocytopenia
		• Prolonged PT/PTT—does not correct with fresh frozen plasma administration (APLA causes thrombosis in vivo, but is an anticoagulant in vitro)
		• dRVVT for confirmation
			• Can occur as a primary disease, or in association with other inflammatory disorders (most commonly SLE)
			• Lifelong anticoagulation following thrombotic event
			• For patients with antiphospholipid antibodies but no clinical events, no clear concensus or recommendations

ACA = anticardiolipin antibody; APLA = antiphospholipid antibody; CNS = central nervous system; CV = cardiovascular; dRVVT = dilute Russel Viper Venom Test; INH = isoniazid; LA = lupus anticoagulant; PT = prothrombin time; PTT partial thromboplastin time; RNP = ribonuclear protein; SLE = systemic lupus erythematosus.

Table 11-8

The Scleroderma Spectrum

Type	Clinical	Diagnosis	Treatment/Note
Localized Scleroderma	• Morphea: plaques and/or drops ("guttate" pattern) • Linear: affects single dermatome • *En coup de sabre*: involvement of scalp	• +/− RF • +/− ANA • Increased immunoglobulins • Skin biopsy	• Severe disease may adhere skin to underlying structures, causing contractures that require splinting or surgical intervention • Disease usually self-limited, but may be permanently disfiguring

Table 11-8

The Scleroderma Spectrum (continued)

TYPE	CLINICAL	DIAGNOSIS	TREATMENT/NOTE
PSS Scleroderma (previously known as CREST)	Limited systemic sclerosis: • **C**alcinosis (calcium deposits in the skin) • **R**aynaud's phenomenon • **E**sophageal disease • **S**clerodactyly • **T**elangiectasias • **P**ulmonary lesion similar to primary pulmonary hypertension	• Anticentromere antibodies (70%) • +/− ANA • +/− RF • Skin biopsy	• PFTs +/− imaging +/− bronch in dyspnea to detect early fibrosing alveolitis—may be preventable with immunosuppression • PPIs if reflux • ACE inhibitors in renal crisis to control hypertension • MTX for arthritis, myositis • Avoid high doses of prednisone as can precipitate renal crisis • Physical therapy • Aggressive treatment of complications
	Diffuse systemic sclerosis: May have all of above plus: • Severe skin fibrosis ("fish mouth," ↓ joint mobility) • Pulmonary fibrosis, secondary pulmonary hypertension (poor prognosis) • Hypertension in renal crisis can cause renal failure and death • GI disease (impaired motility, "watermelon stomach") • Cardiac disease (heart block, congestive heart disease, pericardial effusion)	• Antiscleroderma 70 antibody (40%) • Anti-RNP antibody (also seen in mixed connective tissue disease and SLE) • +/− ANA • +/− RF • Skin biopsy	
Raynaud's Phenomenon	• Vasospastic attacks preceded by cold exposure or emotion • Fingers • Color changes: white–> blue–> red • Numbness/pain • Can be seen in pheochromocytoma, carcinoid syndrome, hyperviscosity, cold agglutinins	• +/− ANA	• Cold avoidance • Smoking cessation • Calcium channel blockers • If limb threatening: digital sympathectomy • Nailfold capillaroscopy may predict risk of developing systemic disease

ACE = angiotensin-converting enzyme; GI = gastrointestinal; MTX = methotrexate; PFTs = pulmonary function tests; bronch = bronchoscopy; PPI = proton pump inhibitor; PSS = progressive systemic sclerosis.

Table 11-9
Vasculitides

Disease	Vessel Size	Epidemiology/Clinical	Diagnosis	Treatment/Note

Takayasu Arteritis	Large	*Epidemiology:*
		• Rare, more common in Asia
		• Predominantly young women (<40), F:M = 9:1
		Clinical:
		• Affects aorta and major branches
		• Fever, sweats, fatigue, weight loss (*inflammatory stage*) precede pulseless stage
		• Ischemic complications (*pulseless stage*):
		  - Myocardial ischemia
		  - Pulmonary hypertension
		  - Carotid/vertebral artery involvement → neurologic disease
		  - Neurovascular hypertension
		  - Occlusion of upper extremity arteries → arm claudication
			• Angiography
			• MRI/MRA
			• Elevated ESR/CRP (75%)
			• Pathology: granulomatous panarteritis
				• CS
				• MTX and mycophenolate mofetil are steroid sparing agents
				• ASA, antiplatelet agents
				• Cyclophosphamide for severe cases
				• Angioplasty/vascular surgery for advanced disease

GCA /(Temporal Arteritis)	Large	*Epidemiology:* • F > M, Northern European descent • >50 years old Clinical: • Affects large extracranial arteries to head and neck	• Temporal artery biopsy—may need bilateral sampling • 90% negative predictive value if sample > 1 cm	• Immediate steroid treatment (before biopsy) as delay can lead to blindness • Biopsy will remain positive 3–4 weeks after initiation of steroid treatment

GCA /(Temporal Arteritis) (cont.)		<ul><li>Fever, weight loss, night sweats</li><li>New-onset headache</li><li>50% with PMR (pain and stiffness in neck, shoulders and pelvic girdle)</li><li>Jaw claudication</li><li>Scalp tenderness</li><li>Visual symptoms (blurring, diplopia, amaurosis)</li><li>Claudication</li><li>AION secondary to ophthalmic or posterior ciliary artery occlusion can cause irreversible blindness</li></ul>	<ul><li>Angiography or MRI/ MRA to document large artery involvement</li><li>ESR >50</li><li>Elevated CRP</li><li>Anemia</li><li>Pathology: granulomatous arteritis</li></ul>	<ul><li>Initial dose of prednisone = 60 mg/day</li></ul>
PAN	Medium	<ul><li>Epidemiology:<ul><li>M > F</li><li>Average age of onset 50 years old</li></ul></li><li>Clinical:<ul><li>Associated with hepatitis B, hairy cell leukemia</li><li>Fever, weight loss, night sweats</li><li>Arthralgias, myalgias</li><li>Skin: livedo reticularis, ulcers, nodules</li><li>Mononeuritis multiplex</li><li>Mesenteric ischemia (intestinal angina)</li><li>Cardiac involvement: MI and/or CHF</li><li>Renin-mediated hypertension</li><li>Lungs are spared</li><li>NO glomerulonephritis</li></ul></li></ul>	<ul><li>Anemia, thrombocytosis, leukocytosis</li><li>Elevated ESR</li><li>Microscopic hematuria</li><li>Mesenteric/renal angiography: microaneurysms</li><li>Biopsy (skin or combined sural nerve/gastrocnemius muscle)</li><li>Pathology: fibrinoid necrosis, nongranulomatous</li></ul>	<ul><li>High dose or pulse steroids in severe cases</li><li>Resistant cases: cyclophosphamide</li><li>In hepatitis B associated cases: plasma exchange × 6 weeks plus concurrent CS × 2 weeks and then antiviral treatment (lamivudine)</li></ul>

(continued)

343

Table 11-9
Vasculitides (continued)

DISEASE	VESSEL SIZE	EPIDEMIOLOGY/CLINICAL	DIAGNOSIS	TREATMENT/NOTE
MPA	Small	• Differs from PAN in that it mainly affects the lungs (pulmonary capillaries) and kidneys • Most common cause of pulmonary-renal syndromes • Can present with hemoptysis secondary to alveolar hemorrhage • Mononeuritis multiplex	• P-ANCA+/MPO+ (70%) • Pathology: necrotizing vasculitis, nongranulomatous	• Oral/IV cyclophosphamide and CS
WG	Small	• Epidemiology: - Young and middle-aged adults, but can occur at any age • Clinical: - Vasculitis of upper respiratory tract, lungs, and kidney - Epistaxis, nasal crusting, refractory "sinusitis" - Saddle-nose deformity and nasal septum perforation - Subglottic stenosis - Arthralgias - Necrotizing, crescentic glomerular nephritis can lead to renal failure - Palpable purpura, ulcers	• C-ANCA+/PR3+ (80–90%) • Elevated ESR • Active urine sediment • Anemia • CXR/CT: pulmonary nodules, cavitation, hemorrhage • Biopsy (upper airways, lung, kidneys): necrotizing, granulomatous vasculitis	• Oral/IV cyclophosphamide and CS • MTX and CS if limited/nonlife threatening disease • TMP-SMX for *Pneumocystis jiroveci* prophylaxis during immunosuppressive treatment
CSA	Small	• Epidemiology: - May present at any age, 30–40 mean age of onset • Clinical: - Atopy (nasal polyps, allergic rhinitis) - Difficult to control asthma - Cutaneous vasculitis - Mononeuritis multiplex - Glomerulonephritis - Gut involvement	• Peripheral blood eosinophilia (80%) • CXR: fleeting infiltrates • Skin/lung biopsy: eosinophilic, necrotizing, granulomatous vasculitis • P-ANCA+/MPO+ (50%)	• Very responsive to steroids • Cyclophosphamide for severe disease (renal, GI, CV, pulmonary hemorrhage)

	Size	Clinical Features	Labs	Treatment
Cryoglobulinemic Vasculitis	Small	• Associated with hepatitis C • Recurrent palpable purpura, usually on the legs • Skin ulcerations • Arthralgias • Sicca symptoms • Glomerulonephritis • Mononeuritis multiplex • Mesenteric vasculitis	• Can be RF+ • ↓ C4 > ↓ C3 • Serum cryoglobulins present	• Antiviral therapy (IFN-alpha + ribavirin) if HCV associated • Oral/IV cyclophosphamide and CS • Plasmapheresis if severe
HSP or Anaphylactoid Purpura	Small	• IgA-mediated leukocytoclastic vasculitis • 90% cases in child hood • More likely to have a chronic course in adults • Often antecedent URI Classic tetrad: 1. Palpable purpura (usually on lower extremities, may be widespread in younger patients) 2. Colicky abdominal pain–mesenteric ischemia 3. Arthritis 4. Nephritis (IgA nephropathy)	• Increased ESR • Guaiac + stools • Renal/skin biopsy: +IgA immunofluorescence • UA active sediment: hematuria, proteinuria, casts • Elevated serum IgA (50%)	• Supportive • CS in severe cases • Avoid NSAIDs • Renal failure is number one cause of mortality

AION = anterior ischemic optic neuropathy; ASA = acetylsalicylic acid; CSA = Churg-Strauss angiitis; CSF = congestive heart failure; CXR = chest x-ray; GCA = giant cell arteritis; HCV = hepatitis C virus; HSP = Henoch-Schönlein purpura; IFN = interferon; MI = myocardial infarction; MPA = microscopic polyangiitis; MPO = myeloperoxidase; MRA = magnetic resonance angiography; PAN = polyarteritis nodosa; PMR = polymyalgia rheumatica; CS = corticosteroids; TMP-SMX = trimethoprim-sulfamethoxazole; URI= upper respiratory infection; UA = urinalysis; WG = Wegener granulomatosis.

Table 11-10

Inflammatory Myopathies

DISEASE	DEFINITION/CLINICAL	DIAGNOSIS	TREATMENT/NOTE
PM	• Inflammation of striated muscle • Chronic multiorgan disease • Symmetric trunk and proximal muscle weakness • Dysphagia or respiratory difficulties may be present • Interstitial lung disease (30–50%)	• Elevated CPK, aldolase, lactate dehydrogenase, or transaminases (from muscle breakdown) • MRI: edematous areas proximal to affected muscles • EMG reveals small amplitude spike and waves • Muscle biopsy reveals lymphocytic inflammation around blood vessels • If Jo-1 Ab present, high suspicion for interstitial lung disease	• CS • Physical therapy • Monitor respiratory and swallowing function • Methotrexate if profound muscle weakness, or for steroid-sparing effect • Immune globulin • Suspect underlying weakness, especially if elderly
DM	• Inflammation of skin and striated muscle • Chronic multiorgan disease • Symmetric trunk and proximal muscle weakness • Dysphagia or respiratory difficulties • Classic "heliotrope" rash (violet-colored eyelids +/– periorbital edema) • The rash does *not* spare the nasolabial folds (in contrast to the rash of SLE) • Gottron's papules (scaly rash of extensor surfaces and knuckles) • Nailfold capillary changes • Rare: skin findings without muscular component "amyopathic DM"	• Elevated CPK, aldolase, lactate dehydrogenase, or transaminases (from muscle breakdown) • MRI: edematous areas proximal to affected muscles • EMG: small amplitude spike and waves • Muscle biopsy: perifascicular inflammation • If Jo-1 Ab present, high suspicion for interstitial lung disease	• CS • Physical therapy • Monitoring of respiratory and swallowing function • Methotrexate • Immune globulin • Suspect for underlying weakness, especially if elderly • If underlying malignancy, treatment of cancer may eliminate myositic manifestations
IBM	• Slowly progressive inflammatory myopathy • Chronic and insidious • Weakness may be asymmetric • Weakness may be proximal and distal • Primarily affects elderly men • Dysphagia (20%) • Muscle atrophy • Diminished deep tendon reflexes	• Muscle biopsy: intracellular vacuoles filled with eosinophilic material	• Resistant to treatment • Suspect underlying weakness, especially if elderly

PM = polymyositis; CPK = creatine phosphokinase; EMG = electromyography; CS = corticosteroids; DM = dermatomyositis; IBM = inclusion body myositis.

Table 11-11

Periodic Fever Syndromes

Disease	Etiology	Epidemiology/Clinical	Diagnosis	Treatment/Note
FMF	• *MEFV* gene (codes for pyrin) mutations • Recessive inheritance	Epidemiology: • More common if Jewish, Arab, Turkish, Italian descent Clinical: • Attacks last 1–3 days • Fever • Abdominal pain • Pleurisy • Erysipeloid erythema • Monoarthritis of knee or ankle • AA amyloidosis most serious complication	• Clinical evaluation • Genetic test available, but not required in typical cases	• Daily oral colchicine for prevention of attacks and amyloidosis
TRAPS	• *TNFRSF1A* gene (codes for p55 TNF receptor) • Dominant inheritance	Clinical: - Fever, abdominal pain, pleurisy, arthralgias, monoarthritis, rash • Differences from FMF: - Centrifugal, migratory rash - Duration of attacks longer (up to 6 weeks) - Conjunctival involvement/ periorbital edema - Myalgias • AA amyloidosis in 15%	• Often familial • Diagnosis established by genetic testing	• Etanercept • CS (more effective than in FMF) • Colchicine has poor response

(continued)

Table 11-11

Periodic Fever Syndromes (continued)

DISEASE	ETIOLOGY	EPIDEMIOLOGY/CLINICAL	DIAGNOSIS	TREATMENT/NOTE
HIDS	• *MVK* (mevalonate kinase) mutation • Recessive inheritance	• Fever, rash, arthralgias, cervical lymphadenopathy (tender) Differences from FMF: • Attacks last 3–7days (intermediate between FMF and TRAPS) • Diffuse maculopapular rash that can affect palms and soles • Joint involvement more symmetric than in FMF and TRAPS • Aphthous/vaginal ulcers • NO pleurisy • NO amyloidosis risk	• Clinical • Elevated serum IgD (does not correlate with disease activity) • Mevalonic aciduria • Genetic test available	• No satisfactory treatment • NSAIDs for fever • Colchicine • CS • IVIG • Etanercept
MWS	• *CIAS1* (cryopyrin) mutation	Clinical: • Fever, rash, arthritis, abdominal pain • Attacks last 1–2 days Differences from FMF: • Sensorineural hearing loss • Optic disk swelling • Urticarial rash • AA amyloidosis in 25%	• Familial • Elevated ESR • Elevated WBC • Genetic test available	• No established treatment • NSAIDS for fever, arthralgias • CS • IL-1 blockade (Anakinra)

FMF = familial mediterranean fever; AA = amyloid A; TRAPS = tumor necrosis factor receptor-associated periodic syndrome; HIDS = hyperimmunoglobulinemia D with periodic fever syndrome; IVIG = intravenous immunoglobulin; MWS = Muckle-Wells syndrome.

Table 11-12
Miscellaneous Rheumatologic Disorders

Disease	Definition/Epidemiology/Clinical Presentation	Diagnosis	Treatment/Note
Fibromyalgia	Epidemiology: • Affects 1–2% of the population • F > M Clinical: • Diffuse pain, but trigger points extremely sensitive • Difficulty sleeping • Overlap with chronic fatigue syndrome, depression	• Pain elicited with pressure on trigger points • Absence of inflammatory markers	• Behavioral therapy • Aerobic exercise • Tricyclic compounds at low doses • Fluoxetine • Support groups

Relapsing Polychondritis	Definition:
	• Inflammation and destruction of cartilage and connective tissue
	Epidemiology:
	• Peak incidence 40–50
	• F = M
	Clinical:
	• Auricular chondritis
	• Nasal/respiratory tract chondritis: saddle nose deformity, hoarseness, cough, dyspnea
	• Migratory polyarthritis:
	  - Asymmetric
	  - Small and large joints
	  - Nonerosive
	• Ocular inflammation common; all layers can be involved
	• Middle ear involvement: hearing loss, vertigo
	• Obstructive lung disease
	• Aortic insufficiency secondary to aortitis
		• Biopsy (gold standard): revealing plasma and mononuclear cell infiltration
		• ESR elevation
		• Hypergammaglobulinemia
		• Check PFTs, as obstructive lung disease can be clinically silent
			• Acute attacks may subside spontaneously
			• 40% associated with autoimmune disease
			• NSAIDs effective for mild symptoms
			• High-dose CS and azathioprine or cyclophosphamide for more severe disease
			• MTX for long-term steroid-sparing treatment, or for severe disease

(continued)

Table 11-12

Miscellaneous Rheumatologic Disorders (continued)

DISEASE	DEFINITION/EPIDEMIOLOGY/CLINICAL PRESENTATION	DIAGNOSIS	TREATMENT/NOTE
Behçet Syndrome	Definition: • Systemic vasculitis affecting vessels of any size Epidemiology: • Most common in Old Silk Route (Turkey, Middle East, China, Korea, Japan) Clinical: • Monoarthritis or asymmetric oligo or polyarthritis • Recurrent painful genital and oral ulcers • Uveitis that can lead to blindness • Erythema nodosum, folliculitis • Aortic aneurysms • Pulmonary artery-bronchial fistulae • CNS complications: meningoencephalitis, white matter lesions • GI involvement in Japanese patients	• Clinical • Biopsy of ulcer • Positive pathergy test • Associated with HLA-B51 allele	• Colchicine trial • Low-dose CS or thalidomide for oral/genital ulcers • Azathioprine • Cyclophosphamide/cyclosporine or infliximab for ocular inflammation
Sjögren Syndrome	Definition: • Chronic dysfunction of exocrine glands secondary to lymphoplasmacytic infiltration Epidemiology: • 40–60 is peak age of onset • F > M Clinical presentation: • Can be primary or secondary to other autoimmune diseases • Thick pulmonary secretions • Xerostomia (leads to tooth decay, mouth candidiasis), xerophthalmia (leads to keratoconjunctivitis), and immune system dysfunction • Dysphagia • Atrophic gastritis • Vaginal dryness • Interstitial lung disease, interstitial nephritis, Raynaud's phenomenon, vasculitis, arthritis can all occur • Parotid swelling	• Clinical • +anti-Ro (SS-A) in 55%, anti-La (SS-B) in 40% • + ANA in 95% • + RF in 75% • Biopsy of minor salivary gland or lip can confirm diagnosis	Supportive: • Artificial tears • Gum • Lemon drops • Cholinergic treatment for xerostomia • NSAIDs, CS, DMARDs for systemic manifestations • 50% increased risk of lymphoma and Waldenstrom's

Table 11-13
Infectious Arthritis

Disease	Etiology/Epidemiology	Clinical Presentation	Diagnosis	Treatment/Note

Bacterial Arthritis (nongonococcal)	• Hematogenous seeding
	• 75–80% gram positive
	• Elderly: may have gram negative
	• Common sources:
	  - Skin infections
	  - Pyelonephritis
	  - Endocarditis
	• Rare direct inoculation:
	  - _Pasteurella multocida_ from cat bite
	  - _Pseudomonas aeruginosa_ from dirty nail puncturing sole of shoe
	• Predisposing conditions:
	  - Age > 60
	  - surgery
	  - Artificial joints
	  - Preexisting joint disease
	  - Immunosuppressed state
		• 80–90% monoarticular
		• Red, warm, swollen, tender joint (usually large joint, e.g., knee)
		• Fever
		• May appear toxic
			• Synovial fluid analysis:
			  - ↑WBC count (>50,000)
			  - Poly predominance
			  - Gram stain
			  - Culture
			• The presence of crystals in the synovial fluid does not rule out infection
			• Blood cultures (50% positive)
			• ↑ESR, CRP
			• WBC count in synovial fluid may be falsely lowered to < 10,000 if early in course, or already receiving antibiotics
			• Baseline plain films allow monitoring of progression
				• IV antibiotics for two weeks, then oral for 4–6 weeks
				• Drainage/lavage of joint via arthroscopy or daily aspirations
				• If infected prosthesis: removal of implants, plus 6 weeks antibiotics
				• 10% mortality

Gonococcal Arthritis	• _Neisseria gonorrhoeae_ (gram-negative diplococcus) • Most common of acute bacterial arthritis • Sexually active young adults, especially females	• Migratory polyarthralgia that becomes a mono or oligoarthritis • Genitourinary symptoms or pharyngitis usually absent • Erythematous macules on extremities that become pustules (40%) • Tenosynovitis present	• Synovial fluid Gram stain, culture • Genitourinary, rectal, throat cultures helpful • Blood cultures rarely positive	• Third-generation cephalosporin • Initiate treatment based on clinical suspicion, as culture is difficult and takes at least 24 hours

(continued)

Table 11-13
Infectious Arthritis (continued)

Disease	Etiology/Epidemiology	Clinical Presentation	Diagnosis	Treatment/Note
Viral Arthritis	• Parvovirus B19	• Arthralgias predominate rather than arthritis • In adults no facial rash, can mimic RA • Usually self-limited	• History of exposure (e.g., patient is a teacher) • Anti-B19 IgM antibodies	• NSAIDs

Lyme Disease	• Tick-borne spirochete *Borrelia burgdorferi*	• Multisystem inflammatory disease
		• Early localized: flu-like illness
		  - Erythema chronicum migrans
		• Early disseminated: days to months after tick-bite
		  - Migratory polyarthritis and myalgias
		  - Cardiac disease (heart block, myopericarditis)
		  - Neurologic disease (cranial nerve palsies, meningitis, neuroradiculitis)
		• Late disseminated: months to years after tick-bite
		  - Chronic oligoarthritis (usually knee)
			• Clinical
			• History of tick exposure in endemic areas
			• ELISA testing
			• Western blotting to confirm diagnosis
			• PCR of synovial fluid
				• Prevention: protective clothing, tick repellents, prompt tick removal
				• Antibiotic treatment early in disease is curative and prevents serious disease sequelae
				  - Doxycycline or amoxicillin × 2 weeks
				  - Ceftriaxone for more serious disease
				• Late arthritis:
				  - Rule out persistent infection
				  - NSAIDs
				  - Rarely DMARDs

ELISA = enzyme-linked immunosorbent assay; PCR = polymerase chain reaction.

Table 11-14

Acute Rheumatic Fever

EPIDEMIOLOGY	ETIOLOGY	CLINICAL PRESENTATION	DIAGNOSIS	TREATMENT

• Incidence has decreased since introduction of antibiotics
• Rheumatic heart disease occurs 10–20 years after original attack and is a major cause of valvular disease worldwide
	• Delayed, nonsuppurative sequela of a pharyngitis caused by infection with GAS	• Jones criteria
		  - Major:
		    ∘ Carditis
		    ∘ Polyarthritis (migratory)
		    ∘ Erythema marginatum
		    ∘ Sydenham's chorea
		    ∘ Subcutaneous nodules
		  - Minor:
		    ∘ Fever
		    ∘ Arthralgia (NOT arthritis)
		    ∘ Prolonged PR interval
		    ∘ Elevated acute phase reactants
		• Clinical signs occur 2–3 weeks after pharyngitis
		• Most common cardiac lesion: mitral regurgitation
		• Poststreptococcal reactive arthritis possible
			• Evidence of a preceding strep infection:
			  - Positive throat culture
			  - Positive rapid antigen
			  - Elevation of antistreptolysin O, antihyaluronidase, or antiDNAase B antibody
			  - History of scarlet fever
			AND
			• Two major OR one major and two minor Jones criteria
				• Salicylates for arthritis, mild carditis
				• Consider steroids for severe carditis
				• Benzodiazepines/haloperidol for chorea
				• Lifelong prophylaxis to prevent further streptococcal infections, usually with penicillin

GAS = group A *Streptococcus*.

Chapter 12

Perioperative Care

Table 12-1

Preoperative Testing

TEST	COMMON INDICATION	COMMENT
ECG	• Men >40 years • Women >50 years	• Useful as a baseline Consider in younger patients if: • Diabetes • Cardiovascular disease • Pulmonary disease • Thyroid disease
Serum Electrolytes	• >65 years old	Consider in younger patients if: • Renal disease • Cardiovascular disease • Diabetes • Diuretic use • Steroid use
Serum Glucose	• >65 years old	Consider in younger patients if: • High risk for diabetes
Hemoglobin/ Hematocrit	• >65 years old	Consider if: • Menstruating woman
PT/PTT	• Not routinely indicated	Consider if: • Liver disease • Cancer • Bleeding disorder • Use of anticoagulation • Neurosurgical procedure
Platelets	• Not routinely indicated	Consider if: • Bleeding disorder
CXR	• Not routinely indicated	Consider if: • Cardiovascular disease • Pulmonary disease • Cancer
Urinalysis	• Not routinely indicated	Consider if: • Genitourinary procedure planned • Prosthetic placement planned • Diabetes • Renal disease
Echocardiogram	• Not routinely indicated	Consider if: • CHF and no echocardiogram within 6 months • History of aortic stenosis
Pulmonary Function Test	• Not routinely indicated	Consider if: • Pulmonary disease

CXR = chest x-ray; CHF congestive heart failure; COPD = chronic obstructive pulmonary disease; ECG = electrocardiogram; PT = prothrombin time; PTT = partial thromboplastin time.

Table 12-2

General Approach for Preoperative Cardiac Evaluation for Nonemergent Surgery

- The goal of preoperative evaluation for noncardiac surgery is to assess the patient's perioperative risk of MI, heart failure, and death
- Elective surgery should be deferred to allow cardiac evaluation, for 30 days following MI, or until decompensated heart failure is treated
- Although emergency surgery carries a high risk, by definition it cannot be delayed. Therefore, stratify cardiac risk postoperatively and maximize postoperative care
- There are multiple guidelines for preoperative cardiac evaluation and most suggest a stepwise approach

STEP	DETAILS	
1	Determine if coronary revascularization occurred within past 5 years • If no recurrent signs/symptoms, proceed with surgery • If recurrent signs/symptoms, consider coronary evaluation	
2	Assess clinical predictors, risk of surgery, and activity level (METS) (see Tables 12-3, 12-4, and 12-5)	
3	If major clinical risk factors	• Consider canceling surgery/delaying until cardiac status maximized • Consider coronary angiography
	If intermediate clinical risk factors	• Consider noninvasive cardiac testing if high-risk surgery OR if METS <4
	If low clinical risk factors	• Consider noninvasive cardiac testing if high-risk surgery AND METS <4
4	If noninvasive cardiac testing performed (as indicated above), review results	• If low-risk result, proceed to surgery • If high-risk result, consider coronary angiography
5	If coronary evaluation/angiography performed (as indicated above), review results	• Subsequent care dictated by results*

*PTCA and CABG may be appropriate if indicated independently of the need for surgery. All patients should have postoperative risk stratification and risk factor reduction. Consider periopertive beta-blockade in patients without contraindications if high-risk surgery or high-risk clinical predictors.

CABG = coronary artery bypass graft; METS = metabolic equivalent; MI = myocardial infarction; PTCA = percutaneous transluminal coronary angioplasty.

Data from: Eagle KA, Berger PB, Calkins H, Chaitman BR, Ewy GA, Fleischmann KE, Fleisher LA, Froehlich JB, Gusberg RJ, Leppo JA, Ryan T, Schlant RC, Winters WL Jr. ACC/AHA guideline update for perioperative cardiovascular evaluation for noncardiac surgery update: a report of the American College of Cardiology/American Heart Association Task Force on Practice Guidelines (Committee to Update the 1996 Guidelines on Perioperative Cardiovascular Evaluation for Noncardiac Surgery), 2002. American College of Cardiology Web site. Available at: http://www.acc.org/clinical/guidelines/perio/update/periupdate_index.htm.

Table 12-3

Clinical Predictors of Increased Perioperative Cardiovascular Risk (MI, Heart Failure, and Death)

CLINICAL RISK CATEGORY	TYPE OF RISK FACTOR	KEY RISK FACTORS
Major	• Clinical	• Acute MI (within 7 days) or unstable angina
	• Cardiac evaluation	• Decompensated heart failure • Evidence of important ischemic risk by symptoms or noninvasive study • Significant arrhythmia • Severe valvular disease
	• History	• Recent MI (>7 days, but <30 days)
Intermediate	• Clinical	• Mild angina
	• Cardiac evaluation	• Compensated heart failure
	• History	• MI (by history or pathologic Q wave on ECG) • Heart failure (compensated or prior heart failure) • Diabetes mellitus (especially insulin dependent) • Renal insufficiency (creatinine >2.0)
Minor	• Clinical	• Advanced age • Poor performance status
	• Cardiac evaluation	• Abnormal ECG • Nonsinus rhythm
	• History	• Stroke • Uncontrolled systemic HTN • Low functional capacity

HTN = hypertension.

Data from: Eagle KA, Berger PB, Calkins H, Chaitman BR, Ewy GA, Fleischmann KE, Fleisher LA, Froehlich JB, Gusberg RJ, Leppo JA, Ryan T, Schlant RC, Winters WL Jr. ACC/AHA guideline update for perioperative cardiovascular evaluation for noncardiac surgery update: a report of the American College of Cardiology/American Heart Association Task Force on Practice Guidelines (Committee to Update the 1996 Guidelines on Perioperative Cardiovascular Evaluation for Noncardiac Surgery), 2002. American College of Cardiology Web site. Available at: http://www.acc.org/clinical/guidelines/perio/update/periupdate_index.htm.

Table 12-4

Estimated Energy Requirements for Various Activities

MET	EXAMPLE
1 MET	• Eat and dress self
4 METS	• Climb up one flight of stairs
>10 METS	• Strenuous sport (swimming or singles tennis)

MET = metabolic equivalents of work.
Data from: Fletcher GF, Balady G, Froelicher VF, Hartley LH, Haskell WL, Pollock ML. Exercise standards: a statement for healthcare professionals from the American Heart Association. American Heart Association Exercise Standards. Available at: http://www.americanheart.org.

Table 12-5

Cardiac Risk Stratification for Noncardiac Surgical Procedures

SURGICAL RISK CATEGORY	EXAMPLES OF TYPE OF OPERATION	ESTIMATED COMBINED INCIDENCE OF CARDIAC DEATH AND NONFATAL MI
High	• Emergent operations • Major vascular surgery • Prolonged procedures with fluid shifts/blood loss	• Often >5%
Intermediate	• Carotid endarterectomy • Abdominal and thoracic surgery • Prostate and orthopedic surgery	• Usually <5%
Low	• Endoscopy • Superficial procedures, including cataract and breast surgery	• Generally <1% • Further preoperative cardiac testing generally not required

Data from: Eagle KA, Berger PB, Calkins H, Chaitman BR, Ewy GA, Fleischmann KE, Fleisher LA, Froehlich JB, Gusberg RJ, Leppo JA, Ryan T, Schlant RC, Winters WL Jr. ACC/AHA guideline update for perioperative cardiovascular evaluation for noncardiac surgery update: a report of the American College of Cardiology/American Heart Association Task Force on Practice Guidelines (Committee to Update the 1996 Guidelines on Perioperative Cardiovascular Evaluation for Noncardiac Surgery), 2002. American College of Cardiology Web site. Available at: http://www.acc.org/clinical/guidelines/perio/update/periupdate_index.htm.

Table 12-6

Perioperative Blood Pressure Management Issues

ISSUE	CONDITION
Indication for Treatment of HTN	• Evidence of myocardial ischemia • CHF • Cerebral ischemia • Aortic dissection • MAP 20 mm Hg above baseline in diabetics • Sustained BP of >180/100 mm Hg for >3 hours
Perioperative Beta-Blockers	• Indications for beta-blockers: angina, arrhythmia, high-cardiac-risk patients undergoing vascular surgery, patients already on beta-blocker • Consider beta-blockers: any vascular surgery, intermediate- or high-risk surgery with high or intermediate-cardiac-risk factors • Metoprolol twice a day allows easy titration to achieve a pulse between 50 and 60 beats/min • If possible, start beta-blocker days to weeks prior to surgery

CHF = congestive heart failure; MAP = mean arterial pressure; BP = blood pressure; min = minutes; mm = millimeters; Hg = mercury.

Table 12-6

Perioperative Blood Pressure Management Issues (continued)

ISSUE	CONDITION

Predictors of Postoperative HTN	• Immediately postoperation:
	  - Pain
	  - Hypothermia
	  - Hypoxia
	  - Volume overload
	  - Cessation of positive pressure ventilation (increased preload with subsequent HTN)
	    48 hours postoperation:
	  - Fluid mobilization
	  - Medication withdrawal

Predictors of Postoperative Hypotension	• Acute:
	  - Vasodilation
	  - Myocardial depression
	  - Volume depletion
	  - Anesthesia
	• Delayed (>2 days):
	  - Acute pulmonary embolism
	  - Sepsis

Contraindications to Perioperative Beta-Blockade	• Poorly controlled reactive airways disease • Left ventricular ejection fraction <30% • Bradyarrhythmia with pulse <55/min without pacemaker • Second- or third-degree heart block without pacemaker • Systolic BP <100 mm Hg • Carotid sinus sensitivity • Clonidine may be helpful if cannot tolerate beta-blocker

BP = blood pressure; MAP = mean arterial pressure, HTN = hypertension.

Table 12-7

Indications for Perioperative Anticoagulation

INDICATION/CONDITION	DETAIL

Postsurgery DVT prophylaxis	• Early ambulation
	• Depending on risk factors (see Chapter 9, Hematology) and type of surgery consider:
	  - SQ low-dose heparin
	  - LMWH
	  - Intermittent pneumatic compression

Risk of DVT by location of surgery	• (Higher) knee > hip > neurosurgical > general surgery (lower)

(*continued*)

Table 12-7

Indications for Perioperative Anticoagulation (continued)

INDICATION/CONDITION	DETAIL
Absolute contraindications for postoperative anticoagulation	• LMWH absolutely contraindicated immediately after epidural anesthesia
Rule of thumb for preoperative management of patients on anticoagulation	• If INR 2–3 stop warfarin 4 days before surgery in order to achieve goal INR <1.5 for most surgeries (normal range for neurosurgery) • Check INR day before surgery and consider low-dose vitamin K SQ if INR >1.8

DVT = deep venous thrombosis; INR = international normalized ratio; LMWH = low molecular weight heparin; SQ = subcutaneous.

Table 12-8

Prevention of Postoperative Pulmonary Complications

TIME POINT	INTERVENTIONS TO CONSIDER
Preoperative	• Stop smoking >3weeks (ideally >8 weeks) before surgery to allow return of normal ciliary function • Treat respiratory infections and, if possible, delay surgery until infection resolved • Bronchodilator therapy if history of COPD or asthma • If patient has kyphosis consider undiagnosed restrictive lung disease • Patients with vital capacity <1 L have high chance of prolonged intubation postoperatively
Intraoperative	If known pulmonary disease or high risk for pulmonary complications: • Limit surgery to <3 hours when possible • Use spinal or epidural anesthesia instead of general anesthesia • Use laparoscopic procedures or limit extent of surgery when possible
Postoperative	• Incentive spirometry to decrease atelectasis • Early ambulation • Continuous positive airway pressure • Control pain • Limit sedation • Monitor oxygen saturation if known pulmonary disease • Chest PT/cough encouragement • Maintain normothermia

PT = physical therapy; COPD = chronic obstructive pulmonary disease; L = liter.

Table 12-9

Summary of Perioperative Issues by Organ System

CATEGORY	COMMON ISSUE
Gastroenterology	• Postoperative ileus may be secondary to pain, anesthesia, or inactivity • Consider ulcer prophylaxis if mechanical ventilation for more than 48 hours or coagulopathy
Rheumatology	• Consider stress dose steroids to decrease risk of flare of rheumatologic disease. • For patients with rheumatoid arthritis consider preoperative cervical spine films/MRI to rule out C1–C2 subluxation
Diabetes	• Maximize control of blood sugars before surgery • Avoid oral hypoglycemics on the day of surgery • If receiving insulin, give one-half of the dose of medium-acting insulin on the day of surgery with D5 in IVF. Continue all (or nearly all) glargine insulin the night before or morning of surgery to allow for basal insulin • Monitor for atypical symptoms of MI (such as nausea), development of pressure ulcers (especially on feet), and slow wound healing • Ensure that renal function has normalized before restarting metformin
Adrenal Disease	• Consider stress dose steroids if the patient has been on prolonged corticosteroids within the past year • Adrenal reserve may be abnormal for >1 year following a course of prednisone 20 mg daily for 2–4 weeks (or equivalent). In these patients, consider ACTH stimulation test

ACTH = adrenocorticotropic hormone; C1–C2 = cervical vertebraes 1–2; D5 = dextrose 50%; IVF = intravenous fluid; MRI = magnetic resonance imaging.

Table 12-10

Perioperative Chemoprophylaxis

CLINICAL SITUATION	ANTIBIOTIC OPTION
Coverage for skin flora	• Cefazolin
High likelihood of MRSA infection	• Vancomycin
Gastrointestinal and gynecologic surgeries	• Second-generation cephalosporin
Cephalosporin allergy	• Clindamycin
Genitourinary surgery	• Fluoroquinolones
Risk factors for wound infection: • Abdominal surgery • Duration of surgery >2 hours • Contaminated surgery	
• Consider *Clostridium difficile* in any patient with diarrhea and treat promptly if found	

MRSA = methicillin-resistant *staphylococcus aureus.*

Ophthalmology

Vision Impairment

Definition and Etiology: Blindness is legally defined as the best eye having no better than 20/200 vision despite corrective lenses. Patients with a visual field constricted to a 20-degree angle or less are also considered legally blind. In order to obtain a driver's license, most states require 20/40 vision in either one or both eyes. The etiologies of visual impairment are broad. Age-related macular degeneration is the most common cause of vision impairment and impairs central vision. Treatment of macular degeneration with laser photocoagulation can help preserve vision. Cataracts, glaucoma, and diabetic retinopathy can also cause visual impairment. See Table 13-1 for causes of acute visual loss. See Table 13-2 for details of cataracts. See Table 13-3 for discussion of glaucoma.

Epidemiology: More than 6 million people are visually impaired, but do not fit the legal definition of blindness.

Clinical presentation: Visual impairment is often gradual. Patients with acute or transient vision loss should be evaluated urgently by an ophthalmologist.

Diagnosis: Visual acuity and visual fields testing and fundoscopic examination. Refer to an ophthalmologist if vision is worse than 20/40 in either eye.

Acute Visual Loss

Definition and Etiology: The distinction between monocular and binocular visual loss can help locate the site of the problem. Monocular transient visual loss suggests a disorder anterior to the optic chiasm (the optic nerve or the eye). Etiologies include ocular disorders and ischemia. Binocular transient visual loss suggests a posterior disorder of the optic chiasm or visual cortex.

Anesthesia Considerations in Ophthalmologic Operations

In general, most ophthalmologic operations utilize monitored anesthesia care (MAC) rather than general anesthesia: the patient is awake but mildly sedated. If a patient cannot lie flat in one position for the duration of the procedure, MAC cannot be used. Bradyarrhythmias and hypertension are common during cataract surgery.

Table 13-1

Acute Loss of Vision: Etiology, Clinical Presentation, and Treatment

	DEFINITION AND ETIOLOGY	CLINICAL PRESENTATION	DIAGNOSIS AND TREATMENT
Unilateral causes			
Retinal Detachment	• Detachment of the retina (tissue-paper thin layer that captures light and lines in the inside of the eyeball) • Highly myopic (near-sighted) patients are at increased risk for retinal detachment	• Painless, unilateral acute loss of vision • Floaters, flashes, or a half-moon shadow • Vision progressively worsens as more retina peels off • Occurs in 50% of patients with CMV retinitis	• Visual acuity, visual fields, and fundoscopic examination • Immediate ophthalmology consultation • Rule out nonocular causes • Treatment includes laser, scleral buckle, and vitrectomy • If the macula is still attached, the prognosis is better and prompt treatment can improve outcomes
Retinal Vascular Occlusion	• Decreased flow in the retinal arteries or veins caused by: - Transient ischemic attack of the retina (amaurosis fugax) - Giant cell arteritis - Sickle cell disease - Anterior ischemic optic neuropathy	• Painless, unilateral acute loss of vision (usually partial field) • Intermittent vision loss/blurry vision that waxes and wanes according to perfusion of the tissue • Visual loss due to thromboembolic events generally lasts 1–15 minutes • Thromboembolic events likely from the carotids	• Visual acuity, visual fields, and fundoscopic examination • If giant cell arteritis suspected, treatment (steroids) should not be delayed until a temporal artery biopsy can performed • Check ESR if patient older than 50 and/or giant cell arteritis suspected • Ophthalmology consultation to confirm diagnosis • Systemic workup to identify (and treat) underlying cause (diabetes, hypertension, hypercoagulability, autoimmune/collagen-vascular disease, cardiac or carotid source of emboli)

(continued)

Table 13-1

Acute Loss of Vision: Etiology, Clinical Presentation, and Treatment (continued)

	DEFINITION AND ETIOLOGY	**CLINICAL PRESENTATION**	**DIAGNOSIS AND TREATMENT**
Ocular Disorders	• Acute glaucoma • Hemorrhage in the anterior chamber (hyphema) • Optic neuritis	• Acute glaucoma. Unilateral, painful eye. See dedicated Table 13-3 • Optic neuritis. Unilateral, painful eye. Pain worse with eye movements	
Bilateral Causes			
Papilledema	• Optic nerve swelling due to increased intracranial pressure • Chronic papilledema may be due to idiopathic intracranial hypertension or dural venous sinus occlusion	• Transient (seconds) visual obscurations occur (unilateral or bilateral), but visual loss a late presenting sign • Symptoms usually reflect the underlying intracranial hypertension (headache, nausea, and vomiting) • If chronic, the blind spot may increase in size as the fibers around the optic disc are affected	• On fundoscopic examination, the outer edge of the optic nerve blurs into the surrounding retina (normally looks like a pink donut with distinct outer edges) • Acute papilledema requires emergent evaluation for causes of increased intracranial pressure (mass, obstructive hydrocephalus, etc.) • Treat the underlying cause of increased intracranial pressure • If chronic, acetazolamide and restrictive diets may help
Nonocular Disorders	• Stroke (to visual cortex) • Visual auras related to migraines	• Visual loss due to auras can last 10–30 minutes	

CMV = cytomegalovirus; ESR = erythrocyte sedimentation rate.

Table 13-2

Cataracts: Etiology, Clinical Presentation, and Treatment

Cataract	Etiology	Epidemiology	Clinical Presentation	Treatment
Age-Related Cataracts	• The lens is made of replicating cells and is enclosed by a capsule. The cells in the middle were made during embryonic development while the cells toward the outside are made later in life. When the lens becomes too crowded with cells it becomes cloudy	• Most people have some degree of cataract by age 60 • Risk factors include trauma, radiation, steroid use, diabetes, and hypo-thyroid disease	• Symptoms: change in color perception, decreased visual acuity, monocular diplopia, and glare • Patients with uveitis, diabetes, or those taking systemic steroids tend to progress more quickly • On examination, the pupils may be opaque or white	• Can be removed when vision loss impairs patient function and/or quality of life

Table 13-3

Glaucoma: Etiology, Clinical Presentation, and Treatment

GLAUCOMA	ETIOLOGY	CLINICAL PRESENTATION	TREATMENT
Acute Angle-Closure Glaucoma	• The drainage of the aqueous humor is impaired as the iris physically impedes on the trabecular meshwork • Intraocular pressure rapidly rises to very high levels • Precipitants include papillary dilation from a dark room or anticholinergics • 10% of all glaucoma cases • Risk factor: age	• Acute onset (hours to days) of a red, painful eye and visual loss • Patient may report halos • Nausea, vomiting • Cornea becomes hazy white and edematous from the extremely high intraocular pressure • Pupil is frozen in a middilated position and does not react well to light • Affected eyeball is firm to palpation	• Immediate treatment with eyedrops to lower eye pressure: beta-blocker (e.g., timolol, caution if asthma or COPD), alpha-agonist (e.g., brimonidine), and steroid (prednisolone 1%) • Urgent ophthalmology consult • Systemic treatment includes acetazolamide and osmotic diuresis with mannitol • Definitive treatment is laser peripheral iridotomy • If pressure lowered, some patients regain vision • Untreated acute angle-closure glaucoma can result in permanent visual loss within 2–5 days
Chronic Open-Angle Glaucoma	• Mild to moderately elevated intraocular pressures • Blockage in the small drainage pathways of the trabecular meshwork. The angle is not affected • Affects 2% of U.S. population • Risk factors: age, near sightedness, African American, family history	• Painless and initially asymptomatic • Gradual loss of vision over years, with peripheral vision lost first • Diagnostic findings: (1) moderately elevated intraocular pressures, (2) optic nerve cupping, (3) visual field changes	• Topical medications: beta-blockers, alpha-adrenergics, and carbonic anhydrase inhibitors (contraindicated in sulfa allergy or sickle cell disease) • If not controlled medically, laser or surgical approaches may be useful • Untreated, will cause blindness in 15–25 years

COPD = chronic obstructive pulmonary disease.

Table 13-4
Ophthalmologic Infections: Etiology, Clinical Presentation, and Treatment

INFECTION	ETIOLOGY	CLINICAL PRESENTATION	TREATMENT
Hordeolum and Chalazion	• Blocked oil glands, commonly known as a "stye" causing inflammation on the eyelid margins • Hordeolum: acute phase: painful, erythematous, and tender • Chalazion: chronic phase: painless granuloma	• Untreated lesions may resolve on their own or progress to a chalazion • Causative agent usually *Staphylococcus aureus* • Large chalazion overlying the cornea can induce visual disturbances	• Warm compresses to the affected area multiple times a day • Ophthalmologic antibiotic/steroid combination • If the lesion persists despite compresses and antibiotic, may need an incision and drainage
Preseptal Cellulitis	• Infection of the superficial skin of the periorbital region (eyelids and cheek area) that does not cross the septum into the orbital area	• Warmth, tenderness, and edema of the superficial periorbital skin • No diplopia, proptosis, blurry vision, or pain on eye movement	• If mild: oral amoxicillin/clavulanate • If moderate or severe: IV ceftriaxone • Consider CT or MRI if severe, or if it progresses despite antibiotic treatment
Orbital Cellulitis	• Infection within the orbital cavity • Most common cause is spread from sinus infection	• Diplopia • Proptosis • Blurry vision • Painful, restricted eye movements • Eye pain	• Immediately involve ophthalmology • IV antibiotics • If immunocompromised also give antifungal agents
Endophthalmitis	• Inflammation of the intraocular cavities • Endogenous: hematogenous spread of an infection from a distant infection (often endocarditis) • Exogenous: direct inoculation of the eye as a complication from surgery, trauma, or a foreign object	• Blurry vision • Eye pain and erythema • Hypopyon (pus in the anterior chamber) • Absent red reflex • May have proptosis and decreased ocular motility if involves the orbit	• Immediately involve ophthalmology • IV antibiotics for at least 2 weeks with doses used for meningitis; and antibiotics directly injected into the eyeball • Culture the blood, the eye, and any other possible sources of infection • If the visual acuity is poor, may need a vitrectomy • Under normal circumstances, the blood-ocular barrier prevents infection

CT = computed tomography; MRI = magnetic resonance imaging.

Table 13-5

Irritative Ophthalmologic Issues

Eye Irritation	Etiology	Clinical Presentation	Treatment
Dry Eyes (Keratoconjunctivitis Sicca)	• Decreased tear production and/or increased tear evaporation from: - Aging - Medications (antihistamines, general anesthetic and topical beta-blockers) - Sjögren syndrome - Facial nerve palsy - Exophthalmos (Graves' disease) - Decreased blinking (Parkinson disease) - Contact lenses - Herpes simplex keratitis	• Gritty sensation, itching, redness, light sensitivity, inability to produce tears, excessive mucous secretion • Increased reflex tearing triggered by the irritation of dryness (a confusing symptom for patients) • Worse in dry weather or windy conditions	• Ophthalmologic lubrication with artificial tear drops, gels, or ointments • Attempt to correct the underlying etiology
Pterygium or Pinguecula	• Benign growths in the conjunctiva that can encroach on the cornea	• May become intermittently irritated and inflamed	• Sunglasses, ophthalmologic lubrication • Topical ophthalmologic NSAIDs • If threatens to grow over the pupil, consider excision. However, tends to grow back frequently
Bacterial Conjunctivitis	• Causative agents: - *Staphylococcus* - *Streptococcus* - *Haemophilus influenzae* - *Moraxella* - *Pseudomonas* (if contact lenses)	• Moderate amount of pus • Severe, purulent conjunctivitis may be due to *Neisseria* or *Chlamydia* (need ophtho referral and IV antibiotics)	• Topical ophthalmologic antibiotic (sulfacetamide, tobramycin, or ciprofloxacin) • Prevent spread by washing hands, towels, and bedding
Viral Conjunctivitis	• Most common cause of red eye • Causative agent: - Adenovirus	• Profuse tearing with scant discharge • Associated upper respiratory infection • Palpable/tender preauricular lymph nodes • No pain or impaired vision • Often unilateral	• Artificial tears

Allergic Conjunctivitis	• Causative agents:
	  - Seasonal allergies
	  - Dust
	  - Animal hair, etc.
		• Pruritic, bilateral, recurrent erythematous conjunctiva
		• Other allergic symptoms: runny nose, sneezing, etc.
			• Topical ophthalmologic antihistamine or mast cell inhibitor (i.e., olapatadine; Patanol)
			• Systemic antihistamines

Corneal Abrasion	• Abrasion of the cornea, not penetrating into the eyeball • Often the patient can recall the incident	• Foreign body sensation (even though no object present) • Erythema, tearing • Possible blurry vision • Visible sloughed edges of the abrasion • Opacity of normally clear cornea • Fluorescein stain lights abrasion up green when examined under cobalt blue light	• Mild: artificial tears • Moderate: topical ophthalmologic antibiotic • Central abrasion: see ophthalmology within 24 hours • Contact lens wearer: no contact lenses until the abrasion heals • Ocufloxacin to cover *Pseudomonas* • Flip eyelids to look for a foreign body and flush the eye, especially for vertical abrasions suggesting abrasion during blinking

Uveitis	• Inflammation of the uveal tract: iris, ciliary body (makes intraocular fluid), and the choroid (lies beneath the retina)
	• Nongranulomatous uveitis:
	  - HLA-B27 conditions:
	    ○ Ankylosing spondylitis
	    ○ Reiter syndrome
	    ○ Psoriasis
	    ○ Ulcerative colitis
	    ○ Crohn disease
	    ○ Herpes zoster
	    ○ Herpes simplex
	    ○ Behçet disease
	• Granulomatous uveitis:
	  - Sarcoid
	  - Tuberculosis
	  - Syphilis
	  - Toxoplasmosis
		• Photophobia
		• Eye pain (more discomfort from anterior uveitis than from posterior uveitis)
		• Erythema of the eye
		• Blurry vision
		• Granulomas in conjunctiva or large "mutton fat" precipitates on the corneal endothelium
			• A screening workup for systemic disease is indicated for bilateral, granulomatous, or recurrent uveitis of unknown etiology
			• The first episode of unilateral, nongranulomatous uveitis does not necessarily require a battery of screening tests

NSAIDs = nonsteroidal anti-inflammatory drugs.

Table 13-6

Ophthalmologic Screening

REASON FOR SCREENING	SCREENING FOR	SCREENING FREQUENCY
Diabetes	• Retinopathy	• Yearly • Every 6 months if have mild retinopathy
Family History of Glaucoma	• Glaucoma	• Yearly
HIV	• HIV retinopathy • CMV retinitis	• Every 6–12 months • Every 3 months if CD4< 200
Age > 40	• Glaucoma • Cataracts • Visual acuity	• Every 3–5 years

Chapter 14

Dermatology

Table 14-1

Lumps and Bumps—Verrucous Lesions, Corns, and Calluses

LESION	EPIDEMIOLOGY/ETIOLOGY	CLINICAL	DIAGNOSIS	TREATMENT/NOTE

Common Wart	• Benign skin tumor associated with HPV
	• Common wart: HPV 2, 4, 27, 29
	• Flat wart: HPV 3, 10, 28, 49
	• Plantar wart: HPV 1
	• Transmitted via direct contact or autoinoculation
	• Widespread if patient immunocompromised or has hereditary epidermodysplasia verruciformis
		• Types
		  1. *Verruca vulgaris*: raised, round papules with a rough surface
		  2. *Verruca plana*: small flat, hyperpigmented lesions
		  3. *Plantar warts*: painful scaly lesions on sole of feet
		• Location: fingers, dorsum of hands, elbows, and knees
			• Clinical
			• Plantar warts interrupt the normal skin lines of the foot (vs. calluses/corns)
			• May see thrombosed capillaries ("seeds") after scraping with a surgical blade
				• Two-thirds spontaneously resolve within 2 years
				• Pare down wart
				• Liquid nitrogen
				• Electrodessication and curettage
				• Daily use of 10–17% salicylic acid
				• Occlusive tape

Genital Wart
Condyloma acuminata
	• 50% of sexually active individuals infected with HPV. Only 1–2% with clinical lesions
	• Risk factors:
	  1. High number of sexual partners/ frequency of intercourse
	  2. Partner with external genital lesions
	  3. Sexual partner's number of partners
	  4. Infection with other STDs
		• Soft, flesh colored lesions that can become large and pedunculated (cauliflower-like); can lead to obstruction
		• Location: perineum, vagina, anus, penis, scrotum, mouth
			• Clinical
			• Application of acetic acid causes lesions to turn white and can facilitate identification and may help define extent of infection
				• Liquid nitrogen
				• CO_2 laser therapy
				• Weekly applications of 25% podophyllin
				• Imiquimod 5% cream
				• Anogenital neoplasia associated with increased risk of cervical and anal carcinoma
				• Pap smear, colposcopy, anoscopy for internal warts
				• Prophylactic vaccine now available, protects against HPV 6, 11, 16, 18

Genital Warts (cont.)	• Genital wart (benign): HPV 6 and 11 • Anogenital neoplasia: HPV 16, 18, 31, 33, 35 • HPV 16, 18 highest risk for cervical carcinoma • HPV can be transmitted to a newborn through the birth canal		
Corns/ Calluses	• Chronic repetitive pressure or friction forces result in keratotic papules (corns) and plaques (calluses) • Osseous structure may predispose a patient to sites of increased cutaneous friction or shear stress (hallux valgus, "rocker bottom foot")	• Location: dorsal aspects of pedal PIP/DIP joints (hard) and between toes (soft) • Painful symptoms such as burning may be present • Complications: bursitis, blistering, and ulceration → septic arthritis, osteomyelitis	• Clinical • Unlike verrucae, no pinpoint hemorrhage, papilliform surface, or interruption of skin lines	• Prevention: reduce or eliminate mechanical forces (occupational habits, shoes) • Paring followed by felt dispersion padding • Keratolytics • Surgery to correct osseous deformities

DIP = distal interphalangeal; HPV = human papilloma virus; PCR = polymerase chain reaction; PIP = proximal interphalangeal; STDs = sexually transmitted diseases.

Table 14-2

The Pigmented Lesions—Congenital, Acquired, and Dysplastic Nevi

Lesion	Epidemiology/Etiology	Clinical	Diagnosis	Treatment/Notes
Congenital Melanocytic Nevi	• Groups of melanocytes clustered at the dermis, forming a plaque	• Size: variable • Color: uniform, darkens with age to brown-black color • Border: well-demarcated edge, symmetric	• Clinical examination • Refer to dermatology if lesions suspicious for malignancy • Biopsy required for lesions that are suspicious for malignancy • Wood's lamp: accentuates epidermal hyperpigmentation	• Surgical removal of entire congenital nevi is controversial • Large lesions (>20 cm) have 5–15% risk of transformation to melanoma • Signs of malignant transformation require biopsy: **(ABCDEs)** (see Table 14-3)
Acquired Melanocytic Nevi (Pigmented/ Common Mole/Typical Nevi)	• Groups of melanocytes initially clustered at dermal-epidermal junction (*junctional nevi*), progressing to include both epidermal and dermal components (*compound nevi*), and eventually exclusively in the dermis (*intradermal nevi*) • Early childhood sun exposure may increase number of nevi • More common in fair skinned	• Course: first appear in infancy, peaking in number during late adolescence • Color: brown or black • Border: round, smooth, and regular • Location: sun-exposed areas • *Halo nevi* = surrounding skin hypopigmented	• Clinical examination	• Increased melanoma risk if >50 to 100 nevi • Signs of malignant transformation require biopsy: **(ABCDEs)** (see Table 14-3) • Each typical nevi with up to 0.03% lifetime risk of transformation to melanoma

| Dysplastic: Atypical Nevi | • Disordered proliferations of variably atypical melanocytes, either de novo or within a compound nevus
• Potential precursors of melanoma
• A marker of increased risk for melanoma in "normal" skin
• Autosomal dominant transmission in familial melanoma/dysplastic nevus syndrome | • Course: arise later in childhood than common nevi and continue to develop with age
• Share some clinical characteristics of melanoma (color variable, border fuzzy, larger size), but generally stable and asymptomatic
• Location: often in sun-protected areas | | • Routine follow-up with serial photography every 6 months
• Signs of malignant transformation require biopsy: **ABCDEs** (see Table 14-3)
• Lifetime risk of dysplastic nevi developing melanoma is 18% |

LESION	EPIDEMIOLOGY/ETIOLOGY	CLINICAL	DIAGNOSIS	TREATMENT/NOTES
Malignant Melanoma	• Malignant melanocytes in nests that expand radially within epidermis and then vertically to dermis and beyond • 50% de novo, 50% arise from dysplastic nevus • Risk factors: 1. New or changing mole 2. Increasing age 3. Family history 4. Dysplastic nevus 5. Large congenital nevus (>20 cm) 6. Multiple nevi 7. White race 8. Severe childhood sunburns 9. Immunosuppression • Lifetime risk of developing melanoma: - General: nearly: 2% - Dysplastic nevi: 18% - Familial atypical multiple mole melanoma (FAMM): nearly 100%	• Types (frequency) 1. Superficial spreading (70%)—trunk and extremities 2. Nodular (20%)—initial growth vertical 3. Lentigo maligna/melanoma-in-situ (5%) face, ear, back of hand 4. Acral lentiginous (2–10% overall, but 35–90% of melanomas in nonwhites)—digits, nailbed, feet • Location: occur anywhere on skin and mucous membranes. Most common on back (men) and legs (women)	• Full body skin examination including scalp, mucous membranes, genital area, nails, and palpation of lymph nodes • Signs of malignancy requiring biopsy or removal: **A**symmetry **B**order (irregular) **C**olor (variegated) **D**iameter (>6 mm) **E**nlargement/Elevation • Total thickness excisional biopsy of entire lesion is indicated when melanoma is suspected	• Always need to do re-excision to achieve 2 cm margins when melanoma diagnosed • Prognosis and staging based on Breslow thickness • Sentinel lymph node dissection for palpable nodes or melanoma depth >1 mm and <4 mm • Adjuvant therapies: interferon alpha-2b increases survival in patients with regional lymph node involvement • Follow-up every 3–6 months including CXR, CT scan, and LDH for advanced stages • Amelanotic melanoma has minimal pigmentation and poor prognosis secondary to delayed diagnosis

Basil Cell Carcinoma (BCC)	• Locally invasive neoplasm of nonkeratinizing cells from basal layer of epidermis
	• Most common cancer (25% of all cancers diagnosed in the United States)
	• Risk factors
	  1. Fair complexion
	  2. Childhood sunburns
	  3. Exposure to ionizing radiation
	  4. Immunosuppression (organ transplant recipients have five times risk)
	  5. Nevoid BCC syndrome
		• Classic: "pearly" or waxy papule with rolled border, central depression and telangiectasias
		• Types:
		  1. Nodular
		  2. Superficial
		  3. Morpheaform
		  4. Pigmented
		• Easily missed lesions in "danger zones" include nasolabial folds, and posterior auricular skin
			• Clinical
			• Shave biopsy to confirm diagnosis
				• Electrodessication and curettage in areas of low recurrence (trunk and extremities)
				• Excision or Mohs' micrographic surgery for high risk areas of recurrence (head and neck)
				• Cryosurgery, radiation
				• Metastases are rare
				• Frequent follow-up necessary

Actinic Keratosis *Precursor to SCC*	• Associated with cumulative damage to keratinocytes by UVB radiation • Onset in middle age, especially in people with outdoor occupations/hobbies • 1%/year evolve to SCC	• Rough, dry, scaly yellow to brown papules and plaques on sun-exposed skin • Location: face, ears, neck, forearms, dorsal hands, lower legs, and scalp of bald men	• Clinical • Punch biopsy to rule out squamous cell cancer	• Prevention: daily sun protection • Cryotherapy with liquid nitrogen is mainstay • Topical 5-fluorouracil, retinoids for extensive lesions

(continued)

Table 14-3
The Skin Cancers—Melanoma, Basal Cell, and Squamous Cell, Including Precancerous Actinic Keratosis Lesions (continued)

LESION	EPIDEMIOLOGY/ETIOLOGY	CLINICAL	DIAGNOSIS	TREATMENT/NOTES
Squamous Cell Carcinoma (SCC)	• Locally invasive neoplasm of keratinizing cells that shows anaplasia, rapid growth, and metastatic potential • Second most common cancer • Risk factors: 1. Fair complexion 2. History of radiation 3. Burn scars, ulcers 4. Arsenic ingestion 5. Chronic inflammatory dermatoses 6. HPV infection 7. Immunosuppression	• Lesion: superficial, discrete, hard, lesion rising from an erythematous base • Arises within actinic keratoses • Risk of perineural invasion	• Clinical • Punch biopsy to confirm diagnosis and to evaluate depth of lesion	• Excision or Mohs' micrographic surgery for invasive SCC • Electrodessication and curettage, cryotherapy for noninvasive SCC • Radiation • Topical modalities: Imiquimod, 5-fluourouracil • Increased risk of metastasis if arises on mucosa or sites of chronic inflammation • 2–5% metastasize • Frequent follow-up needed

BCC = basal cell carcinoma; CT = computed tomography; CXR = chest x-ray; LDH = lactate dehydrogenase; SCC = squamous cell carcinoma; UVB = ultra violet.

Table 14-4
The Itchy Lesions: General Pruritus, Atopic Dermatitis, and Urticaria

Lesion	Epidemiology/Etiology	Clinical	Diagnosis	Treatment/Notes
Pruritus	• Common primary dermatologic diseases: - Xerosis (dry skin) - Atopic dermatitis - Allergic dermatitis (medication) - Contact dermatitis (soap) - Nummular eczema - Dermatophyte infections - Urticaria - Lichen planus, lichen simplex chronicus - Bullous pemphigoid - Dermatitis herpetiformis	Systemic causes (15% of patients): • Endocrine: hyper/hypothyroidism, diabetes • Renal: chronic failure • Malignancy: lymphoma, leukemia, multiple myeloma • Hematologic: iron-deficiency anemia polycythemia vera (exacerbated by hot water) • Liver: cholestasis, primary biliary cirrhosis • Drugs: morphine, codeine, aspirin, alcohol • Infectious: scabies, pediculosis corporis, HIV, parasites • Psychiatric: parasitosis delusions, depression • Pregnancy	• History and clinical examination • Consider lab tests/further workup to rule out systemic causes if etiology unclear	• Identify underlying cause and treat • Topical agents that contain menthol, phenol, camphor, pramoxine may provide symptomatic relief • Topical steroids if primary skin lesions are present • Oral antihistamines • Phototherapy if intractable
Atopic Dermatitis	• Acute, subacute, or chronic allergic disorder with genetic and immunologic components ("the itch that rashes") • Associated with personal or family history of atopy triad: atopic dermatitis, allergic rhinitis, asthma	• Lesion: tiny, pruritic, erythematous papules. Can also be crusted, weeping and scaly plaques • Chronic rubbing → pigment changes and lichenification • Superinfection with *Staphylococcus aureus* or HSV (eczema herpeticum) common	• Clinical • Bacterial/viral culture if appears superinfected • Increased serum IgE (85%)	• Avoid suspected allergens • Emollients, humidity, less frequent bathing • Topical steroids/antibiotics • Nonsteroidal topicals: tacrolimus, pimecrolimus (side effects include local burning, flu-like symptoms)

(continued)

Table 14-4

The Itchy Lesions: General Pruritus, Atopic Dermatitis, and Urticaria (continued)

LESION	EPIDEMIOLOGY/ETIOLOGY	CLINICAL	DIAGNOSIS	TREATMENT/NOTES

Atopic Dermatitis (cont.)	• Exacerbating factors:
	  1. Dehydration from frequent bathing or low humidity
	  2. Infections
	  3. Emotional stress
	  4. Hormonal changes
		• Course: more than 50% of patients develop allergic rhinitis and/or asthma	• See above	• Antihistamines
				• Oral antibiotics/antivirals for superinfection
				• Short course of systemic steroids if intractable
				• Phototherapy if severe

Urticaria (Hives)	• Mediated by IgE, complement, and vasoactive amines • Type I hypersensitivity (IgE) most frequent cause • Common inciting agents: foods, drugs, contact allergy, insect bites, and infections (bacterial and viral) • Also: cold, cholinergic (exercise, hot baths, emotions), sun, physical exercise • Usually a cause is not identified	• Triple response: vasodilatation (erythema), increased vascular permeability (wheal), axon reflex (flare) • Lesion: extremely pruritic, slightly raised lesions that appear suddenly • Lesion: red with white halo, or white with red halo. Not vesicular • Course: Lesions last 2–12 hours before resolving, changing shape, and/or shifting to new sites (migrating)	• Clinical • Check for dermatographism • If involves subcutaneous tissue evaluate for angioedema. Check complement levels • If chronic (>6 weeks), evaluate for chronic infection (hepatitis, sinusitis), connective tissue disorders or autoimmune disorders	• Avoidance of known triggers • Antipruritics for symptomatic relief • Antihistamines • In angioedema consider epinephrine • Corticosteroids not proven to be beneficial

HSV = herpes simplex virus.

Table 14-5

The Bad Lesions: Erythema Multiforme (EM), Minor and Major Steven-Johnson (SJS), Toxic Epidermal Necrolysis, Pemphigus Vulgaris, and Bullous Pemphigoid

Lesion	Epidemiology/Etiology	Clinical	Diagnosis	Treatment/Notes

EM *Minor*	• Male > female
	• Unclear etiology, likely an autoimmune phenomenon
	• Common triggers:
	  1. Medications (sulfas, anticonvulsants, allopurinol)
	  2. Infection (HSV, myco-plasma, *Streptococcus*)
	  3. Connective tissue disorders
	  4. Idiopathic (>50% of cases)
		• Classic "target lesions": erythematous rash with central clearing. May be macular, papular, and/or vesicular
		• No bullae
		• Lesions located on extremities. Limited mucosal involvement
		• Lesions develop over 10+ days, last 5–7 days and resolve spontaneously
			• Clinical
			• Morphology of the rash is diagnostic
			• Biopsy reveals perivascular mononuclear infiltrate, edema of the upper dermis
				• Supportive
				• For recurrent EM, consider prophylactic antiviral therapy with acyclovir

EM *Major*	• See above	• Lesions identical to EM minor, but often become bullous, necrotic, and slough off. Severe and extensive • Two or more mucous membranes involved: oral, genital, and conjunctiva. Genitourinary, gastrointestinal, and respiratory tract lesions less common • Associated illness: prodromal fever, fluid and electrolyte imbalance, vomiting, diarrhea, arthralgias	• Clinical • More severe than EM minor	• Supportive • Early withdrawal of suspected drugs • Steroids are controversial; appear most beneficial in early stages • Aggressive fluid and electrolyte management • Urgent ophthalmology evaluation to prevent corneal scarring • Gynecology/urology consultation to prevent genital mucosal scarring • Course: 5–25% of cases are fatal

(*continued*)

Table 14-5

The Bad Lesions: Erythema Multiforme (EM), Minor and Major Steven-Johnson (SJS), Toxic Epidermal Necrolysis, Pemphigus Vulgaris, and Bullous Pemphigoid (continued)

LESION	EPIDEMIOLOGY/ETIOLOGY	CLINICAL	DIAGNOSIS	TREATMENT/NOTES
SJS/TEN	• SJS is a severe variant of EM major • TEN is a severe variant of SJS • Age: >40 years • Risk factors: SLE, HIV • 80% of TEN, and 50% of SJS cases associated with medications • Drugs implicated: sulfa, allopurinol, anticonvulsants, penicillins, other antibiotics • Symptoms occur 1–3 weeks after first drug exposure (faster if a medication rechallenge)	• Acute inflammation involving the skin, mucous membrane, bowel and respiratory epithelium • SJS: full-thickness epidermal necrosis and detachment of <10% of the body surface • TEN: >30% of body surface involved • Lesions begin on the face and upper extremity and spread to the lower body • Lesions resemble second-degree burns • Lesions preceded by an influenza-like illness, skin tenderness, and conjunctival burning/itching • Respiratory failure • Conjunctivitis • Diarrhea, bowel obstruction	• Clinical • Nikolsky sign • Biopsy of active lesion: separation at the dermal-epidermal junction	• Same management as EM major • Early IVIG may be useful • Admission to intensive care or burn unit • Mortality approaches 30%

PV	• Serious acute/chronic autoimmune bullous disease of skin and mucous membranes • Age of onset: 40–60 years • IgG antibodies to epidermal desmoglein 3 results in loss of normal intercellular adhesion and clinical bullae formation	• Painful round to oval vesicles and flaccid bullae (erosions if rupture) • Bullae rupture easily • Distribution usually starts in oral mucosa • Nikolsky sign: superficial layers of skin separate from lower layers with minimal pressure • Clinical variants with antibodies to different antigens, including drug-induced and paraneoplastic	• Clinical • Biopsy: loss of intercellular cohesion in lower part of epidermis, with split just above the basal cell layer. Immunofluorescence reveals IgG and C3 intercellularly in epidermis • Serum IgG autoantibody titers correlate with disease activity	• Fatal if not treated • Systemic corticosteroids are mainstay • Concomitant immunosuppressive agents help spare steroids: mycophenolate mofetil, azathioprine, methotrexate, cyclophosphamide • Antibiotics for bacterial infections, correct fluid and electrolyte imbalances
BP	• Chronic autoimmune bullous disease • Age of onset: 60–80 years • IgG antibodies to basement membrane antigens (BP-Ag1, BP-Ag2) correlate more closely with deeper-seated bullae than those seen in PV	• Large tense bullae on normal or erythematous base, may contain serous, hemorrhagic fluid • Bullae rupture less easily than PV • Distribution: axillae, medial thighs, groin, abdomen • Mucous membrane involvement less common, less severe/less painful compared to PV	• Clinical • Biopsy: neutrophils at dermal-epidermal junction, subepidermal bullae, immunofluorescence reveals IgG and C3 deposits along the basement membrane zone • Antibasement membrane serum IgG in 70% (levels do not correlate with disease activity)	• Systemic corticosteroids, alone or in combination with mycophenolate mofetil/azathioprine • For mild cases, topical steroids alone may be beneficial • May go into permanent remission

EM = erythema multiforme; SJS = Stevens-Johnson syndrome; TEN = toxic epidermal necrolysis; SLE = systemic lupus erythematosus; IVIG = intravenous immunoglobulin; PV = pemphigus vulgaris; BP = bullous pemphigoid.

Table 14-6
Acne and Psoriasis

Lesion	Epidemiology/Etiology	Clinical	Diagnosis	Treatment/Notes

Acne	• Inflammation of pilosebaceous units as a result of complex interaction between androgens, *Propionibacterium acnes*, abnormal keratinization, and sebum
	
	• Exacerbating factors:
	  1. Endocrine disorders
	  2. Mechanical trauma
	  3. Emotional stress
	  4. Occlusion (e.g., mechanical, creams, lotions)
	  5. Drugs (lithium, dilantin, corticosteroids, androgens)
	  6. Sweating/chemical exposure
	
	• Mostly affects adolescents but comedonal acne persists into adulthood in 5–10%
	
	• Relationship with diet is controversial
		• Hallmark is comedo, open or closed
		
		• Also papules, pustules, cystic nodules, sinuses, atrophic or hypertrophic scars
		
		• Distribution: face, neck, chest, back, upper arms, buttocks
		
		• May flare with menses
		
		• SAPHO syndrome:
		  Synovitis, **A**cne, **P**ustulosis, **H**yperostosis, **O**steitis
			• Clinical
			
			• Females: if history of irregular menses or hirsutism, evaluate for hyperandrogenism and polycystic ovary syndrome (free testosterone, DHEA-S, FSH/LH)
				• Mild acne (pustular or comedal)
				  - Topical antibiotics
				  - Benzoyl peroxide
				  - Topical retinoids
				• Moderate acne (or not responsive to above therapy)
				  - As above, plus oral antibiotic therapy
				  - Consider oral contraceptive pills
				• Severe acne (nodulocystic or resistant pustular)
				  - Oral isotretinoin:
				  Significant side effects: teratogenetic, dryness, increased triglycerides/cholesterol, hepatotoxicity, night blindness, pseudotumor cerebri, depression
				• Evaluate after 2–3 months, as follicles mature every 2 months
				• Oral contraceptives and spironolactone are effective for hormonal acne

Psoriasis	• Etiology unknown, role for antecedent infections, T-cell mediation
	• Genetic predisposition
	• Affects 2–3% of population
	• Trigger:
	  1. Physical trauma (Koebner phenomenon)
	  2. Infections
	  3. Stress
	  4. Drugs (lithium, beta-blockers, systemic interferon, antimalarials)
	• Types:
	  1. Localized plaque
	  2. Widespread plaque
	  3. Guttate: "droplike" plaques, associated with streptococcal infections
	  4. Pustular
	  5. Palmoplantar
		• Red papules or plaques with thick silvery adherent scale
		• Removal of scale results in punctate hemorrhages (Auspitz sign)
		• Location: scalp, ears, elbows, knees, umbilicus, and gluteal cleft
		• Pitting of nail or separation of nails from nail bed, subungual hyperkeratosis, oil spots
		• Seronegative arthritis in 5–8%: asymmetric small joint oligoarthritis most common
			• Clinical	• Emollients
				• Topical corticosteroids
				• Topical calcipotriene
				• Oral retinoids for palmoplantar psoriasis
				• Systemic therapies: methotrexate, cyclosporin A
				• Phototherapy (PUVA—**psoralen plus ultraviolet A**)
				• Immunologic systemic therapies: TNF-alpha inhibitors
				• Sudden onset may be associated with HIV infection
				• First presentation may be erythroderma

Seborrheic Dermatitis	• Etiology unknown, may be related to response to colonization with the lipophilic yeast *Malassezia furfur* • May overlap with psoriasis • Increased frequency and severity in HIV (80% of HIV patients) and parkinsonism	• Greasy, yellow scale on erythematous plaques in hair-bearing parts of the body: scalp, eyebrows, eyelashes, beard, chest, ears, nasolabial folds, and axillae • Pruritus is variable	• Clinical • If rash is severe, consider HIV testing	• Selenium sulfide, zinc pyrithione, ketoconazole, or tar-based shampoos • Mild topical corticosteroids • Topical ketoconazole • Chronic condition that requires maintenance treatment

DHEA-S = dehydroepiandrosterone; FSH = follicle-stimulating hormone; LH = luteinizing hormone; TNF = tumor necrosis factor.

385

Table 14-7

Skin Infestations

Lesion	Epidemiology/Etiology	Clinical	Diagnosis	Treatment/Notes
Pediculosis	• Infestation by blood sucking lice: *Pediculus humanus capitis* (head lice), *Pediculus humanus corporis* (body lice), *Phthirus pubis* (pubic lice) • Transmission via direct person-to-person contact or indirect contact through fomites • Head lice seen in all ages and socioeconomic groups • Body lice associated with poor living conditions, indigence, refugee-camp populations • Pubic lice sexually transmitted	• Papules, pruritus, excoriations • Lice and nits are visible to naked eye • Frequently coexists with scabies • Secondary infections *with S. aureus*, *Streptococcus Pyogenes* common	• Head lice: live adult lice, nymphs, or nits adherent to hair close to scalp. Visual inspection without combing overlooks 75% of infestations • Body lice: lice and eggs found in seams of clothing • Pubic lice: live adult lice, nymphs, or nits in pubic area, axillae, or eyelashes	• Topical insecticides: permethrin, or pyrethrin, or malathion • Must be applied appropriately, and may need to repeat treatment • Examine and treat household contacts • Wash fomites (no direct evidence) • Resistance is emerging worldwide to permethrin, pyrethrins, and malathion • Systemic therapy with Ivermectin • No need to stay home from work or school once treated
Scabies	• Infestation by the mite *Sarcoptes scabiei* which burrow into epidermis • Pruritus results from hypersensitivity to mite feces • Transmission via skin-to-skin contact or through fomites • Seen in all ages, especially the impoverished and immobilized • Norwegian scabies: massive infestation with disabling pruritus	• Generalized severe pruritus with papules, excoriations • Distribution: wrists, periumbilical, genital region, buttocks, axillae, nipples • Burrows prominent in web spaces	• Clinical • Mite prep: place drop of mineral oil on burrow and scrape onto slide for microscopic examination	• Permethrin 5% cream • If mite cannot be isolated, empiric therapy based on clinical judgment • Treat household contacts at same time, even if asymptomatic • Decontaminate clothing and bedding • Pruritus can persists for several weeks after therapy. Treat symptomatically

Table 14-8

Pustular Skin Infections

Lesion	Epidemiology/Etiology	Clinical	Diagnosis	Treatment/Notes

Impetigo	• Superficial infection of the skin with *S. aureus* or group A *Streptococcus*
	• May occur in patients with compromised skin barrier
	• Predisposing factors:
	  1. Crowded conditions
	  2. Poor hygiene
	  3. Neglected minor trauma
	  4. Heat and humidity
		• Lesion: fragile vesicles/pustules (nonbullous impetigo) or bullae (bullous impetigo) that rupture and leave a "honey-colored" crust
		• Variable pruritus, lymphadenopathy
		• Most common on extremities and face, especially periorifice
		• Resolves in days to weeks, even if untreated
			• Clinical
			• Wound culture with sensitivities may be performed
				• Empiric treatment with oral antibacterial therapy such as cephalexin, erythromycin, or dicloxacillin (effective in 90% of cases)
				• Topical mupirocin for uncomplicated localized disease
				• Recurrent impetigo: eradicate *S. aureus* in chronic nasal carriers (20% of individuals): mupirocin twice a day for 5 days each month
				• Complications are rare
				• Impetigo from Strep species may in rare cases be followed by scarlet fever or acute poststreptococcal glomerulonephritis
				• Healing occurs without scarring

Folliculitis	• Infection of upper portion of hair follicle by bacteria (*S. aureus*, *Pseudomonas*), fungi (*Candida* species), or viruses
	• Predisposing factors:
	  1. Shaving/plucking/waxing
	  2. Topical corticosteroids
	  3. Diabetes mellitus
	  4. Immunosuppression
	• *Pseudomonas* can cause "hot tub folliculitis"
	• Patients with HIV can get eosinophilic folliculitis
		• Pustules, papules surrounded by an erythematous halo
		• Tendency to recur
			• Clinical
			• Wound bacterial/fungal/viral cultures
			• KOH prep
				• Correct underlying predisposing factor
				• Hot compresses and topical antibiotics
				• May progress to furuncle/carbuncle

(*continued*)

Table 14-8

Pustular Skin Infections (continued)

LESION	EPIDEMIOLOGY/ETIOLOGY	CLINICAL	DIAGNOSIS	TREATMENT/NOTES
Furuncles/ Carbuncles	• Deep-seated tender nodules that evolve from *S. aureus* folliculitis • Predisposing factors: as above for folliculitis	• Furuncle lesion: fluctuant tender nodule with central necrotic plug. May be surrounded by cellulitis • Carbuncle lesion: adjacent coalescing furuncles with contiguous deep abscesses	• Clinical • Wound cultures • If febrile and with constitutional symptoms, consider blood cultures	• Incision, drainage, and systemic antibiotics • Eradicate *S. aureus* nasal carriage as above • Prevent recurrence with povidone—iodine soap or benzoyl peroxide wash

KOH = potassium hydroxide.

Table 14-9

The Tineas

Lesion	Etiology	Clinical	Diagnosis	Treatment/Notes
Tinea corporis "Ringworm"	• *Microsporum* spp • *Trichophyton* spp • Transmission: autoinoculation, contact with animals or contaminated soil • Predisposing factors: - Immunosuppression - atopic diathesis	• Affects all ages • Lesion: erythematous, annular, scaling lesion with central clearing ("ring") • Location: trunk, legs, arms, and/or neck, excluding the feet, hands, and groin • Asymptomatic or mild pruritus	• Clinical • KOH microscopic examination shows septated hyphae • Fungal culture • Wood's lamp: *Microsporum* spp fluoresces green	• Treatment depends on the severity • Local lesions may only require topical antifungal treatment: imidazoles (clotrimazole), allylamines (terbinafine), ciclopirox • More extensive infections or infections involving scalp and nails require oral griseofulvin, terbinafine, itraconazole, or fluconazole
Tinea pedis "Athlete's foot"	• *Trichophyton* spp • *Epidermophyton* spp • Most common dermatophyte infection • Predisposing factors: - Occlusive footwear - Excessive sweating - Hot humid weather	• Lesion types: - Macerated interdigital - Moccasin distribution - Inflammatory/bullous • Compromised skin barrier due to tinea pedis is common portal of entry for lymphangitis/cellulitis, especially in diabetic patients	• Same as tinea corporis • Greenish hue suggests *Pseudomonas aeruginosa* superinfection	• Topical antifungals for 2–4 weeks • Systemic antifungals indicated for extensive infection, and topical failures • Keep feet dry, wear shower shoes, aluminum chloride hexahydrate 20% (Drysol) to reduce sweating

(*continued*)

Table 14-9
The Tineas (continued)

LESION	ETIOLOGY	CLINICAL	DIAGNOSIS	TREATMENT/NOTES

Tinea cruris "Jock itch"	• *Epidermophyton* spp
	• *Trichophyton* spp
	• Predisposing factors:
	  - Warm environments
	  - Obesity
	  - Tight clothing
	  - Tinea pedis
		• Lesion: sharply demarcated, pruritic erythematous scaly plaques
		• Location: medial thighs, groin, pubic area (penis and scrotum rarely involved)
			• As with tinea corporis	• Topical antifungal treatment is usually sufficient
				• Wear loose clothing

Onychomycosis	• *Trichophyton* spp
	• *Candida albicans*
	• Molds
	• Predisposing factors:
	  - Occlusive footwear
	  - Immunocompromise
	  - Diabetes
	  - HIV
		• Lesion type classified by location:
		  - Distal and lateral subungual
		  - Superficial white
		  - Proximal subungual
		• Course: does not resolve spontaneously
			• Clinical diagnosis should be confirmed by laboratory testing
			• Clip nail back and scrape for KOH
			• Fungal culture or histology of nail clipping with PAS stain to detect fungal elements
				• Good foot hygiene
				• Systemic therapy if fingernail involvement, functional limitation, pain, source of recurrent epidermal dermatophytosis, quality of life issues
				• Oral itraconazole pulse therapy (70% cure rate)
				  - Watch for CHF
				• Oral terbinafine daily for 6–12 weeks (80% cure rate)
				  - Watch for hepatotoxicity
				• Topical lotions and lacquers less effective than oral treatment

| Tinea versicolor (Pityriasis versicolor) | • *Malassezia furfur* (yeast) | • Lesion: Hypopigmented/ hyperpigmented oval, fine-scaling lesions
 • Nonpruritic
 • Location: neck, chest, and back. Most noticeable on sun-exposed areas | • Clinical
 • Wood's light examination
 • KOH microscopic examination reveals a "spaghetti and meat-balls" pattern (hyphae and spores) | • Topical 2.5% selenium sulfide
 • Tendency to recur
 • Monthly itraconazole 200 mg can decrease rate of recurrence |

CHF = congestive heart failure; PAS = periodic acid-Schiff; spp = species; KOH = potassium hydroxide.

Sports Medicine

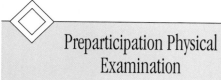

Preparticipation Physical Examination

The goal of the preparticipation physical examination is to identify conditions that might disqualify an athlete from or interfere with sports participation, endanger an athlete, or worsen as a result of physical activity.

Table 15-1

Sports Preparticipation Examination

EXAMINATION COMPONENT	FOCUS
Past/Present Medical Conditions	• Cardiac and pulmonary diseases • Musculoskeletal diseases and injuries • Menstrual history
Family History	• Sudden cardiac death • Cardiac disease
Review of Symptoms	• Pulmonary symptoms at rest and with exercise • Cardiac symptoms at rest and with exercise • Musculoskeletal symptoms at rest and with exercise
Social History	• Use of performance enhancing drugs • Use of sunscreen if sport played out • Disordered eating • Body image
Physical Examination	• Cardiac examination • Pulmonary examination • Musculoskeletal examination

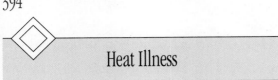

Heat Illness

Heat illnesses are mostly preventable conditions associated with dehydration, suboptimal conditioning, and/or exercising in a hot environment.

Table 15-2
Heat Illnesses

HEAT ILLNESS	SYMPTOMS	SIGNS	TREATMENT
Heat Cramps	• Severe muscle pain, usually in lower extremities • Patient may collapse	• Muscle cramping usually in the hamstrings and calves • Body temperature is within normal limits	• Stretch affected limb • Oral fluids • Rest in a cool environment • Remove excess clothing
Heat Exhaustion	• Extreme fatigue • Dizziness • Nausea • Vomiting • Patient may collapse	• Rapid pulse • Staggering/swaying gait • Fainting • Moderately increased body temperature	• Rest • Oral fluids • Ice packs • Remove excess clothing • Elevate feet above head • More severely affected patients may need IV fluids
Heat Stroke	• Extreme fatigue • Dizziness • Nausea • Vomiting • Patient may collapse • May be unable to communicate	• Rapid pulse/low BP • Delirium or altered consciousness • Possible coma/seizures • Elevated body temperature to greater than 104°F • Warm, flushed skin • Lack of significant perspiration • All organ systems can be affected and end organ damage can occur	• Medical emergency • ABCs • Transport to hospital • Aggressive cooling (ice, wet towels, fan) • Remove excess clothing • Intravenous fluids • Monitored setting

ABCs = airway control, breathing, and circulation; BP = blood pressure.

Infectious Diseases in Sports Medicine

Infectious Mononucleosis

Definition: Mononucleosis is usually a self-limited illness of young adults.
Etiology: Caused by the Epstein-Barr virus.
Epidemiology: Outbreaks can occur when people live in close contact: military recruits or college dorms.
Clinical: Symptoms can include fever, sore throat, lymphadenopathy, muscle soreness, and splenic enlargement. However, many infections are unrecognized.
Treatment: In order to reduce the risk of splenic rupture, patients should refrain from heavy lifting, vigorous activity, and contact sports until the spleen is no longer palpable for 3–4 weeks after symptom onset. Alternatively, an athlete can return to sport if symptom-free and an imaging study shows the spleen to be of normal size.

HIV

There have been no documented cases of HIV transmission from sports activities. Universal precautions should be used whenever bodily fluids are encountered in a sports setting, such as bleeding in wrestling.

Herpes Gladiatorum

Definition: Herpes gladiatorum is a cutaneous infection caused by the herpes simplex virus (either type 1 or type 2).
Etiology: HSV-1 is spread via direct skin contact with contagious sores or with fomites such as sports equipment.

Epidemiology: Wrestlers and rugby players are the athletes at highest risk.
Clinical: The characteristic lesions are grouped vesicles on an erythematous base. The illness may cause no other symptoms, or may cause fever, localized lymphadenopathy, malaise, myalgias, and pharyngitis.
Treatment: Athletes with active infections should not participate in sports until the lesions are crusted over and dry. Bandaging an active infection is insufficient. Treatment with antivirals early in the course can shorten the duration of the infection (consider acyclovir for 10 days or valcyclovir 2 days for herpes labalis). In athletes with frequent outbreaks, daily prophylactic antivirals may be helpful.

Orthopaedics

Most orthopaedic injuries are related to acute trauma (fracture) or chronic overuse (tendonitis). The most common musculoskeletal injuries are muscle strains and ligament sprains. Although long-term treatment for each condition should be individualized, most injuries can be initially treated with PRICE: Protection, Rest, Ice, Compression, Elevation.

Nonsteroidal anti-inflammatory drugs (NSAIDs) can play an important role in reducing inflammation, but their utility in many overuse conditions has come into question. Tissue studies show fewer inflammatory mediators are involved with musculoskeletal injuries than previously thought. Many tendon injuries termed "tendonitis," may be more accurately termed "tendonosis," to reflect the pathology of chronic tissue injury/breakdown rather than inflammation. Controlled and gradual stretching and strengthening program may be more effective for these conditions than "rest" and anti-inflammatory agents.

Table 15-3
Knee Pain: Definition, Symptoms, Physical Examination, Diagnosis, and Treatment

	DEFINITION	SYMPTOMS	PHYSICAL EXAMINATION	DIAGNOSTIC TESTING	INITIAL TREATMENT
Prepatellar Bursitis	• Inflammation of the prepatellar bursa	• Pain and swelling anterior knee	• Tenderness • Warmth/erythema • Extra-articular effusion, superficial to patella	• Clinical diagnosis • Consider bursal aspiration	• NSAIDs/ice • Relative rest • Ace wrap • Antibiotics commonly given because super-infection difficult to assess
Patellar Tendonitis	• Inflammation of the patellar tendon	• Anterior knee pain with activity	• Tenderness over patellar tendon (between distal patella and tibial tubercle)	• Clinical diagnosis	• NSAIDs/ice • Relative rest • Stretch/strength program • Patellar strap
Patellofemoral Arthritis (Chondromalacia patellae)	• Pain associated with knee positions that increase or misdirect mechanical forces between the kneecap and femur	• Anterior knee pain with activity • Knee stiffness with prolonged inactivity	• Retropatellar tenderness • Occasional swelling	• Clinical diagnosis • X-rays may show alignment issues	• NSAIDs/ice • Relative rest • Stretch/strength program • Patellofemoral brace • Consider foot orthotics
Patellar Dislocation	• Dislocation of the patella from its anatomic alignment	• Severe anterior knee pain • Knee swelling	• Visual deformity of anterior knee present • Tenderness • Effusion • Decreased range of motion	• X-rays • Consider MRI to evaluate for chondral injury	• NSAIDs/ice • Relative rest • Consider aspiration for tense effusions • Brace/limit extension • Weight bear as tolerated

Meniscus Tears	• A tear in the shock-absorbing carti-lage (meniscus) of the knee	• Knee pain local-ized medially or laterally • Gradual onset knee swelling • Discomfort with squatting	• Medial or lateral joint line tender-ness • Knee effusion • Pain with knee flexion and twisting	• X-rays to evalu-ate for arthritis • MRI	• Conservative care: rela-tive rest, physical ther-apy, consider cortisone injection • For mechanical or per-sistent symptoms, con-sider arthroscopy for meniscal debridement
Ligament Injuries	• Stretch and/or tear in a liga-ment (a band of fibrous tissue that con-nects two or more bones at a joint)	• ACL injury: audible "pop," knee pain, rapid knee swelling, episodes of knee "giving way"	• Knee effusion • Decreased range of motion • Increased anterior translation of tibia relative to femur (Lachman & Anterior Drawer Tests)	• X-rays • MRI	• NSAIDs/ice • Relative rest • Weight bear as tolerated • Knee brace if unstable • Physical therapy • ACL tears: consider sur-gical reconstruction
		• MCL injury: medial knee pain after twist-ing injury	• Tenderness over MCL • Decreased range of motion • Pain or laxity on stressing of the MCL (Valgus Stress Test)		

(continued)

Table 15-3

Knee Pain: Definition, Symptoms, Physical Examination, Diagnosis, and Treatment (continued)

	DEFINITION	SYMPTOMS	PHYSICAL EXAMINATION	DIAGNOSTIC TESTING	INITIAL TREATMENT
Iliotibial Band (ITB) Syndrome	• Lateral knee pain related to irritation and inflammation of the distal portion of the ITB (a band of tissue that extends from the thigh, over the knee and attaches to the tibia)	• Lateral knee pain with activity • Common in runners, symptoms worse downhill	• Pain over ITB, 3 cm proximal to lateral joint line • Muscle inflexibility • Tight ITB	• Clinical diagnosis	• Stretch/strength program • Knee strap • Consider foot orthotics
Popliteal Cyst (Baker's Cyst)	• Fluid distention of the gastrocnemio-semi-membranosus bursa (posterior to the medial femoral condyle between the tendons of the medial head of the gastrocnemius and semi-membranosus muscles)	• Posterior knee pain	• Popliteal mass or swelling	• Clinical diagnosis • Ultrasound • Rule out DVT	• NSAIDs • Observation • Aspiration usually followed by reacummulation of the fluid • Surgery if large or persistent

ACL = anterior cruciate ligament; DVT = deep vein thrombosis; ITB = iliotibial band; MCL = medial collateral ligament.

Note: Knee pain may be referred pain from a hip injury.

Table 15-4

Shoulder Pain: Definition, Symptoms, Physical Examination, Diagnosis, and Treatment

	DEFINITION	SYMPTOMS	PHYSICAL EXAMINATION	DIAGNOSTIC TESTING	INITIAL TREATMENT
Impingement: (Subacromial Bursitis/ Rotator Cuff Tendonitis)	• Pressure on the rotator cuff from part of the scapula as the arm is lifted	• Shoulder pain worse with overhead activities	• Discomfort with arm motions overhead and behind the back • Rotator cuff weakness secondary to pain	• X-rays may show hooked acromium (loss of subacromial space)	• NSAIDs/ice • Relative rest • Stretch/strength program • Consider cortisone injection • For persistent symptoms, consider surgical debridement
Rotator Cuff Tear	• A tear in one of the four muscles and their tendons that combine to form a "cuff" over the head of the humerus to stabilize the joint	• Shoulder pain, worse with overhead movement and at night • Loss of range of motion and weakness	• More limited active range of motion (ROM) than passive • Significant weakness of rotator cuff	• X-ray may show superior migration of humeral head • MRI	• Relative rest • Stretch/strength program • For persistent pain and/or unacceptable ROM/weakness consider surgical repair
Shoulder Instability (Dislocation, Subluxation, and Laxity)	• Dislocation: complete loss of the humeral articulation with the glenoid fossa as a result of acute trauma • Subluxation: symptomatic partial loss of the articulation. Caused by repetitive trauma • Laxity: asymptomatic partial loss of the glenohumeral articulation.	• Shoulder pain • Shoulder feels "loose/out of place" or "can't move arm" • Posttrauma, often caused by landing on an outstretched arm • Temporary numbness/tingling common	• Dislocation: - Inability to move arm - Shoulder "squared-off" - Humeral head palpable • Subluxation and laxity: - Apprehension with arm in abduction and external rotation - Discomfort with end range of motion - Weakness of rotator cuff	• X-rays may show displaced humerus; anterior displacement most common • MRI to evaluate for associated injuries	• If dislocated → prompt reduction AFTER assessing for neurovascular compromise, then: - Sling for comfort - NSAIDs/ice - Relative rest - Stretch/strength program • For persistent instability, consider surgery

(continued)

Table 15-4

Shoulder Pain: Definition, Symptoms, Physical Examination, Diagnosis, and Treatment (continued)

	Definition	Symptoms	Physical Examination	Diagnostic Testing	Initial Treatment
AC Joint Sprain	• AC joint is the point where the clavicle meets the acromion	• Shoulder pain at AC joint • Decreased shoulder mobility • History of trauma with impact at acromium	• Discomfort to palpation of AC joint • Limited shoulder range of motion secondary to pain • Shoulder weakness secondary to pain	• X-ray may show elevated distal clavicle	• NSAIDs/ice • Sling for comfort • Relative rest • Gradual stretch/strength program • Consider surgery for more severe injuries in active people
Frozen Shoulder	• Also called adhesive capsulitis, it is characterized by pain and loss of motion or stiffness in the shoulder	• Decreased shoulder mobility • More common in diabetics • History of trauma often reported	• Limited active and passive range of motion in the shoulder	• Clinical diagnosis	• Physical therapy for shoulder mobility • For persistent symptoms consider manipulation under anesthesia • Consider early cortisone injection

AC = acromioclavicular; ROM = range of motion.

Table 15-5

Foot and Ankle Pain: Definition, Symptoms, Physical Examination, Diagnosis, and Treatment

	DEFINITION	SYMPTOMS	PHYSICAL EXAMINATION	DIAGNOSTIC TESTING	INITIAL TREATMENT
Achilles Tendonitis	• Inflammation, irritation, and swelling of the tendons of the ankle • Often due to overuse	• Posterior ankle pain	• Discomfort to palpation over distal Achilles tendon • Discomfort with resisted ankle plantar flexion	• Clinical diagnosis	• NSAIDs/ice • Heel lifts • Stretch/strength program
Ankle Sprain	• Stretch and/or tear in a ligament of the ankle	• Ankle pain, usually on the lateral ankle	• Lateral ankle tenderness and swelling • Limitation of motion • Loose ankle ligaments	• X-ray if suspicious for fracture	• NSAIDs/ice • Ace wrap or brace • Gentle range of motion exercises • Gradual strength and proprioceptive training
Shin Splints (Medial Tibial Stress Syndrome)	• Inflammation of the periosteum of the tibia and the muscles that attach to the periosteum	• Anterior shin pain with activity	• Broad area of discomfort to palpation over antero-medial shin • Ankle inflexibility	• Clinical diagnosis • X-ray • Consider bone scan or MRI to evaluate for stress fracture	• NSAIDs/ice • Wrap or anterior panel • Stretch/strength program • New sneakers • Consider foot orthotics
Plantar Fasciitis	• Inflammation of the plantar fascia connecting the calcaneous to the abductor hallucis, flexor digitorum brevis and abductor digiti minimi muscles	• Plantar foot pain, worse with the first morning steps or after prolonged inactivity	• Discomfort over antero-medial calcaneous	• Clinical diagnosis • X-ray may show heel spur	• NSAIDs • Stretch/strength program • Night splints • Consider foot orthotics

(continued)

Table 15-5

Foot and Ankle Pain: Definition, Symptoms, Physical Examination, Diagnosis, and Treatment (continued)

	DEFINITION	SYMPTOMS	PHYSICAL EXAMINATION	DIAGNOSTIC TESTING	INITIAL TREATMENT
Intermetatarsal Neuroma (Morton's Neuroma)	• Thickening of the tissue that surrounds the digital nerve as it passes under the ligament connecting the metatarsals in the forefoot • Develops in response to irritation, trauma, or excessive pressure • Incidence is 8–10 times greater in women than in men	• Burning pain or numbness in ball of foot or interspace between toes (usually third and fourth), worse with activity or narrow shoes	• Discomfort over interspace between toes (usually third and fourth toes) • Discomfort on squeezing foot from the sides • Web space paresthesias	• Clinical diagnosis • X-ray can rule out fracture	• Wide footwear • Avoid high heels • Metatarsal pads • NSAIDs • Consider foot orthotics • Cortisone injection • Consider surgery for resistant cases
Hallux Valgus ("Bunion")	• Tilting of the first metatarsal away from the midline of the body	• Medial forefoot pain, worse with activity	• Increased valgus angle (great toe tilts laterally toward the smaller toes) at the first MTP • Medial enlargement of the first MTP ("bunion") often present	• X-ray shows first metatarsal head deviated medially and dorsally	• Wide footwear • Avoid high heels • NSAIDs • Bunion padding • Consider foot orthotics • Consider surgery for severe cases

MTP = metatarsophalangeal.

Table 15-6

Elbow Injuries: Definition, Symptoms, Physical Examination, Diagnosis, and Treatment

	DEFINITION	SYMPTOMS	PHYSICAL EXAMINATION	DIAGNOSTIC TESTING	INITIAL TREATMENT
Lateral Epicondylitis/ "Tennis Elbow"	• Degeneration, inflammation, or traumatic tear of the tendons that attach to the lateral epicondyle for the muscles that extend or straighten the wrist and fingers • Overuse injury	• Pain over lateral elbow	• Tenderness over lateral epicondyle • Discomfort with resisted wrist dorsiflexion	• Clinical diagnosis	• NSAIDs • Ice massage • Stretch/strength program • Counterforce brace • Consider cortisone
Medial Epicondylitis/ "Golfer's Elbow"	• Degeneration, inflammation, or traumatic tear of the tendons originating at the anterior medial epicondyle for the flexor-pronator muscles • Overuse injury	• Pain over medial elbow	• Tenderness over medial epicondyle • Discomfort with resisted wrist plantar flexion	• Clinical diagnosis	• NSAIDs • Ice massage • Stretch/strength program • Counterforce brace
Olecranon Bursitis	• Inflammation of the bursa overlying the olecranon process at the proximal aspect of the ulna	• Swelling at the tip of the elbow • Mild elbow pain • History of acute or chronic elbow trauma	• Extra-articular swelling, warmth, and erythema over the tip of the elbow • Tenderness over the olecranon	• Clinical diagnosis	• NSAIDs/ice • Ace wrap/ cushioning • Antibiotics commonly given because superinfection difficult to assess

Table 15-7

Wrist Injuries: Definition, Symptoms, Physical Examination, Diagnosis, and Treatment

	DEFINITION	SYMPTOM	PHYSICAL EXAMINATION	DIAGNOSTIC TESTING	INITIAL TREATMENT
DeQuervain's Tenosynovitis	• Inflammation of the tendons in the first dorsal compartment of the wrist (tendons for the abductor pollicis longus and extensor pollicis brevis muscles which abduct the thumb)	• Pain at base of thumb	• Discomfort to palpation at base of thumb over abductor pollicis longus tendon • Pain with resisted thumb abduction or with wrist ulnar deviation (Finkelstein's test)	• Clinical diagnosis	• NSAIDs/ice • Brace with thumb immobilizer • Consider cortisone injection
Carpel Tunnel Syndrome	• Thickening of the nine flexor tendons which run through the carpal tunnel • Thickening leads to compression of (and restricted blood to) the median nerve which also runs through the tunnel	• Wrist pain • Numbness in the first to third digits	• Symptoms are exacerbated by tapping on carpel tunnel (Tinel's sign) and prolonged wrist plantar flexion (Phalen's sign)	• Clinical diagnosis • Nerve conduction studies	• Wrist splint, especially at night • NSAIDs • Cortisone injection • For persistent symptoms, consider surgical release

Table 15-8

Fracture Types

FRACTURE TYPE	DESCRIPTION	COMMENT
Transverse	• Fracture line is at a right angle to the bone's long axis	• Often the result of a direct blow
Oblique	• Fracture line is at an angle to the bone's long axis	• Less common
Spiral	• Fracture line is oblique to the bone's axis and encircles a portion of the shaft	• Caused by a twisting movement about the long axis of a bone, often an unstable fracture
Comminuted	• Fracture site involves more than two fragments	• Often requires surgery
Compound (Open)	• Fracture associated with a skin break	• Always requires antibiotics
Stress	• Crack in the bone cortex from repetitive stress	• Best diagnosed with bone scan or MRI
Pathologic	• Fracture in an area of bone that has been weakened by an underlying process	• Bony metastases or osteoporosis are common underlying bone pathologies

Fractures

Fractures are defined as a break in the bone. The energy of the event and the strength of the bone determine how and where the bone breaks. Excessive force to a bony structure is the etiology. Broken bones are among the most common acute adult injuries. The most common fracture before age 75 is a wrist fracture. After age 75, hip fractures are most common.

Table 15-9

Treatment of Fracture

Initial	• Apply a splint to the fracture site, including joint above and below the fracture to support the bone and to prevent further bony, soft-tissue, nerve, or vessel injury • If skin broken, cover with sterile gauze • Monitor peripheral neurovascular examination as sharp ends of bone may compromise nerves and vessels
X-ray	• Determines if bones are displaced
If patient has a displaced fracture	• Reduce manually or surgically, depending on extent and location
Immobilization after reduction	• May need temporary cast to accommodate soft tissue swelling (2–3 days) • Depending on site and ability to achieve union may need surgical fixation

Low Back Pain

Definition: Back pain in the lumbosacral spine.
Epidemiology: Up to four out of five adults
will experience significant low back pain in their
lifetime. It is one of the most common reasons
for doctor visits and missed days from work.
Symptoms last for more than 2 weeks in less than
20% of cases.
Etiology: Most cases of low back pain are tempo-
rary and respond to conservative treatments. Risk
factors include pregnancy, jobs requiring flexion,
rotation of the trunk with repetitive lifting and
job dissatisfaction. A strain of the back muscles or
sprains of the ligaments attaching the vertebrae are
the most common identifiable causes of back pain.
Less common, but more serious causes include
herniated discs, spinal stenosis, vertebral fractures,
osteoarthritis, infections, and metastases.

Diagnosis: The presence of any of "red flags"
listed in Table 15-11 is suggestive of a serious
pathology leading to back pain. Depending on
the underlying suspected etiology, patients with
a "red flag" should have a rapid evaluation, imaging, treatment, and/or specialty referral. If imaging is indicated, magnetic resonance imaging
(MRI) is usually the test of choice. However, MRI
can be associated with overdiagnosis of anatomic
abnormalities in asymptomatic patients.

Imaging and blood tests are usually unwar-
ranted if a thorough history and examination fail
to show any of the "red flag" warning signs.
Treatment: Functional limitations and recur-
rences can be minimized with exercise, medicines
(anti-inflammatories and muscle relaxers), and
patient education. Acute low back pain is often
responsive to NSAIDs. Sciatica often responds to
conservative treatment.

Table 15-10
"Red Flags" for Back Pain

SIGN OR SYMPTOM	POTENTIALLY SERIOUS ETIOLOGY	COMMENT
Age <20 or >55 at first onset	• Numerous	
History of violent trauma	• Anatomic injury	
History of cancer	• Recurrence of cancer	
History of weight loss	• Cancer or other systemic disease	
Thoracic back pain	• Cancer or other systemic disease	
History of drug abuse	• Infection	
HIV+	• Infection or cancer	
Bowel or bladder dysfunction	• Cauda equine	• Requires emergent evaluation and treatment • Also associated with bilateral leg weakness and severe pain at night
Pain radiating into the legs	• Sciatica	• See Table 15-12
Numbness in legs	• Spinal stenosis	• Pain worse with extension of lumbar spine and improves with flexion • Pain less likely to radiate below buttocks
Persistent pain for >4–6 weeks	• Numerous	

Table 15-11
Sciatica

SIGN OR SYMPTOM	ETIOLOGY	COMMENT
Pain radiating into the legs	• Sciatica	• Radiating pain a poor predictor of a herniated disc • 95% of patients with a herniated disk have radiating pain
Positive straight leg raise	• Sciatica	• Raising the leg on the opposite side producing the characteristic pain • Most common finding predictive of sciatica
Weak plantar flexion	• S1 radiculopathy	• Highly predictive
Wasting of calf muscle and weak ankle dorsiflexion	• S1 radiculopathy	• Generally predictive

Concussion

Definition: Impaired cognition after head trauma.
Etiology: Concussions result from head trauma causing functional brain disturbance, rather than structural injury.
Clinical: Patients experience headache, nausea, vomiting, drowsiness, dizziness, light sensitivity, irritability, and difficulty with concentration and memory. The more concerning symptoms are loss of consciousness and amnesia.
Diagnosis: A clinical diagnosis. Neuroimaging studies are generally unremarkable. Concussion grading scales have not been shown to predict symptom severity or outcome.
Treatment: Symptoms resolve gradually without specific treatment.

Female Athlete Triad

The triad includes: (1) disordered eating, (2) amenorrhea, and (3) osteoporosis. The triad is seen in a wide range of female athletes, from recreational athletes to elite. Severe health consequences include nutritional deficiencies, bone loss, and death.

Ergogenic (Performance Enhancing) Aids

Anabolic-Androgenic Steroids

Steroids are man-made substances related to testosterone and have both anabolic and androgenic effects on the body. Steroid abuse can lead to increased muscle mass, reduced body fat, increased motivation, and decreased fatigue. Adverse consequences include heart attack, stroke, liver tumors, unhealthy cholesterol profile, prostate problems, infertility, gynecomastia, mania, and depression.

Ephedra

Ephedra (ma huang) is a Chinese herb related to ephedrine that is used for performance enhancement and weight loss. Ephedra has been linked to heart attacks, strokes, seizures, and fatalities. It had been banned by many sports organizations, and in April 2004 it became the first dietary supplement to be banned for sale in the United States by the Food and Drug Administration (FDA).

Creatine

Creatine is a nitrogenous amino acid compound found in most body tissues and is needed for adenosine triphosphate (ATP) production during anaerobic exercise. It may provide benefit in short explosive activities. Muscle cramping, nausea, diarrhea, and renal dysfunction are commonly reported side effects. Creatine is legal, although its safety profile is not known.

Caffeine

At high doses, caffeine may enhance the contractility of skeletal and cardiac muscle and help fat metabolism. As a central nervous system (CNS) stimulant, it may improve concentration. Side effects include restlessness, nervousness, insomnia, tremors, hyperesthesia, and diuresis.

Chapter 16

Women's Health

Table 16-1

Osteoporosis

Definition	• Decrease in bone mineral density and compromised bone strength leads to an increased risk of fractures • Most frequently involves the vertebra, hip, and long bones • Affects approximately 55% of Americans 50 years and older • Approximately 1 in 2 women over the age of 50 years will have an osteoporosis-related fracture in her lifetime	
Risk Factors	**Primary osteoporosis:** • Female—80% of cases (also occurs in men) • White and Asian ethnicity (although may affect people with any background) • Family history • Age • Low body weight • Inactivity • Estrogen deficiency (menopause, excessive physical activity causing amenorrhea) • Tobacco use • Alcohol consumption	
	Secondary osteoporosis: • Medications: corticorticoids (most common cause of secondary osteoporosis), anticonvulsants • Endocrine disorders: hyperthyroidism, hyperparathyroidism • Other: celiac disease, chronic renal failure	
Clinical Features	• Kyphosis • Back or bone pain, even after mild trauma	
Diagnosis	• Bone densitometry	
Prevention	• Adequate calcium and vitamin D intake • Exercise • Modification of lifestyle factors (alcohol, smoking, etc.)	
Treatment	**Intervention**	**Notes**
	• Calcium supplementation	• Vitamin D supplementation (improves calcium absorption)
	• Weight-bearing and resistance exercise	• Increases bone formation and decreases risk of falls
	• Bisphosphonates (alendronate, ibandronate, risedronate)	• Decreases risk of both vertebral and nonvertebral fractures • Patient must be able to sit up for at least an hour after taking weekly dose
	• Parathyroid hormone therapy (teriparatide)	• Decreases risk of both vertebral and nonvertebral fractures • Stimulates osteoblastic bone formation • Cost and concern for risk of osteosarcoma limits use

Table 16-1

Osteoporosis (continued)

Treatment (cont.)	Intervention	Notes
	• Selective estrogen receptor modulators (Raloxifene)	• Estrogenic effect on bone, but blocks estrogen effect on breast and uterus • Decreases risk of vertebral fractures • Decreases risk of breast cancer (in contrast to estrogen supplementation)
	• Estrogen therapy	• Use limited by increased risk of cardiovascular disease, breast cancer, and thromboembolic disease

Table 16-2

Guidelines for Cervical, Pelvic, and Breast Screening

Guidelines for Cervical Cancer Screening	• The American College of Obstetrics and Gynecology recommends that Pap smears begin within 3 years of initiation of intercourse but no later than 21 years of age • Women under 30 years should undergo annual cervical cytology screening • Women over 30 years who have had 3 consecutive negative screenings and no identified risk factors may extend the interval between screenings to every 2–3 years • Women with HIV or who are immune compromised should undergo annual cervical cytology screening • Screening can stop at approximately 70 years of age if no risk factors
Guidelines for Pelvic Examination and Screening	• Pelvic examinations are typically recommended and performed with cervical screening and may be able to palpate ovarian or other masses • Vaginal discharge may be analyzed under a microscope to look for yeast, *Trichomonas*, bacterial vaginosis, irritation, and infection • A visual examination may identify genital warts, herpes, and syphilis • The most frequently encountered pelvic infection is genital warts caused by HPV. HPV is the single most important risk factor for cervical cancer • Many authorities recommend Chlamydia and Gonorrhea testing in sexually active adults
Guidelines for Breast Examination and Screening	• All women should have clinical breast examinations annually • Self-breast examination has the potential to detect a palpable mass • Unilateral breast pain and any palpable mass discovered by the patient (even if not palpable by the physician) requires further evaluation • Mammography is the screening modality of choice • Mammography in younger women may be difficult because of dense breast tissue and ultrasound/MRI may be needed to evaluate areas of concern • For women with a history of breast cancer in their family, consider starting screening at least 10 years prior to the age that the family member was diagnosed • Although there is controversy, women aged 40–49 years often have screening mammography every 1–2 years • Women aged 50 years and older should have annual screening mammography

HPV = human papillomavirus; MRI = magnetic resonance imaging.

Table 16-3

Management of Abnormal Pap Smear Results

CONDITION	MANAGEMENT
ASCUS	• Test for HPV • Colposcopy and biopsy if high risk • Women under 30 years of age and no identified risk factors can be closely observed • Repeat Pap smear at 6 and 12 months until two are negative • Estrogen creams may be beneficial
ASC-H **(Cannot Exclude HSIL)** **LSIL**	• Colposcopy and biopsy
HSIL	• Colposcopy and biopsy • Further treatment as needed with LEEP, cryotherapy, laser therapy, conization, or hysterectomy.

ASCUS = atypical squamous cells of undetermined significance; ASC-H = atypical squamous cell; HSIL = high grade squamous intraepithelial lesion; LEEP = loop electrosurgical excision procedure; LSIL = low grade squamous intraepithelial lesion.

Table 16-4

Amenorrhea

CONDITION	DEFINITION	ETIOLOGY	EVALUATION/TREATMENT

Primary Amenorrhea	• Absence of menarche by age 16 in the presence of normal secondary sexual characteristics, or by the age of 14 if there is no visible secondary sexual characteristic development	• Causes of amenorrhea with abnormal pubertal development:
		- Hypergonadotropic hypogonadism (ovarian failure with resultant low estrogen levels and *high* FSH levels)
		  a. Chromosomal abnormalities (XY gonadal dysgenesis)
		  b. Turner syndrome
		- Pituitary pathology (*low* FSH/LH production and resultant low estrogen)
		  a. Craniopharyngioma
		  b. Prolactinomas
		- Hypothalamus disorders
		  a. Stress
		  b. Malnutrition associated with chronic illness or anorexia nervosa
		  c. Genetic syndromes: Laurence-Moon-Biedl, Prader-Willi, and Kallmann syndromes
			• Depends on the etiology

Table 16-4

Amenorrhea (continued)

CONDITION	DEFINITION	ETIOLOGY	EVALUATION/TREATMENT

Primary Amenorrhea (cont.)		• Causes of amenorrhea with normal pubertal development:
		  - Pregnancy
		  - Polycystic ovarian syndrome	

Secondary Amenorrhea	• 6 months of amenorrhea or the absence of 3 consecutive menstrual cycles in patients who have had previously established regular menses	- Testicular feminization
		- Imperforate hymen
		- Acquired ovarian failure (i.e., damage from chemotherapy)
		- Acquired pituitary pathology (prolactinoma and infiltration)
		- Hyperthyroidism
		- Hypothalamic pathology (similar to that seen in primary disease)
		- Hormonal contraceptive use
		- Mayer-Rokitansky sequence: agenesis of the uterus and proximal two-thirds of the vagina, resulting in normal external genitalia, and a blind vaginal pouch
			• First rule out pregnancy
			• Common workup considerations:
			  - TSH level
			  - Prolactin level
			  - Progestin challenge
			  - Discontinue oral contraceptives
			  - MRI to evaluate pituitary gland

FSH = follicle-stimulating hormone; LH = luteinizing hormone; TSH = thyroid-stimulating hormone.

Table 16-5

Menstrual Disorders

CONDITION	DEFINITION	TREATMENT/NOTES

Dysmenorrhea	• Primary dysmenorrhea:
	  - Crampy abdominal, back, thigh, and/or pelvic pain
	  - No other pelvic pathology
	  - Secondary to excess prostaglandin production
	• Secondary dysmenorrhea:
	  - Crampy abdominal, back, thigh, and/or pelvic pain
	  - Associated with pelvic pathology
	  - Endometriosis is the most frequently associated condition
		• Nonsteroidal anti-inflammatory medications to decrease prostaglandin production
		• Consider oral contraceptive agents
		• Patients who do not respond to initial interventions should undergo more extensive evaluation (i.e., radiologic imaging) to evaluate for underlying disease

Polycystic Ovarian Syndrome (Stein-Leventhal Syndrome)	• A constellation of symptoms:
	  - Irregular menses
	  - Anovulation
	  - Hyperandrogenism
	  - Affected patients are classically obese, hirsute, virilized, and infertile
		• The ovaries are usually, but not invariably, cystic
		• Hyperinsulinism, lipid abnormalities, and increased levels of LH are associated laboratory findings
		• Acanthosis nigricans is often present in insulin-resistant patients
		• Treatment options:
		  - Oral contraceptives
		  - Antiandrogen agents (spironolactone)
		  - Metformin

Menorrhagia	• Prolonged and/or excessive cyclic bleeding	• Endometrial pathology (polyps, cancer, pregnancy) should be excluded • If menorrhagia began with menarche (first menses), consider a bleeding disorder (Von Willebrand, Factor V Leiden)
Metrorrhagia	• Irregular and frequent bleeding	• Endometrial pathology (polyps, cancer, pregnancy) should be excluded
Polymenorrhea	• Cycles less than 21 days	• Anovulation
Oligomenorrhea	• Cycles greater than 35 days	• Pregnancy • Systemic inflammatory illness (rheumatoid arthritis) • Hypothalamic disorder

Table 16-6
Contraception

METHOD	MECHANISM	PRO	CON	NOTES
Hormonal methods: suppress ovulation, increase cervical mucus (making penetration of sperm difficult), and thin the endometrial lining (making implantation difficult)				
Oral Contraceptive "The Pill"	• Estrogen and/or progesterone	• Easy to use • May improve regularity of menses, and decrease incidence of PID gonorrhea, anemia, and ovarian cancer • Failure rate extremely low (<2%)	• No protection against STDs • Increases risk of thromboembolic disease • Complications: cholestatic jaundice and hepatic adenomas	• Absolute contraindications: pregnancy, increased risk for thromboembolic disease, liver disease, complicated valvular heart disease, hypertension, headaches with focal aura, and cerebrovascular and coronary artery disease • Relative contraindications: hyperlipidemia, sickle cell disease, and diabetes (nonvascular disease) • Many drugs, including some antibiotics, sedative hypnotics, and antiepileptic medications interfere with effectiveness
Emergency Contraception	• Hormonal methods are the mainstay of treatment and should be started within 72 hours of the possible conception event	• FDA approved • Easy to purchase • Failure rate: almost 80% reduction in risk of pregnancy after a single act of unprotected sex	• The effectiveness decreases with time since event • Nausea	• Two methods: - The more common method ("the morning after pill") consists of two doses of 0.75 mg levonorgestrel given 12 hours apart - Two doses of combined oral contraception pills with at least 100 μg of ethinyl estradiol and 0.5 levonorgestrel (or 1.5 mg norgestrel) given 12 hours apart
The "Ring"	• Estrogen and progesterone • Plastic ring is inserted inside the vagina by the patient	• Easy to use • Lasts 3 weeks • Possible increased compliance when compared with the pill • Failure rate very low (<2%)	• Some patients find it uncomfortable to place and remove the device • No protection against STD	• Lowest estrogen and progesterone dose available • Same efficacy as lowest dose oral contraceptive

(continued)

Table 16-6
Contraception (continued)

METHOD	MECHANISM	PRO	CON	NOTES
DMPA	• Long-acting, highly effective progestin-only contraceptive	• Failure rate of less than 0.3% when used consistently • Requires little patient effort • Can be used in patients who cannot take estrogen • Given every 3 months	• Irregular menstrual bleeding/amenorrhea common • No protection against STD	• Weight gain, headaches, bloating, mood changes, and depression • Can take as long as 18 months for full fertility to return after discontinuation • Reduction in bone mineral density that is reversible with cessation of DMPA • Consider calcium supplementation
Barrier methods: physically prevent the passage of sperm into the cervix				
Male Condom	• Latex, polyurethane or animal skin sheath placed over the penis	• Decreases the transmission of STDs when used correctly and consistently • No prescription needed	• Requires interruption of activity to put on condom • Failure rate approximately 10%	• Spermicidal condoms are not more effective • Latex/polyurethane condoms provide better STD protection than animal skin condoms
Female Condom	• Polyurethane sheath with two rings. One end is placed inside the vagina and the other end is placed outside the labia	• Same as male condom • May offer women more control	• Same as male condom • Failure rate approximately 20%	• Same as male condom

Method	Description	Advantages	Disadvantages	
Diaphragm/ Cervical Cap	• Dome-shaped rubber cup that fits over the cervix • Spermicide is placed in the diaphragm/cap prior to insertion	• Can be placed up to 6 hours (diaphragm) and 48 hours (cap) prior to intercourse	• Does not protect against STDs • Requires physician for fitting, and a prescription • Failure rate approximately 17%	
Contraceptive Sponge	Polyurethane sponge containing spermicide	• Can be placed up to 24 hours and must be left in place for 6 hours after intercourse • No prescription needed	• Does not protect against STDs • Failure rate as high as 28%	
Other				
Intrauterine Device	• A device composed of copper or progesterone inserted into the uterus, preventing sperm from fertilizing the ova	• Lasts up to 5 years (progesterone) and 10 years (copper) after insertion • Failure rate less than 1%	• Does not protect against STDs • Irregular bleeding common	• Not associated with increased risk of PID, and ectopic pregnancy • Protective against endometrial cancer
Coitus Interruptus	Withdrawal of the penis prior to ejaculation	• May be more acceptable to some patients	• Failure rate as high as 50%	• Ineffective because preejaculatory fluids contain semen

DMPA = depot medroxyprogesterone acetate; FDA = Food and Drug Administration; PID = pelvic inflammatory disease; STDs = sexually transmitted diseases.

Table 16-7

Maternal Conditions and Neonatal Sequelae

IF MOM HAS . . .	BABY IS AT RISK FOR . . .
Systemic Lupus Erythematosus	• Congenital heart block
Insulin-Dependent Diabetes	• SGA (from insulin therapy) • Hypoglycemia/hyperinsulinemia • Polyhydramnios • Preeclampsia • Renal agenesis, duodenal atresia, and TGA
Urinary Tract Infection	• PROM • Sepsis
Obesity	• Macrosomia • Hypoglycemia
Preeclampsia	• Uteroplacental insufficiency and fetal hypoxia • Fetal demise

SGA = small for gestational age; TGA = transposition of the great arteries; PROM = premature rupture of membranes.

Table 16-8

Maternal Habits/Ingestions/Medications and Neonatal Manifestations

MATERNAL EXPOSURE . . .	BABY IS AT RISK FOR . . .
Cigarette Smoke	• IUGR • SGA
Alcohol	• Fetal alcohol syndrome • IUGR • Microcephaly • Central nervous system dysfunction
Marijuana (THC)	• IUGR • Behavioral problems
Cocaine	• IUGR
Carbamazepine	• Spina bifida
Phenytoin	• IUGR • Fifth fingernail or toenail hypoplasia • Neurodevelopmental abnormalities
Valproate	• Spina bifida • Heart defects

(continued)

Table 16-8

Maternal Habits/Ingestions/Medications and Neonatal Manifestations (continued)

MATERNAL EXPOSURE . . .	BABY IS AT RISK FOR . . .
Benzodiazepines, Opiates	• Seizures • Agitation • Tremors • Choreoathetoid movements
Tetracycline	• Enamel hypoplasia • Cataracts • Limb defects
Propranolol	• Hypoglycemia • Bradycardia • Respiratory distress
Coumadin	• Bleeding • Limb defects
Aspirin	• Bleeding
NSAIDs	• Renal failure • Necrotizing enterocolitis
ACE Inhibitors	• Renal failure • Hypotension
Thiazides	• Thrombocytopenia
Vitamin K	• Jaundice
Retinoids	• Congenital heart disease • Midfacial anomalies
Quinine	• Hearing loss • Thrombocytopenia

IUGR = intrauterine growth restriction; NSAIDs = nonsteroidal anti-inflammatory drugs; ACE = angiotensin-converting enzyme.

Table 16-9

Physiologic Changes of Pregnancy

Normal Physiologic Changes of Pregnancy	• Intravascular volume increases by 50% (singleton pregnancy) • Heart rate increases by 10–20 beats/min, with a resultant increase in stroke volume and cardiac output • Systemic vascular resistance decreases • Blood pressure decreases by 5–10 mm Hg in first two trimesters • Plasma volume expands, as does the red cell mass to a minimal extent. Therefore, overall mild decrease in hematocrit • GFR increases 50% above baseline and returns to prepregnancy levels in early postpartum period (therefore, "normal" creatinine may actually be evidence of renal impairment) • Respiratory alkalosis

GFR = glomerular filtration rate.

Table 16-10

Hypertension and Pregnancy

CONDITION	DEFINITION	TREATMENT	CLINICAL NOTES
Chronic Hypertension	• BP >140/90 before conception or 20 weeks' gestation or persisting more than 6 –12 weeks post-partum	• Methyldopa • Beta-blockers (except atenolol) most frequently used • Hydralazine • Calcium channel blockers • ACE inhibitors contra-indicated	• Associated with preterm delivery and SGA infants • Avoid treating mild hypertension, as it results in decreased placental perfusion and fetal growth • Increased risk of developing superimposed preeclampsia
Gestational Hypertension	• BP >140/90 occurring after 20 weeks' gesta-tion, during labor, or within 48 hours of delivery without pro-teinuria	• Treat with above agents if SBP >160 or DBP >100	• Resolves after delivery • More common in multiparas, overweight women, with a + family history • Treatment of mild hyperten-sion is generally avoided, as aggressive blood pres-sure lowering may impair placental perfusion and fetal growth

Table 16-10

Hypertension and Pregnancy (continued)

CONDITION	DEFINITION	TREATMENT	CLINICAL NOTES
Preeclampsia	• Onset usually after 20 weeks' gestation, proteinuria and renal impairment	• Primary: delivery • Seizure prophylaxis with magnesium sulfate • Bed rest • Antihypertensives if SBP >160 or DBP >100	• More common in primigravidas (women pregnant for the first time) • Associated with uric acid >5.5 • Pathologic renal lesion is glomerular endotheliosis (swelling of endothelial cells) • Resolves <6 weeks postpartum

Preeclampsia Superimposed on Chronic Hypertension	• Preeclampsia in woman with preexisting hypertension	• Treat the same as preeclampsia	• Increased frequency of:
			  - Abruptio placentae
			  - Preterm delivery
			  - Neonatal complications/death

HELLP	• **H**emolysis **E**levated **L**FTs (AST/ALT, LDH) **L**ow **P**latelets	• Immediate delivery • Steroids to accelerate fetal lung maturity if needed	• Can present with epigastric or RUQ abdominal pain, nausea/vomiting, malaise • CT abdomen to diagnose hepatic complications • DIC in 20%
Eclampsia	• Preeclampsia with seizures	• Immediate delivery	

AST/ALT = aspartate aminotransferase/alanine aminotransferase; BP = blood pressure; CT = computed tomography; DBP = diastolic blood pressure; DIC = disseminated intravascular coagulation; LDH = lactate dehydrogenase; RUQ = right upper quadrant; SBP = systolic blood pressure.

Table 16-11

Select Cardiac Disorders in Pregnancy and Cardiovascular Disease

CONDITION	RISK TO MOTHER	MANAGEMENT/NOTES
Innocent Murmur	• None	• Early peaking <3/6 systolic present murmur occurs in more than 90% of normal pregnant women (pulmonary outflow murmur)
Regurgitant Valve Disease	• Low	• Generally well tolerated because of the decrease in systemic vascular resistance due to normal pregnancy
Aortic Stenosis	• Moderate to high depending on severity	• Because of the blood volume expansion and resultant increase in stroke volume and cardiac output, fixed obstructive cardiac lesions are poorly tolerated during pregnancy • Careful hemodynamic monitoring during labor • Consider valve repair or pregnancy termination in severe cases
Mitral Stenosis		

(continued)

Table 16-11

Select Cardiac Disorders in Pregnancy and Cardiovascular Disease (continued)

CONDITION	RISK TO MOTHER	MANAGEMENT/NOTES
Dilated Cardiomyopathy	• Moderate to high risk depending on severity	• Moderate disease: - Limit exercise - Low salt diet - Diuretics may be required • Severe disease: - Avoid pregnancy - Manage with hydralazine, digitalis, diuretics - ACE inhibitors contraindicated due to effects on fetus
Previous Peripartum Cardiomyopathy	• Recurrence common • High risk	• Defined as CHF that occurs in the last trimester of pregnancy or <6 months postpartum • If serious episode or persistent left ventricular dysfunction, avoid pregnancy

CHF = congestive heart failure.

Table 16-12

Gestational Diabetes

Definition	• Glucose intolerance in pregnant women with no previous history of diabetes • Affects up to 8% of all pregnant women • High blood sugar in pregnancy is related to overall increased morbidity and mortality of the infant
Risk Factors	• Age over 25 years • Family history • Overweight before pregnancy • African American, Hispanic, American Indian, Asian race
Clinical Features	• Most women are asymptomatic • Symptoms of diabetes: increased thirst, urination, fatigue, and infection
Diagnosis	• Screening typically takes place at 24–28 weeks gestation • Oral glucose tolerance test
Treatment	• Diet • Exercise • Insulin (if needed) • Increases risk (up to 50%) of mother developing diabetes mellitus within 10 years of delivery

Geriatrics

Table 17-1

Tests for Hearing Loss

TEST	PURPOSE	NOTE
Screening	• Assesses for problems during the interview: Ask about hearing dysfunction and perform whisper test	• Whisper test technique: Ask a question while standing 2 ft behind patient and ask patient to answer
Audiometry	• Determines the pattern of loss See Table 17-2 • Documents the decibel loss across frequencies • Assesses if loss is unilateral or bilateral	• Perform if screening is positive
Rinne Test	• Distinguishes normal vs. abnormal ear	• Technique: A vibrating tuning fork (512 Hz) is placed on the mastoid (bone conduction). When the sound is no longer heard, the fork is placed in the air next to one ear (air conduction). In a *normal* ear, air conduction is better than bone conduction and the patient hears a sound when the fork is in the air
Weber Test	• Distinguishes between conductive and sensorineural hearing loss	• Technique: A vibrating tuning fork is placed in the midline of the *forehead*. If the sound is heard better in the impaired ear then the hearing impairment is conductive hearing loss. If the sound is heard better in the normal ear, then hearing impairment is sensorineural hearing loss

vs = versus.

Table 17-2

Hearing Loss

TYPE	DEFINITION/CLINICAL	CAUSE	NOTE
Sensorineural	• Hearing loss due to damage to cochlea or retrocochlear structures	• Medication toxicity (aminoglycoside, loop diuretics, cisplatin chemotherapy) • Acoustic neuroma • Meniere disease • Cranial nerve VIII damage (trauma, hemorrhage, infection) • Worsened with cerumen impaction	• Weber test lateralizes away from impaired ear • Rinne test normal

Table 17-2

Hearing Loss (continued)

TYPE	DEFINITION/CLINICAL	CAUSE	NOTE
Presbycusis (Subtype of Sensorineural Hearing loss)	• Mainly high-frequency hearing loss • Loss of speech discrimination • Increase in the sensation of loudness • Occurs in elderly	• Increased incidence with age • Worsened with cerumen impaction	
Conductive	• Transmission of sound to inner ear is impaired • Bone conduction of sound is better than air conduction	• Osteosclerosis • Rheumatoid arthritis • Paget disease • Worsened with cerumen impaction or external otitis	• Weber test lateralizes toward impaired ear • Rinne test is abnormal in impaired ear
Central Auditory Processing Disorder	• Loss of speech discrimination > loss in hearing sensitivity • Central nervous system has decreased ability to process and interpret sounds	• Often associated with dementia	

Table 17-3

Treatment of Hearing Loss

INTERVENTION	NOTE
Cerumen Disimpaction	• Water or commercial preparation instilled into ear • Allow to remain in contact with cerumen for up to 15 minutes • Hearing may worsen as cerumen expands
Hearing Aid	• Amplification improves speech comprehension
Assistive Listening Devices	• Increases signal-to-noise ratio by placing microphone close to sound source and transmitting sound to listener's ear phones • Useful for central auditory processing disorder
Cochlear Implants	• Used for severe hearing loss • Auditory nerve directly innervated (middle ear bypassed)
Other	Speaker can: • Use lower pitched voice • Speak slowly and distinctly (with pauses at end of phrases) without shouting • Speak toward better ear of listener

Table 17-4

Summary of Pressure Ulcers

Risk Factors	• Exposure of skin to moisture • Restricted mobility • Friction on skin • Patient unable to sense pressure (often due to mental status) • Poor nutrition • Usually develops over bony prominence			
Treatment by Stage	**Stage**	**Definition**	**Treatment Option**	**Note**
	Stage 1	• Skin intact • Color changes of skin evident • May have changes in skin temperature, consistency (firm or boggy), or sensation (pain or itching)	• Occlusive film	• Nutritional support and hydration is important for wound healing • Frequent repositioning of patients can help prevent pressure ulcers from developing and/or progressing • Overlying eschar or slough needs to be removed for accurate staging
	Stage 2	• Partial-thickness (epidermis and dermis) skin loss (abrasion, blister or shallow crater)	• Hydrocolloid sheet • Foam dressing • Alginate	
	Stage 3	• Full-thickness skin loss to the fascia, but not through (deep crater)	• Hydrocolloid sheet • Foam dressing • Alginate • Silver dressings if infected • Consider wound debridement	
	Stage 4	• Full-thickness skin loss with destruction: necrosis, damage to underlying structures (muscle, bone)		

Table 17-5

Minimizing Potential for Drug-Drug and Drug-Disease Interactions in Elderly Patients

INTERVENTION	EXAMPLE/NOTE
Choose nonpharmacologic treatment if possible	• Physical therapy to help alleviate joint pain
Choose one medication for multiple conditions	• Use beta-blocker to treat both hypertension and angina
Consider adverse drug event as cause of new or unexplained medical problems	Common adverse drug events: • Constipation • Delirium • Hypotension/arrhythmia • Renal failure/electrolyte abnormalities
Choose medications with least potential for adverse drug events	• Avoid treating adverse drug events with additional pharmacologic agents
Review prescription and nonprescription medications regularly and eliminate nonessential drugs	
Consider starting new drugs at a low dose and titrate up	• Start at one-half of normal dose and titrate up
If patient takes multiple medications, avoid drugs that inhibit or induce cytochrome P450 hepatic metabolism or are highly bound to albumin	Examples of medications to be used with caution in elderly: • Ceftriaxone • Diazepam/lorazepam • Phenytoin • Warfarin
Address common causes of noncompliance	• Unable to afford medication • Unable to read (literacy or vision) • Difficulty remembering • Difficulty swallowing

Table 17-6
Summary of Falls in the Elderly*

Medical Illnesses Frequently Causing Falls in the Elderly	• Syncope • Stroke/transient ischemic attack • Seizure • Low blood glucose/electrolyte abnormalities • Infection • Low oxygen level (poor cardiac output or pulmonary disease) • Cardiac disease (arrhythmias, valve disease)
Intrinsic Causes of Falls in the Elderly	• Poor balance/proprioception/reflexes • Weakness/debilitation • Arthritis • Gait and balance problems • Visual impairment • Impaired cognition • Depression • Peripheral neuropathy

Extrinsic Causes of Falls in the Elderly	• Medications and drugs:
	  - Alcohol
	  - Sedatives/hypnotics
	  - Narcotics
	  - Antidepressants
	  - Antihypertensives/antiarrhythmics
	  - Diuretics

Environmental Causes of Falls in the Elderly	• Poor lighting • Loose carpets • Clutter/obstacles
Screening for Risk of Falling	• "Get Up and Go Test": observe patient rising from seated position on chair, walk across room, turn and sit in a chair • Cause is often multifactorial • Any person with recurrent falls should be assessed for falls risks
Interventions	• Treat underlying medical disorders • Prevention • Home safety check to identify and fix environmental causes • Rehabilitation • Hip protectors • Screen for and treat osteoporosis to minimize damage of falls
Rehabilitation Options	• Strengthening • Balance training (physical therapy or Tai Chi) • Gait training (helpful in neurologic and joint disease) • Assistive devices (evaluation by physical or occupation therapy)

*Falls account for nearly two-thirds of deaths related to unintentional injuries. Five percent of elderly who fall require hospitalization. Thirty-five percent of people aged > 65 fall each year.

Table 17-7

Preparing for End-of-Life Care

- Elicit patient's goals for end of life and mutually define goals of care
- Discuss advance directives about resuscitation, hospitalizations, chemotherapy use, antibiotic use, nutrition, and pain management
- With patient's consent, involve family members, health care proxy/person with durable power of attorney for health care, social work, religious leaders, and other medical providers in end-of-life discussions
- Consider referral to hospice if prognosis is less than 6 months
- For elderly patients who are not terminal, discuss resuscitation status prior to any major surgery

Table 17-8

Select Issues in Palliative Care

ISSUE	GOAL OF TREATMENT/TREATMENT OPTION/NOTE

Pain	• Goal: relieve suffering
	• Relief of pain often a primary concern for patients and their families
	• Start with nonsteroidal anti-inflammatory drugs unless pain severe
	  - Narcotics for severe pain or as second-line therapy
	• General guideline for narcotic dosing:
	  - Regular schedule of long-acting agents for baseline pain control
	  - Rescue doses of short-acting agents for break through pain and as pretreatment for activities known to cause pain
	  - No ceiling on dosage: patient may become tolerant and require higher doses
	  - Many delivery routes available: oral, intravenous, transdermal, buccal, epidural
	  - Treat side effects: constipation, sedation
	• Adjuvant therapies for pain control:
	  - Corticosteroids
	  - Antidepressants (neuropathic pain)
	  - Radiation or bisphosphonates (bone pain)
	  - Anxiolytics and relaxation techniques (anxiety)
	• Select narcotic conversions:
	  - Morphine PO 30 mg similar to morphine IV 10 mg
	  - Fentanyl transdermal 25 µg/h similar to morphine PO 45 mg/day

(continued)

Table 17-8

Select Issues in Palliative Care (continued)

ISSUE	GOAL OF TREATMENT/TREATMENT OPTION/NOTE

Respiratory	• Goal: relief of dyspnea and sensation of air hunger
	• Address underlying causes of dyspnea: effusions, excessive secretions, low hemoglobin (aggressiveness of treatment determined by goals of care)
	• Treatment options:
	  - Address underlying causes of dyspnea: effusions, excessive secretions, low hemoglobin (aggressiveness of treatment determined by goals of care)
	  - Bronchodilators
	  - Narcotics
	  - Decrease anxiety: relaxation techniques, anxiolytics

Excessive Secretions	• Goal: reduce work of breathing
	• Patient may be too weak to cough up secretions or to swallow them
	• Treatment options:
	  - Elevate head of bed
	  - Encourage patient to move out of bed to chair
	  - Frequent suctioning
	  - Transdermal scopolamine
	  - Atropine drops

Anxiety	• Goal: decrease anxiety about dying process
	• Treatment options:
	  - Discuss patient's concerns and address physical symptoms causing anxiety (pain and dyspnea)
	  - With patient's consent, involve family, friends, counselors, and religious leaders
	  - Relaxation techniques: have familiar objects in room
	  - Anxiolytics: haldol, lorazepam, hydroxyzine

Constipation	• Goal: minimize constipation
	• Narcotics frequently associated with constipation. Start anticonstipation regimen if narcotics are used
	• Treatment options:
	  - Medications: senna, docusate sodium, enemas
	  - Hydration

Nausea	• Goal: minimize discomfort associated with nausea
	• Treatment options:
	  - Small meals
	  - Medications: prochlorperazine, haldol, lorazepam, transdermal scopolamine, ondansetron, dronabinol

Sedation	• Goal: maximize quality of time patient is able to spend with family and friends
	• Treatment options:
	  - Titrate narcotics to maximize pain control while minimizing sedating side effects
	  - Divide daily activities into small units with a rest in between
	  - Medications: methylphenidate

Chapter 18

Allergy and Immunology

Introduction

Role of the Immune System

The basic function of the immune system is to recognize and defend the host (self) from foreign substances or organisms (nonself). An *antigen* is a molecule that elicits an antibody response. Examples of antigens include bacterial cell wall proteins and penicillin. Normally, "self" molecules do not elicit an immune response. Malfunction of the immune system can result in a variety of disorders ranging from immunodeficiency to autoimmunity and anaphylaxis.

Organization of the Immune System

The immune system can be divided into two basic categories, innate and adaptive.

The *innate* immune response is nonspecific, and is often the first line of defense against an offending agent. Examples of the innate immune system include primary barriers to infection (hair, skin, cilia, gastric acid), the complement system, and the primary cellular line of defense (neutrophils, macrophages, eosinophils, and mast cells).

The *adaptive* immune response is specific; in that it recognizes a particular antigen, produces a precise reaction, and then retains memory of the antigen for future interactions. Adaptive immunity is further divided into B cell (*humoral*) and T cell (*cellular*) components. Humoral immunity generally defends against bacterial infection, whereas cellular immunity defends against viruses, fungi, and parasites.

Immunoglobulins

Immunoglobulins (Ig) are secreted by B cells, usually in response to specific antigens. There are five types. IgG is the most prevalent Ig found in the serum, followed (in order) by IgA, IgM, IgD, and IgE.

Table 18-1

Summary of Immunoglobulins

	BASIC STRUCTURE	CHARACTERISTICS	NOTES
IgG	• Monomer • Four subclasses	• The most prevalent Ig • Enhances phagocytosis • Activates complement • Serum half-life = 23 days	• Accounts for 20% of total serum protein • Increased levels indicate late primary or current reactivated disease • Crosses the placenta
IgA	• Dimer • Two subunits held together by a "j" chain	• Found in most secretions and body fluids: (breast milk, saliva, mucous) • Most prevalent in epithelial cells	• Produced by the fetus • Does not cross the placenta
IgM	• Pentamer • Five subunits held together by a "j" chain	• First response to a primary infection • Found in serum, mucosal surfaces, and breast milk • Serum half-life = 5 days	• Increased levels indicate current or recent primary infection, can also be seen in reactivation of some diseases • Does not cross the placenta
IgD	• Monomer	• Membrane-bound receptor on B cells	• Minimal clinical significance
IgE	• Monomer	• The least prevalent Ig • Involved with allergic and hypersensitivity reactions	• Produced by the fetus • Does not cross the placenta

Immune Deficiencies

Table 18-2

Signs and Symptoms of Immune Deficiency

- Recurrent fever
- Recurrent abscesses
- Chronic diarrhea
- Dermatitis
- Chronic atelectasis
- Recurrent/unusually severe presentations of common illnesses (i.e., pneumonia, sinusitis, meningitis), or isolation of unusual organisms
- Infection with opportunistic pathogen
- Failure to thrive
- Malnutrition
- Short stature

Immunocompromise

Immunocompromised individuals may be at risk of disseminated disease after administration of live attenuated vaccines, such as the MMR (measles, mumps, and rubella), varicella, oral polio, oral typhoid, smallpox, and yellow fever vaccines. Immunization with nonlive vaccines is safe, yet may not be as effective as for immunocompetent patients.

B Cell Disorders

B cells develop in the bone marrow and differentiate into plasma cells that ultimately secrete Ig. B cell disorders include problems in quantity (decreased numbers), and in function (normal amounts, but poor Ig production/function). B cell deficiencies often manifest as opportunistic and serious bacterial infections. B cell function can be tested by checking titers to organisms that the patient has been immunized against (i.e., *Streptococcus pneumoniae*, *Haemophilus influenzae* type B, tetanus, or diphtheria).

T Cell Disorders

T cells develop and mature in the thymus. T cell deficiencies manifest with severe or recurrent viral, fungal, mycobacterial, and protozoal diseases. Congenital T cell disorders present in childhood. The most common acquired T cell disorder is caused by HIV infection.

Disorders of Phagocytes

Neutrophils and macrophages are involved in both the innate and adaptive immune responses. They function to kill pathogens intracellularly, and present antigen. Defects in neutrophil function can lead to bacterial and fungal infections; in chronic granulomatous disease, defects in NADPH (nicotinamide adenine dinucleotide phosphate) oxidase prevent use of the respiratory burst to kill catalase-positive bacteria and fungi. Defects in macrophage signaling (interferon-gamma and IL [interleukin]-12) lead to susceptibility to intracellular microbes such as mycobacteria, *Salmonella*, and *Listeria*.

Complement Deficiencies

The complement system is a series of heat-labile plasma proteins that, when activated, bind and opsonize pathogens and induce inflammation. Absence of early complement components results in susceptibility to gram-positive bacteria and autoimmune disease, due to inability to clear immune complexes. Defects in alternative or terminal complement components may lead to *Neisseria* infections. Low CH50 may indicate consumption, as occurs in active rheumatologic disease. Patients with absence of a complement component will have near-absent or undetectable complement activity (CH50 or AH50).

Table 18-3

Immune Deficiencies Presenting in Adulthood

CONDITION	ETIOLOGY	PRESENTATION	NOTES
Common Variable Hypogammaglobulinemia	• Deficient Ig production • Normal B cell quantity • Most frequently diagnosed primary immunodeficiency in adults	• Decreased IgA, IgG, +/− IgM • Recurrent pyogenic infections: especially sinusitis, pneumonia • Diarrhea (*Giardia* infections common) • Presents in adolescence/early adulthood • Hypertrophic lymphoid tissue	• Recurrent respiratory infections often lead to bronchiectasis • ↑ Risk of autoimmune disease and malignancy (lymphoma) • Treat with antibiotics and monthly IVIG
Selective IgA Deficiency	• The most prevalent primary immunodeficiency • Decreased production of IgA	• Often asymptomatic • Infections of the respiratory, GI, and urogenital tracts	• Increased risk of autoimmune disease and malignancies • Possible anaphylactic reactions when administered blood products containing IgA • IgA cannot be replaced
Specific Antibody Deficiency	• Inability to produce antibodies against specific pathogens, such as *S. pneumoniae*	• Recurrent pyogenic infections: pneumonia, sinusitis • Absent or low antibody titers after vaccination	• Treat with antibiotics and monthly IVIG
Chronic Granulomatous Disease	• X linked (majority), usually presents in childhood • Defect in phagocyte NADPH oxidase	• Infections with catalase + organisms (*Staphylococcus aureus, Escherichia coli, Serratia, Salmonella, Candida, Aspergillus, Nocardia*) • Repeated skin infections • Fever • Lymphadenopathy • Obstructive granulomas	• Oxidative burst testing (DHR flow cytometry, NBT dye reaction) • Treatment with interferon-gamma and prophylactic antibiotics (i.e., TMP/SMX)

Table 18-3

Immune Deficiencies Presenting in Adulthood (continued)

CONDITION	ETIOLOGY	PRESENTATION	NOTES
MPO Deficiency	• Autosomal recessive • Complete absence of MPO from neutrophils • The most common disorder of neutrophils	• Usually asymptomatic • Mild bacterial infections • Mild fungal infections, especially *Candida* in diabetics	• Absence of neutrophil MPO • Abnormal phagocyte function - Treat with antibiotics when clinically indicated
Complement Deficiency	• Near or complete absence of a given complement component	• Defects in early pathway components (C1q/r/s, C2, C3, C4) associated with autoimmunity • Defects in alternative and terminal components associated with *Neisseria* infections	• Initial tests: CH50 and AH50 • MBL deficiency is the most common deficiency among complement disorders

DHR = dihydrorhodamine; GI = gastrointestinal; IVIG = intravenous immunoglobulin; MBL = mannose-binding lectin; MPO = myeloperoxidase; NBT = nitroblue tetrazolium; TMP/SMX = trimethoprim/sulfamethoxazole.

Allergic Disorders

The most common allergic disorders include atopic dermatitis (AD), asthma, and allergic rhinitis (AR) and conjunctivitis. They occur in 20–30% of the population, and are IgE and mast cell-mediated type I hypersensitivity reactions. Allergic contact dermatitis, on the other hand, is a type IV cell-mediated disorder. There is a large genetic component to allergic disorders. If one parent has an atopic disorder, the risk of the child having an atopic disease is 30%. If both parents have a history of atopic disorders, the child has a 50–70% risk of atopic disease. Eosinophilia and elevated IgE levels may be an associated finding of any atopic disease.

Allergy testing

A variety of methods are used to evaluate a patient for allergies. Identification and avoidance of allergens is the most important component of the management of allergic disorders.

Skin testing: Identifies allergen-specific IgE. Diluted allergen is introduced into the skin (either percutaneous or intradermal) and interacts with mast cell-bound IgE. Cross-linking of IgE antibodies causes histamine release, resulting in a wheal and flare reaction within 15–20 minutes of testing. This test is usually performed on the volar aspect of the arms or upper back.

Antihistamines (including H₂ blockers) and tricyclic antidepressants can produce false negative results, and should be withheld for at least 48–72 hours prior to testing. Topical steroids used at the injection site can also suppress skin test results. Inhaled corticosteroids and short-term systemic corticosteroids do not have any effect on skin testing. Skin testing should not be performed directly on actively eczematous skin.

In vitro testing: Measures serum levels of allergen-specific IgE. Commonly used methods include the radioallergosorbent test (RAST) and enzyme-linked immunosorbent assay (ELISA). These tests are generally not as sensitive as skin testing in defining clinically pertinent allergens, and are indicated for patients who are not candidates for skin testing. Examples include patients who suffer from severe skin disease, cannot discontinue medications that interfere with skin testing, or have experienced severe anaphylaxis (skin testing can, in rare cases, cause anaphylaxis).

Patch testing is used to identify patients with contact dermatitis (i.e., from latex or nickel). A suspected agent is applied to the skin with an occlusive dressing and the area is evaluated 72–96 hours after application. The test is positive when the agent interacts with sensitized Langerhans cells in the skin, with subsequent T cell activation, resulting in erythema, induration, and vesiculation of the involved area.

Common Allergic Disorders

Asthma: *Discussed in Chapter 2, Pulmonology.*
Allergic Rhinitis (AR) and Conjunctivitis: This disease occurs when allergens encounter nasal and conjunctival mucosa, bind to IgE antibody, and cause degranulation of superficial mucosal mast cells and basophils. This results in increased vascular permeability, tissue edema, congestion, and, eventually, nasal obstruction.

Frequent symptoms include rhinorrhea, sneezing, watery eyes, and nasal or ocular pruritus. Infraorbital edema and cyanosis ("allergic shiners") develop due to obstruction of vascular drainage, and chronic disease may be complicated by nasal polyposis and anosmia, sinusitis, and otitis media.

Perennial AR occurs with constant exposure to the offending agent; common causes include indoor allergens such as dust mites, cockroaches, animal dander, and indoor molds. *Seasonal* AR (commonly referred to as "hay fever") usually involves sensitivity to pollens or outdoor mold spores. Although pollen seasons have geographic variability, tree pollen is typically responsible for symptoms in the spring, grass pollens in late spring through early summer, and weed pollens in late summer through early fall. Flowers are not typical causes of AR, although inhalation of their pollen particles may have an irritant effect on nasal and conjunctival mucosa.

In AR, nasal swabs often demonstrate eosinophils. Treatment includes identification and avoidance of offending agents, intranasal steroids, antihistamines, antileukotrienes, and allergen-specific immunotherapy. Other options include nasal cromolyn (safe in pregnancy) or ipratropium, and nasal decongestants. Topical nasal decongestant sprays are not recommended for long-term use, as tachyphylaxis and rebound nasal congestion occur. Recommended environmental control measures include removal of offending allergens from the home if possible, maintaining indoor humidity below 50% to limit dust mite and mold growth, use of impermeable mattress and pillow covers, washing bedding weekly in hot water (≥130°F), and minimization of stuffed animals, carpets, and upholstered furniture.

Table 18-4

Differential Diagnosis of Allergic Rhinitis

DIAGNOSIS	TYPES/CAUSES
Infectious Rhinitis	• Viral • Bacterial
AR	• Seasonal • Perennial • Other intermittent (i.e., occupational)
Drug-Induced Rhinitis (Rhinitis Medicamentosa)	• Overuse of topical nasal decongestants • Cocaine • Antihypertensives • Antipsychotics • Aspirin and NSAIDs • Oral contraceptives
Hormonal Rhinitis	• Pregnancy • Puberty • Hypothyroidism
Idiopathic Nonallergic (Vasomotor) Rhinitis	• Chemical irritants • Strong smells • Changes in temperature, humidity
Gustatory Rhinitis	• Ingestion of hot, spicy foods or alcohol
Atrophic Rhinitis	• Age
Nasal Polyps	• Aspirin sensitivity (Samter's triad) • Cystic fibrosis • Churg-Strauss syndrome • Allergic fungal sinusitis
Anatomic Factors	• Deviated septum • Hypertrophic turbinates • Foreign body • Tumors
Granulomatous Disease	• Wegener's granulomatosis • Sarcoid
Ciliary Defects	• Primary ciliary dyskinesia
Cerebrospinal Fluid Rhinorrhea	• Trauma • Postsurgical • Tumors • Hydrocephalus

Atopic Dermatitis (AD): This disease is best described as a chronic, relapsing inflammatory Th2-cell-mediated skin disorder most frequent in patients with a personal or family history of atopic disease. AD may be associated with high circulating levels of IgE. In older children and adults, flexural surfaces are most often involved. Clinically, patients will have a pruritic rash that is erythematous, crusted, or scaly in nature. Chronic irritation results in lichenification (thickening) of skin, and pigmentation changes (either hyper- or hypopigmentation). Treatment consists of identification and avoidance of offending agents, emollients, topical corticosteroids, and calcineurin inhibitors (tacrolimus and pimecrolimus), and treatment of superinfections. Excoriation is frequent, and superinfection may occur.

Urticaria: Urticaria is pruritic, erythematous, raised cutaneous wheals that blanch with pressure, caused by mast cell degranulation and subsequent blood vessel dilation and edema. Urticaria is a common manifestation of allergic reactions to foods, drugs, infections, insect stings, or environmental allergens, and can be a symptom of anaphylaxis. However, chronic urticaria (>6 weeks) without obvious triggers may be idiopathic. IgG antibodies against the high affinity IgE receptor, FcεRI, have been found in 30–40% of patients with chronic idiopathic urticaria, and IgG antibodies against IgE in another 10%. Rarely, urticaria is caused by vasculitis. Treatment consists of aggressive use of antihistamines (both H_1- and H_2-blockers), and sparing use of systemic corticosteroids for severe flares.

Urticaria may also be caused by physical stimuli, such as scratching (dermatographism), pressure, cold, vibration, sunlight, cholinergic stimuli, and exercise. Exercise-induced, cold, and solar urticaria may be accompanied by anaphylaxis.

Angioedema: Angioedema is characterized by localized subcutaneous swelling caused by extravasation of fluid into interstitial tissues due to inflammatory mediators, dilation of blood vessels, and increased vascular permeability. This may be mediated by mast cells, complement, and/or bradykinin. Angioedema is generally not pruritic but may be painful or burning. It is rapid in onset, asymmetric, does not occur in dependent areas, usually resolves within hours, and most commonly involves the face, oropharynx, and extremities. Among patients with urticaria, angioedema occurs in 40% of these patients. The most common cause of acquired angioedema in the adult population is the use of angiotensin-converting enzyme (ACE) inhibitors. Rarely, acquired angioedema may be caused by lymphoma.

Hereditary angioedema (HAE) is an autosomal dominant disorder caused by either the absence, or dysfunction, of the regulatory complement component *C1 inhibitor* (C1-INH), which normally acts to degrade activated C1 and proteases that lead to kinin formation. Patients with HAE invariably have low C4 levels; those with type I HAE have low levels of C1-INH antigen; those with type II HAE have normal or elevated levels of C1-INH antigen, but low levels of C1-INH function. C2 levels decrease during acute attacks; C1q levels are normal. Treatment includes prophylaxis with the attenuated androgens, danazol (200–400 mg/day) and stanozolol (2–4 mg/day), which increase hepatic synthesis of C1-INH and C4. Fresh frozen plasma may be used as preoperative and preprocedural prophylaxis. Acute exacerbations may be spontaneous or caused by trauma, and are not associated with urticaria. Symptoms may include life-threatening laryngeal edema, and abdominal edema causing pain, vomiting, and bowel obstruction. Treatment of acute episodes should include airway protection and epinephrine, although epinephrine is not as effective in this situation, as it is for treatment of angioedema in anaphylaxis. Tracheostomy may be necessary, as laryngeal obstruction causes endotracheal intubation to be technically difficult.

Acquired angioedema may also be associated with low levels of C4; lymphoproliferative diseases and other malignancies may cause excessive complement activation and consumption of C1-INH and C1q; autoantibodies against C1-INH have also been reported. In both cases, C1q levels will also be decreased.

Table 18-5
Complement Levels in Angioedema

				C1-INH	
	C1Q	**C4***	**C2***	**Antigen**	**Function**
Inherited:					
Type I	Normal	Low	Low	Low	Low
Type II	Normal	Low	Low	Normal or Elevated	Low
Acquired:					
Complement consumption	Low	Low	Low	Low	Low
Autoantibody	Low	Low	Low	Low	Variable

*C4 and C2 are always low during acute attack in HAE; in a majority of patients, they are chronically low as well.

Hypersensitivity Reactions

Table 18-6
Summary of Hypersensitivity Reactions

TYPE	ETIOLOGY	PRESENTATION	TREATMENT/NOTES
Type I (Anaphylaxis, IgE Mediated)	• IgE mediated • Histamine, heparin, leukotrienes, mast cells • Can be caused by insect stings, peanuts, and medications	• AR and conjunctivitis • Hives/flushing • Bronchoconstriction • Laryngeal edema • Hypotension/shock	• ABCs • IM epinephrine • Histamine antagonists • Corticosteroids
Type II (Cytotoxic, Ig Mediated)	• IgG, IgM mediated • Involves activation of complement • Cellular lysis • Transfusion reactions	• Hemolytic anemia • ITP	• Corticosteroids
Type III (Immune-Complex Mediated)	• IgG, IgM mediated • Formation of antigen/antibody complexes	• Acute glomerulonephritis • Serum sickness	• Corticosteroids
Type IV (Delayed, T Cell Mediated)	• T lymphocyte mediated • Does not involve antibodies	• Contact dermatitis (Poison ivy, poison oak, allergic contact dermatitis) • Graft-versus-host disease	• TB skin testing is an example of delayed-type hypersensitivity • Corticosteroids

ABCs = airway, breathing, circulation; ITP = immune thrombocytopenic purpura; TB = tuberculosis.

Anaphylaxis: Anaphylaxis is an immediate hypersensitivity reaction involving more than one organ system (systemic) caused by IgE-mediated release of mediators from mast cells and basophils, and is a potentially life-threatening condition.

Table 18-7

Signs and Symptoms of Anaphylaxis

- Flushing, pruritus
- Urticaria and/or angioedema
- Oropharyngeal and laryngeal edema
- Rhinitis, conjunctivitis
- Bronchospasm, cough, and respiratory failure
- Abdominal pain, nausea, vomiting, diarrhea
- Hypotension, arrhythmias, and cardiovascular collapse
- Sense of impending doom

The cornerstone to treatment of anaphylaxis after placing the patient in a recumbent position is the administration of epinephrine, 0.2–0.5 mL of a 1:1000 dilution (0.2–0.5 mg) intramuscularly, repeating every 5 minutes as needed. Treatment also includes airway management, oxygen, intravenous fluids, inhaled beta-agonists, antihistamines, and systemic corticosteroids. Refractory hypotension may warrant vasopressors and glucagon infusion, if beta-blockade is present. Elevated serum tryptase levels obtained 1–4 hours after the event may be helpful to establish a diagnosis of anaphylaxis, although a normal tryptase level does not exclude the diagnosis. Tryptase levels may also be constitutively elevated in systemic mastocytosis. Plasma histamine is elevated for only 30–60 minutes after anaphylaxis; histamine metabolites will subsequently appear in the urine, so 24-hour urinary histamine may be measured.

Systemic mastocytosis is a rare condition with symptoms that may mimic anaphylaxis, including flushing, pruritus, dizziness, syncope, abdominal discomfort, nausea, and diarrhea. It is also associated with musculoskeletal pain, neuropsychiatric symptoms, and skin lesions (urticaria pigmentosa). Respiratory symptoms, however, are

rare. The diagnosis is made by demonstrating an increase in mast cell mediators in serum (tryptase) or urine (histamine), and an increase of abnormal mast cells in the bone marrow. The most common form of cutaneous mastocytosis, urticaria pigmentosa, takes the form of brown macules that wheal and flare when scratched (Darier's sign). Diagnosis is made by skin biopsy.

Drug Hypersensitivity

Table 18-8

Mechanisms of Adverse Drug Reactions

- Overdosage
- Pharmacologic side effect
- Altered metabolism, drug-drug interactions
- Secondary/indirect effects (e.g., disturbance of microbial flora from antibiotics; Jarisch-Herxheimer reaction in syphilis treatment)
- Genetic predisposition (e.g., G6PD deficiency)
- Immunologic reactions:
  - I. Immediate hypersensitivity (IgE mediated)
  - II. Antibody-dependent cytotoxicity (e.g., hemolytic anemia with penicillin)
  - III. Immune complex mediated
  - IV. Delayed T cell mediated (e.g., contact dermatitis, morbilliform rashes, erythema multiforme/Stevens-Johnson syndrome)
- Direct mast cell activation

G6PD = glucose-6-phosphate dehydrogenase.

The majority of adverse drug reactions are due to pharmacologic side effects or dose-related toxicity. Drug reactions that are confirmed by skin testing to be IgE mediated (e.g., penicillin) are amenable to desensitization, if the agent is needed. A few patients with cell-mediated reactions (e.g., sulfa allergy in HIV) can be desensitized, but history of Stevens-Johnson or toxic epidermal necrolysis is a strict contraindication. Although urticaria and angioedema are usually signs of an IgE-mediated mechanism, they may also occur with shifts in biochemical pathways as occurs in aspirin and NSAID sensitivity, and angioedema due to ACE inhibitors. Aspirin sensitivity can be associated with asthma and nasal polyposis (Samter's triad); patients with chronic urticaria and angioedema will often flare with aspirin or NSAID use as well.

Some agents can directly activate mast cells to release histamine. Examples include opiates, vancomycin, and muscle relaxants. Reactions to radiocontrast media are not due to iodine but, rather, their high osmolarity triggering histamine release. Pretreatment with corticosteroids and antihistamines often prevents further reactions; use of nonionic iso-osmolar agents is also recommended.

Food Allergy

This group of disorders results from an abnormal immunologic response. The most common food allergens are proteins found in cow's milk, eggs, soy, wheat, peanuts, tree nuts, fish, and shellfish. This disorder should be distinguished from food *intolerance*, which is nonimmunologic in nature (i.e., lactase deficiency, resulting in milk intolerance).

Symptoms are variable and involve several systems:

- Cutaneous: Fish, shellfish, peanuts, and tree nuts are the most common causes of food-related urticaria and angioedema in adults. Food allergy may also contribute to AD.
- GI: Cow's milk, eggs, soy, and wheat are the most common causes of GI immune-mediated disorders. Symptoms include nausea, vomiting, abdominal pain, diarrhea, steatorrhea, enterocolitis, malabsorption, and allergic eosinophilic gastroenteropathy.
- Respiratory and generalized anaphylaxis: Upper and lower respiratory tract symptoms, and anaphylaxis with cardiovascular collapse, have been reported with a variety of foods. Peanuts, tree nuts, and shellfish are the most frequently implicated. Cutaneous and GI manifestations may be present as well. Asthma and failure to use epinephrine early are both risk factors for fatal food-induced anaphylaxis.

The only definitive treatment is identification and avoidance of offending agents. Patients who have a history of an anaphylactic reaction should be given an auto-injectable epinephrine kit, and taught its vital role in saving lives.

Individuals with *oral allergy syndrome (OAS)* have specific IgE to airborne allergens (i.e., tree pollens) that cross-react with proteins in fresh fruit, causing rapid onset symptoms of pruritus, tingling, and angioedema almost exclusively of the oropharynx. OAS patients can generally ingest these foods after cooking, and are at minimal risk of anaphylaxis.

Latex Allergy

Up to 3% of the general population may have an allergy to latex. Patients with spina bifida, health care workers, and those with a history of multiple surgeries (especially urinary tract surgery) are especially at risk. Contact dermatitis, immediate hypersensitivity (anaphylaxis), and irritant dermatitis (from occluded skin under the impermeable latex) are all possible manifestations. A radioallergosorbent test (RAST) is available with high specificity but low sensitivity. Identification of the allergy and avoidance of latex is the best therapy.

Hymenoptera Allergy

Stings from honeybees, bumblebees, yellow jackets, hornets, wasps, and fire ants can cause local and/or systemic reactions. Up to 5% of the population is at risk of anaphylaxis from insect stings. Systemic reactions include generalized urticaria, angioedema, laryngeal edema, bronchospasm, GI symptoms, and cardiovascular collapse. Patients who have a history of systemic reaction should be evaluated by an allergist for skin testing with venoms. For those with positive skin tests, venom immunotherapy has been proven to decrease the incidence and severity of subsequent reactions. All patients should be given an autoinjectable epinephrine kit, however, as immunotherapy does not completely eliminate the risk of future reactions.

Chapter 19

Neurology

Table 19-1

Summary of Primary Headaches

TYPE (DURATION)	DESCRIPTION OF PAIN	ASSOCIATED SIGN AND SYMPTOM	TREATMENT	NOTES

Migraine (4–72 hours)	• Unilateral is more frequent than bilateral
	• Throbbing or pulsating
	• Moderate to severe
		• Nausea, vomiting
		• Photophobia, phonophobia
		• Visual or sensory aura
		• Nasal congestion
		• Aggravated by activity
		• Inhibits or prohibits normal daily activities
			• Prophylactic:
			  - Sleep hygiene *(may be most effective)*
			  - Beta-blockers
			  - Anticonvulsants
			  - TCAs
			• Abortive:
			  - Caffeine/aspirin/acetaminophen
			  - Triptans (5-HT agonists)
			  - Ergot derivatives
			• Rescue:
			  - Morphine
				• >2 headaches/week
				• Efficacy of prophylaxis may take several months
				• Sleep disorders should be excluded in all patients with chronic headaches
				• Menstrual-related migraine may benefit from low-dose estrogen or magnesium therapy

Tension (30 minutes–7 days)	• Bilateral
	• Squeezing or pressure
	• Mild or moderate
		• No nausea or vomiting
		• Inhibits but does not prohibit daily routine
			• Prophylactic:
			  - TCAs
			  - SSRIs
			• Abortive:
			  - Ibuprofen
				• Prophylaxis indicated for >2 headaches/week

Cluster (15–180 minutes, once to many times a day for 2 weeks to a month)	• Unilateral:
	  - Orbital
	  - Supraorbital
	  - Temporal
	• Sharp or stabbing
	• Severe
		• Ipsilateral:
		  - Lacrimation
		  - Rhinorrhea
		  - Miosis/ptosis
		  - Eyelid edema
		• Restlessness during the headache
		• Fatigue after the headache resolves
			• Prophylactic:
			  - Prednisone taper
			  - CCB
			  - Divalproex
			  - Topiramate
			• Abortive:
			  - Oxygen
			  - Triptans
			  - Dihydroergotamine
				• Most require prophylactic treatment due to intensity and repetitive nature
				• Triptans are contraindicated in patients with coronary artery disease

CCB = calcium channel blocker; SSRI = selective serotonin reuptake inhibitor; TCA = tricyclic antidepressants.

Table 19-2

Summary of Secondary Headaches

TYPE	KEY POINTS	DIAGNOSIS	TREATMENT	NOTES
Giant Cell Arteritis	• Affects patients > 50 years old • New onset of progressive, throbbing headache • May experience jaw claudication and amaurosis fugax (transient blindness in one eye)	• Elevated ESR and CRP • Temporal artery biopsy	• Prednisone	• Start therapy early • Risk of visual loss
		See Rheumatology section (Chapter 11) for additional details		
Pseudotumor Cerebri	• Idiopathic intracranial hypertension • More common in young obese woman • Daily headaches worse with cough, sneezing, or supine position	• Papilledema • Visual field abnormalities • May have cranial nerve VI palsy • MRI to exclude structural disease • High opening pressure on lumbar puncture	• Acetazolamide (*decreases CSF production*) • Weight control	• Close follow-up is needed since there is risk of visual loss
Trigeminal Neuralgia	• Paroxysmal pain involving divisions of trigeminal nerve • Touching area may produce pain • May be caused by compression of the 5th cranial nerve by adjacent vessels	• MRI indicated to rule out other causes	• Anticonvulsants • Baclofen	• Refractory cases may require surgery to decompress trigeminal ganglion
Medication Overuse Headaches	• May mimic migraine and tension headaches • Analgesic rebound: use of analgesics more than 2–3 days a week may cause intractable headache • Treatment: complete withdrawal of the overused medication (e.g., analgesics, opioids, ergotamine, or triptans)			

CN = cranial nerve; CSF = cerebrospinal fluid; ESR = erythrocyte sedimentation rate; CRP = C reactive protein; MRI = magnetic resonance imaging.

Table 19-3

Delirium Versus Dementia

	DELIRIUM	DEMENTIA
Onset	• Acute	• Chronic
Course	• Fluctuating	• Stable
Duration	• Hours to weeks	• Months to years
Attention	• Fluctuates	• Normal
Perception	• Hallucinations are frequent	• Usually normal
Sleep/Awake	• Disrupted	• Fragmented

Note	• Common causes:
	  D drugs
	  E emotion (mania or depression)
	  L low oxygen
	  I infection
	  R retention (urine/feces)
	  I ictal states (after a seizure)
	  U under nourished
	  M metabolic (thyroid function/
	    organ failure)
	  S stroke
		• Features:
		  - Memory impairment
		  - Aphasia *(language disturbance)*
		  - Apraxia *(impaired skilled or symbolic movement despite intact motor function)*
		  - Agnosia *(failure to recognize or identify entities despite intact sensory function)*
		  - Disturbance in executive functioning *(planning, organizing, sequencing, abstracting)*
		• Cognitive deficits cause a significant impairment in social or occupational functioning and represent a significant decline from a previous level of functioning

Table 19-4
Summary of Dementia

Type (% of Dementia Cases)	Etiology	Clinical Presentation	Diagnosis	Treatment	Notes
Vascular (VaD) (30%)	• Multiple small cerebral infarcts (or sometimes hemorrhages) resulting in neuronal and axonal impairment	• Onset within 3 months of stroke or with stroke-like time course • Progressive decline • Cognitive slowing, apathy, and poor problem solving abilities	Clinical: • MMSE has low sensitivity • CT and MRI show vascular lesions • Dementia must present within 3 months of stroke	• Primary prevention of stroke may prevent vascular dementia • Adjunctive drugs for depression, psychosis, and sleep disorders are useful	• Therapy for AD may benefit patients with mixed disease

Alzheimer's (AD) (55%)	• Deposition of beta-amyloid protein in extracellular plaques
	• Intracellular accumulation of neurofibrillary tangles
	• Cholinergic deficit
		• Progression from mild cognitive impairment to AD about 10–15% per year
		• Memory impairment marks onset
		• Progresses over 8–10 years
		• Risk factors:
		  - ↑ age
		  - Genetic (presenilin mutations)
		  - HTN
		  - Menopause
			• Clinical
			• Broad-based cognitive and recent memory impairment
			• CT and MRI rule out other diseases
			• PET can show a pattern of decreased glucose absorption that is strongly suggestive of AD
			• Neuropsychological examination
			• Consider alternative diagnosis if no early memory loss or course is not insidious/chronically progressive
				• Cholinesterase inhibitors (donepezil, galantamine, rivastigmine) have modest benefit
				• Glutamate agonists (Memantine)
				• Trials have not demonstrated improvement in memory loss or prevention of progression to AD from mild cognitive impairment
					• Ginkgo biloba has been associated with mild improvement of cognition
					• Inherited AD manifests before age 65

Frontotemporal (<10%)	• 50% of all cases are inherited • Mutations involve abnormalities of the microtubule-binding tau protein (an axonal protein involved in microtubule assembly)	• Insidious onset and gradual decline of executive function (decision making, prioritizing, planning) • As opposed to AD, early executive and personality changes with emotional blunting, loss of insight and decline in social interactions	• Clinical • CT and MRI may show focal atrophy	• Supportive • Trazodone may alleviate agitation, irritability, depression, and eating disorders • Prohibit patients from driving and making financial decisions early in disease (due to impaired judgment)
Lewy Body Disease (<10%)	• Intraneuronal Lewy bodies in cerebral cortex	• Gradually progressive dementia • Fluctuations in cognitive function • Well-formed visual hallucinations • Spontaneous motor features of Parkinson's	• Clinical • High index of suspicion is needed • PET may show Lewy bodies	• Supportive • Psychiatric symptoms may respond to cholinergic augmentation • Cholinesterase inhibitors associated with reduction of behavioral symptoms

(continued)

Table 19-4

Summary of Dementia (continued)

Type (% of Dementia Cases)	Etiology	Clinical Presentation	Diagnosis	Treatment	Notes
Creutzfeldt-Jakob	• Most frequent prion disease	• Insidious onset over weeks to months with rapid progression • Transmissible • Myoclonus • Visual or cerebellar sign • Pyramidal or extrapyramidal motor signs • Akinetic mutism	• EEG with periodic sharp wave • CSF positive for 14-4-3 protein	• Supportive	• Death usually occurs in 3–6 months
Reversible Dementia	• Pseudodementia (depression) • Medications (corticosteroids) • Alcohol withdrawal • Metabolic disorders (B$_{12}$ deficiency) • Disorders affecting the brain (chronic subdural hematoma, normal pressure hydrocephalus)	• Presentation mimics dementia • Does not have features characterizing delirium: acute onset, hallucinations, fluctuating attention • Clinical diagnosis	• Evaluate offending agent	• Remove offending agent	

CT = computed tomography; EEG = electroencephalogram; MMSE = mini-mental status examination; PET = positron emission tomography.

448

Table 19-5

Brain Ischemia and Brain Hemorrhage

CONDITION	KEY POINTS	TREATMENT

TIA	• Sudden ischemic neurologic deficit that resolves completely in less than 24 hours
	• Etiology: 75% embolic and 25% thrombotic
	• Workup:
	  - Rule out metabolic causes of mental status changes
	  - Evaluate for source of emboli (carotid ultrasound, echocardiogram to rule out atrial clot or PFO [need bubble study]; ECG to rule out atrial fibrillation)
	  - CT/CTA, MRI/MRA to evaluate brain parenchyma and rule out narrowing/obstruction of cerebral arteries
		• Depends on the pathophysiology of the ischemic event
		• Antiplatelet therapy (aspirin, clopidogrel)
		• Carotid endarterectomy in patients with >70% ipsilateral stenosis
		• Risk of stroke after TIA: 5% within 2 days; 25% within 3 months

Ischemic Stroke	• Workup:
	  - Rule out metabolic causes of mental status changes
	  - Carotid duplex scanning if carotid artery stenosis or occlusion suspected
	  - Echocardiogram if cardiogenic embolism is suspected
	  - CT/MRI to identify territory of brain affected *(imaging may be normal within the first 48 hours)*
		• Maintain euvolemia
		• TPA
		  - Effective (decreases disability) for ischemic stroke if given less than 3 hours after onset of symptoms
		  - If time of onset cannot be determined, TPA is contraindicated
		  - Risk of hemorrhage
		• Aspirin
		  - Indicated in most ischemic stroke patients, especially if extracranial atherosclerosis
		• Antihypertensive medications
		  - Only used acutely if diastolic BP above 120 mm Hg and/or systolic BP above 220 mm Hg or the patient has active ischemic coronary disease, heart failure or aortic dissection

STROKE TERRITORIES AND CLINICAL MANIFESTATIONS

ANTERIOR CEREBRAL	MIDDLE CEREBRAL	POSTERIOR CEREBRAL
• Infrequent • Contralateral hemiparesis • Incontinence • Apathy • Confusion • Poor judgment • Mutism • Grasp reflex[*] • Gait apraxia[*]	• Frequent • Contralateral hemiparesis • Dysarthria • Hemianesthesia • Contralateral homonymous hemianopia[†] • Aphasia • Apraxia	• Contralateral homonymous hemianopia • Unilateral cortical blindness • Memory loss • Unilateral 3rd cranial nerve palsy • Hemiballismus[‡]

(continued)

Table 19-5

Brain Ischemia and Brain Hemorrhage (continued)

Condition	Key Points	Treatment
Intraparenchymal Hemorrhage	• Usually a bleed from arterioles or small arteries in the brain parenchyma • Symptoms usually increase gradually over minutes or a few hours • Associated with HTN • CT/MRI demonstrate intraparenchymal bleed	• Avoid anticoagulants • HTN should be treated if mean arterial pressure is >130 mm Hg • Coma patients need intracranial pressure monitoring • Large hematomas may require surgical evacuation
Subarachnoid Hemorrhage	• Rupture of an aneurysm (usually berry aneurysm) or AVM • Patients complain of "worst headache of my life" • Noncontrast CT usually shows a clot • Bloody or xanthochromic spinal tap	• Avoid anticoagulants • HTN should be treated if mean arterial pressure is >130 mm Hg • Nimodipine to prevent vasospasm • Coma patients need intracranial pressure monitoring • Surgical clipping/coiling of the aneurysm remains the surgical choice • If clinical signs of acute hydrocephalus occur, ventricular drainage should be considered
Subdural Hematoma	• Venous bleeding (delay in onset of symptoms) • Appears as a crescent-shaped, high-attenuation lesion on CT scan • Most cases result from a fall or an assault	• Avoid anticoagulants • Coma patients need intracranial pressure monitoring • Clot size and midline shift determine need for evacuation
Epidural Hematoma	• Arterial hemorrhage into the potential space superficial to the dura • Skull fracture is found in most cases • CT shows biconvex (lens shaped) collection with high attenuation • Patients usually have a lucid phase followed by rapid deterioration ("talk and die")	• Avoid anticoagulants • Coma patients need intracranial pressure monitoring • Clot size and midline shift determine need for surgical evacuation

*Apraxia is the inability to execute a voluntary motor movement despite being able to demonstrate normal muscle function

†Hemianopia: loss of vision for one half of the visual field

‡Hemiballismus: sudden, violent, spasmodic movements involving particularly the proximal portions of the extremities on one side of the body (caused by a destructive lesion of the contralateral subthalamic nucleus or its neighboring structures or pathways)

AVM = arteriovenous malformation; BP = blood pressure; CTA = computed tomography angiogram; HTN = hypertension; PFO = patent foramen ovale; MRA = magnetic resonance angiogram; TIA = transient ischemic attack; TPA = tissue plasminogen activator.

Table 19-6

Systemic Abnormalities Causing Generalized Seizures

CATEGORY	DETAILS
Electrolyte Abnormalities	• Hyponatremia • Hypocalcemia • Hypomagnesemia
Glucose Abnormalities	• Hypoglycemia
Organ Failure	• Uremia • Hepatic failure • TTP • Sepsis
Intoxication	• Penicillins • Local anesthetics • Tricyclic antidepressants • Lithium • Theophylline (narrow therapeutic window) • Amphetamine • Cocaine • Phenylcyclidine
Withdrawal	• Alcohol • Benzodiazepines • Barbiturates
Endocrine	• Hypoparathyroidism
Stroke	• Seizures may occur 3–12 months after stroke

TTP = thrombotic thrombocytopenic purpura.

Table 19-7

Distinguishing Generalized Tonic-Clonic Seizure from Syncope

FEATURE	SEIZURE	SYNCOPE
Precipitating Factor	• Generally none	• Emotional stress • Valsalva maneuver
Premonitory Symptoms	• None or vague	• Tunnel vision • Lethargy • Nausea • Diaphoresis
Posture at Onset	• Any posture	• Generally standing

(*continued*)

Table 19-7

Distinguishing Generalized Tonic-Clonic Seizure from Syncope (continued)

FEATURE	SEIZURE		SYNCOPE
Transition to Unconsciousness	• Immediate		• Gradual over seconds • Usually preceded by premonitory symptoms
Duration of Unconsciousness	• Minutes		• Seconds
Duration of Tonic and/or Clonic Movements	• 30–60 seconds		• If present, <15 seconds
Facial Appearance	• Cyanotic		• Pallid
Postevent Confusion/ Lethargy	• Minutes to hours		• If present, <5 minutes
Tongue Biting	• Occasional		• Rare
Incontinence	• Occasional		• Occasional
Elevated CPK	• Frequent		• Occasional
SEIZURE DETAILS	ABSENCE SEIZURE	COMPLEX PARTIAL SEIZURE	
Duration	• Seconds	• Minutes	
Automatisms	• Rare	• Frequent *(lip smacking)*	
Postictal State	• None	• Frequent	
EEG Pattern	• 3 cycles/second in all leads (generalized)	• Focal area of abnormal spikes and waves	

CPK = creatine phosphokinase.

Table 19-8

Antiepileptic Medications and Side Effects

MEDICATION	TYPE OF SEIZURE	SELECT SIDE EFFECTS
Ethosuximide	• Absence	• Rash • Bone marrow suppression
Carbamazepine	• Partial and generalized tonic-clonic	• Aplastic anemia, leukopenia • Hepatotoxicity • Hyponatremia • Vertigo
Gabapentin	• Partial and generalized tonic-clonic	• GI upset
Phenobarbital	• Partial and generalized tonic-clonic	• Depression • Sedation • Confusion
Phenytoin	• Partial and generalized tonic-clonic	• ↓ Ca • Gum hyperplasia • Rash • Osteomalacia
Topiramate	• Broad spectrum	• Weight loss • Sedation • Metabolic acidosis • Word-finding difficulties
Valproic Acid	• Broad spectrum	• Hepatotoxicity • Thrombocytopenia • Polycystic ovarian syndrome • Weight gain

GI = gastrointestinal.

Table 19-9

Suggested Strategies for Treating Status Epilepticus

STAGE (IN ORDER OF PROGRESSION)	TREATMENT OPTIONS
Initial Seizure Activity	• Diazepam IV (over 2–5 minutes) or lorazepam IV *(bolus)*
Early Status Epilepticus	• Lorazepam IV bolus (if not given earlier)
Established Status Epilepticus • *continuous seizure activity or ≥2 sequential seizures without full recovery of consciousness*	• Phenobarbital continuous IV infusion or • Phenytoin continuous IV infusion or • Fosphenytoin continuous IV infusion
Refractory Status Epilepticus • *seizure activity that continues after first- and second-line therapy has failed*	• General anesthesia with either: - Propofol bolus, followed by continuous infusion or - Thiopental boluses every 2–3 minutes until seizures are controlled, followed by a continuous infusion

Table 19-10

Movement Disorders and Tremors

• Movement disorders are generally divided into two categories:
  - Hypokinetic: Parkinson's
  - Hyperkinetic: rest tremor, essential tremor, chorea, dystonia

TREMOR TYPE	DESCRIPTION	CLASSIC CONDITIONS
Resting	• Usually a "pill rolling" type tremor • Present only at rest	• Parkinson's
Postural	• Present when limbs are voluntarily maintained against gravity	• Physiologic tremor • Essential tremor • Enhanced physiologic tremor
Kinetic	• Occurs during voluntary movement	• Cerebellar tremor

Table 19-11

Hypokinetic Movement Disorders

CONDITION	ETIOLOGY	KEY POINTS	TREATMENT	COMMENTS

Parkinson Disease	• Degeneration of dopaminergic neurons in the substantia nigra of the midbrain
	• Risk factors:
	  - Age
	  - Male gender
	  - Family history
		• Clinical diagnosis: at least two of following:
		  - Bradykinesia
		  - Resting tremor
		  - Postural reflex abnormality
		• Presents in 50–60s
		• Rest tremor is usually the first manifestation
		• Bradykinesia is initially distal and facial *(facial mask)*
		• Rigidity may be:
		  - Cogwheel *(intermittent resistance felt when a limb is passively flexed)*
		  - Lead pipe *(constant resistance felt when a limb is passively flexed)*
			• Levodopa/carbidopa:
			  - Considered mainstay of therapy
			  - Reduces disability and improves quality of life
			  - Chronic use may produce akinesia, dyskinesia, and dystonia
			• Dopamine agonists:
			  - May be used alone in early disease
			  - May reduce levodopa side effects
			• Anticholinergics:
			  - Improves tremor and rigidity
			• COMT inhibitors:
			  - Rarely used due to liver toxicity
				• There are no disease modifying drugs
				• Therapeutic goal is alleviation of symptoms

Parkinsonism	• Clinical features resemble Parkinson disease • Less responsive to therapy			
Drug-induced (Secondary Parkinsonism)	• Most important form of secondary parkinsonism • Caused by many antiemetic drugs, neuroleptic drugs (haloperidol), amiodarone, and valproic acid		• Remove offending drug	

(continued)

Table 19-11

Hypokinetic Movement Disorders (continued)

CONDITION	ETIOLOGY	KEY POINTS	TREATMENT	COMMENTS
Progressive Supranuclear Palsy	• Rare • Parkinsonism • Vertical gaze impairment which progresses to complete paralysis of eye movements • Falls occur early in course (in contrast to Parkinson disease)		• Supportive	• Results in disability within 3–5 years • Progression to death within 10 years
Multiple System Atrophy (Includes Shy-Drager)	• Parkinsonism • Cerebellar ataxia • Parkinsonism corticospinal tract signs • Dysautonomia • Nocturnal stridor		• Supportive	

COMT = catechol *O*-methyltransferase (enzyme that breaks down dopamine).

Table 19-12
Summary of Other Important Movement Disorders

DISEASE	KEY POINTS	TREATMENT
Essential Tremor	• Predominantly postural tremor • Starts in middle age and worsens over time • Family history is typical • Improves with alcohol	• Beta-blockers and primidone may be effective

Focal Dystonia	• Spasms force the body into abnormal, sometimes painful positions or movements:
	  - Blepharospasm (increased blinking frequency)
	  - Torticollis (spasms of the neck muscles, causing the head to twist forward, backward, or sideways)
	  - Writer's cramp
		• Anticholinergic agents
		• Botulinum toxin injection

Huntington Disease	• Presents in the fourth to fifth decades of life
	• Classic triad:
	  - Chorea *(involuntary, dance-like movements)*
	  - Dementia
	  - Family history *(mutations seen in the short arm of chromosome 4 are transmitted in an autosomal dominant fashion)*
	• May also have psychiatric manifestations
	• The disorder progresses, making walking impossible, swallowing difficult, and dementia severe
	• Diagnosis: genetic testing
		• Amantadine and neuroleptics may improve chorea
		• There are no disease modifying drugs
		• Consider genetic testing of family members

Restless Leg Syndrome	• Leg jerks occurring throughout sleep, preventing restful sleep • May have itchy or pulling sensation in legs • Rarely caused by iron deficiency	• Gabapentin may be useful • Dopamine agonist • Levodopa may have a rebound effect and worsen symptoms

Table 19-13

Demyelinating Disorders

CONDITION	KEY POINTS	DIAGNOSIS	TREATMENT

Multiple Sclerosis	• Demyelination of CNS
	• Etiology unknown
	• Disseminated patches of demyelination/ inflammation in the brain and spinal cord
	• Relapsing/remitting course
	• Onset between 15 and 50 years of age
	• Female predominance
	• Large differential diagnosis
		• Clinical:
		  - CNS lesions must occur over time and in different areas (may be documented by clinical, laboratory radiographic evidence)
		  - Symptoms depend on area of CNS involved: *optic neuritis, paresthesias, ataxia, hyperreflexia, spasticity*
		• MRI:
		  - Ovoid lesions perpendicular to lateral ventricles and corpus callosum
		• CSF:
		  - Oligoclonal bands
		  - High IgG/albumin ratio
		  - Elevated IgG synthesis rate
			• Corticosteroids to treat acute exacerbations
			• Plasma exchange if refractory to steroids
			• Immunomodulators IFN-b1a/1b decrease number of exacerbations and their severity
			• Supportive:
			  - Baclofen (for spasticity)
			  - Amantidine/ modafinil (for fatigue)

Guillain-Barré Syndrome	• Autoimmune demyelinating (peripheral) polyneuropathy
	• Associated with preceding infection *(Campylobacter, Lyme, hepatitis, HIV)*
	• Symptoms evolve over 2–4 weeks
		• Clinical:
		  - Progressive weakness
		  - Paresthesias
		  - Autonomic dysfunction
		  - Ophthalmoparesis
		  - Respiratory failure
		• CSF:
		  - Albuminocytologic dissociation: elevation in CSF protein (>0.55 g/L) without an elevation of white blood cells (<10 lymphocytes/mL)
		• EMG:
		  - Demyelinating pattern
			• IV gamma globulin
			• Plasmapheresis
			• Supportive care

CNS = central nervous system; EMG = electromyography; HIV = human immunodeficiency virus; IV = intravenous; IFN = interferon.

Table 19-14

Electrophysiologic Findings of Peripheral Neuropathies

	AXONAL NEUROPATHY	DEMYELINATING NEUROPATHY
Nerve Conduction Studies	• Low amplitude CMAPs or SNAPs in the setting of relatively normal conduction velocities	• Significantly slowed nerve conduction velocities with relatively normal CMAP and SNAP amplitudes with distal stimulation
Needle EMG	• Positive sharp waves, fibrillation potentials, and complex repetitive discharges usually appear within 7–10 days after axonal injury	• Decreased interference patterns

CMAPs = compound muscle action potentials; SNAPs = sensory nerve action potentials.

Table 19-15

Neuropathies

CONDITION	COURSE	TYPE OF NEUROPATHY	SELECTED CAUSES

Polyneuropathy
• Motor:
  - Cramps
  - Fasciculation
  - Weakness
  - Atrophy
• Sensory:
  - Pain
  - Tingling
  - Numbness
	• **Acute-subacute generalized**	• Sensorimotor	• Alcohol/nutritional
			• Toxins (metals)
			• Acute motor and sensory axonal neuropathy syndrome

		• Motor > sensory	• Guillain-Barré syndrome • Acute motor axonal neuropathy syndrome • Porphyria • Diphtheria • Toxins (dapsone, vincristine)
		• Sensory	• Vitamin B_6 toxicity • Toxins (cisplatin) • HIV • Paraneoplastic/autoimmune (anti-Hu associated)
	• **Chronic generalized symmetric** - **most frequent pattern of symmetric neuropathy**	• Sensorimotor	• Diabetes • Uremia • Alcohol/nutritional • Dysproteinemias • Connective tissue diseases

(continued)

Table 19-15
Neuropathies (continued)

CONDITION	COURSE	TYPE OF NEUROPATHY	SELECTED CAUSES
Polyneuropathy (cont.)	• **Chronic generalized symmetric**	• Motor > sensory	• Dysproteinemias • Hypothyroidism • Toxins (amiodarone, cytosine arabinoside, metals, tacrolimus) • Chronic inflammatory demyelinating polyradiculoneuropathy
		• Sensory	• Paraneoplastic/autoimmune (anti-Hu associated) • Vitamin B$_6$ toxicity • Sjögren syndrome • Vitamin E deficiency
	• **Generalized symmetric inherited**	• Sensorimotor	• Charcot-Marie-Tooth disease • Familial amyloidosis
	• **Generalized asymmetric**	• Sensorimotor	• Sarcoidosis • Lyme disease • Diabetes • Vasculitis
Mononeuropathy	• **Acute**		• Trauma (penetrating wounds) • Ischemic
	• **Subacute/chronic**		• Leprosy • Compression/entrapment • Vasculitis • Diabetes
Autonomic Neuropathies • Hyperhydrosis • Anhydrosis • Diarrhea/constipation • Orthostatic hypotension • Impotence	• **Acute**		• Acute pandysautonomia (paraneoplastic and idiopathic) • Guillain-Barré syndrome • Botulism • Porphyria • Toxins *(vincristine, amiodarone, cisplatin, organic solvents, metals)*
	• **Chronic**		• Diabetes • Chronic pandysautonomia (paraneoplastic and idiopathic) • Amyloidosis • Riley-Day syndrome

Table 19-16

Clinical Features of Neuropathies

ETIOLOGY	TYPE OF NEUROPATHY	CLINICAL FEATURE	NOTES
Diabetes	• Mononeuritis multiplex (MM), distal symmetrical polyneuropathy (DSPN), cranial nerve neuropathy (CN)	• Usually causes a slowly progressive sensory > motor DSPN • Increased risk of diabetic foot ulcers	• Evaluation for neuropathy is an important part of the diabetic physical examination • May improve with glucose control
Nutritional Deficiency	• Distal symmetrical polyneuropathy (DSPN)	• Common in alcoholics and other chronically malnourished patients	• Most common deficiencies: vitamins B_1, B_6, and folic acid • B_{12} deficiency: usually masked by the UPN signs from spinal cord disease
Chronic Inflammatory Demyelinating Polyneuropathy	• Demyelinating neuropathy (DN)	• Similar to Guillain-Barré but weakness continues to progress after 4 weeks • CSF may have elevated protein	• Treatment: steroids
Chemotherapy Agents	• Distal symmetrical polyneuropathy (DSPN)	• Usually dose-related • May be sensorimotor (pain and weakness) or just sensory	• Most common agents: vincristine, cisplatin, and taxol
Infections	• Distal symmetrical polyneuropathy (DSPN), mononeuritis multiplex (MM), dermatomal (D), cranial nerve neuropathy (CN)	• HIV, Lyme disease, and leprosy can cause various types of neuropathies • Leprosy involves cooler areas (ears, nose) • VZV (shingles) can cause a dermatomal sensory loss	• HIV neuropathy may be seen in patients with good CD4 counts
Neoplasms	• Mononeuritis multiplex (MM), distal symmetrical polyneuropathy (DSPN)	• Multiple myeloma and MGUS most frequent causes • Consider SPEP if no clear cause of neuropathy	• Common in SCLC
Systemic Diseases	• Distal symmetrical polyneuropathy (DSPN)	• Seen in critical illness, uremia, hepatic disease, hypothyroidism, and porphyria	• Variably reversible with treatment of systemic process

(continued)

Table 19-16

Clinical Features of Neuropathies (continued)

Etiology	Type of Neuropathy	Clinical Feature	Notes
Hereditary Diseases	Distal symmetrical polyneuropathy (DSPN), mononeuritis multiplex (MM)	• Most common cause is Charcot-Marie-Tooth disease, an autosomal dominant (chromosome 17) condition resulting in a slowly progressive demyelinating neuropathy which presents in third decade of life	• Associated with pes cavus *(foot deformity characterized by an abnormally high arch)*

MGUS = monoclonal gammopathy of undetermined significance; SCLC = small cell lung cancer; SPEP = serum protein electrophoresis; UPN = upper motor neuron; VZV = varicella zoster virus.

Table 19-17

Differential Diagnosis of Weakness

Sign	Upper Motor Neuron (UMN)	Lower Motor Neuron (LMN)	Neuromuscular Junction	Primary Muscle Disease
Atrophy	−	↑↑↑	−	↑
Tone	↑	↓	Normal	Normal or ↓
Fasciculations	−	+	−	−
Weakness Pattern	Focal, fine movements	Distal or in a nerve's distribution	Cranial/proximal muscles, fatigable	Generally proximal
Reflexes	↑	− or ↓	Normal	Normal or ↓
Babinski Sign	+	−	−	−

+ = present; − = none; ↑ = mild; ↑↑↑ = marked; ↓ = decreased.

Table 19-18

Motor Neuron Diseases

CONDITION	COURSE	KEY POINTS	TREATMENT
Poliomyelitis	Acute	• Caused by poliovirus • Oral-fecal transmission • Presents as aseptic lymphocytic meningitis • 1/1000 cases present asymmetric flaccid limb paralysis or bulbar palsies without sensory loss	• Prevention: polio vaccine
Amyotrophic Lateral Sclerosis	Chronic	• Male predominance in the sixth decade of life • Cause unknown, 95% of cases sporadic • Degeneration of cortical motor neurons and anterior horn cells • UMN symptoms: muscle weakness, stiffness, slow movements, emotional lability • LMN symptoms: cramps, muscle fasciculations, cramps • Weakness begins distally and ascends (asymmetric) • No sensory signs or pain • Mean survival 2–5years	• Riluzole prolongs survival 2–3 months, but does not improve muscle strength • NPPV when FVC <50% • PEG tube for feeding

FVC = forced vital capacity; NPPV = noninvasive positive pressure ventilation; PEG = percutaneous endoscopic gastrostomy.

Table 19-19

Medical Conditions Associated with Myopathies

ETIOLOGY	KEY POINTS
Hypothyroidism	• Weakness • Muscle hypertrophy • Myxedema • Normal reflexes with delayed relaxation phase
Hyperthyroidism	• Weakness • Muscle atrophy • Fasciculation associated with hyperactive reflexes
Corticosteroid	• Weakness more severe in lower extremities • Proximal muscle atrophy
Statins	• Subacute proximal weakness • Myalgias • Increased risk if renal failure • Discontinuation usually improves symptoms

Table 19-20

Diseases Affecting the Neuromuscular Junction

CONDITION	ETIOLOGY	KEY POINTS	DIAGNOSIS	TREATMENT

Myasthenia Gravis (MG)	• Ab against Ach receptor on muscles	• Peak incidence in women in 20s–30s, later in men
		• Cardinal feature: fatigability
		• Weakness increases with activity and improves with rest
		• Muscles affected:
		  - Cranial muscles (ptosis, diplopia, dysphagia, dysarthria)
		  - Proximal limbs
		  - Neck muscles
		  - Respiratory muscles
		• Medications may exacerbate weakness:
		  - Aminoglycosides
		  - Beta-blockers
		  - Ca blockers
		  - Tubocurarine
			• CT of the chest may demonstrate thymoma
			• Ach receptor Ab serologies positive in 50% of ocular and 90% of generalized MG
			• EMG: muscle response decreases with repetitive stimulation
			• Edrophonium test (short-acting anti-cholinesterase improves weakness)
				• Mild disease:
				  - Acetyl-cholinesterase inhibitors (pyridostigmine)
				• Moderate disease:
				  - Immunosuppression with steroids, azathioprine, and cyclosporine
				• Severe disease/respiratory failure):
				  - IV gamma globulin or plasmapheresis
				  - Thymectomy and immunosuppression

Botulism	• Toxin prevents release of ACh from presynaptic neuron	• Acute intoxication causes:
		  - Descending paralysis
		  - Diplopia
		  - Dysarthria
		  - Dysphagia
		  - Respiratory difficulty
		  - Limb weakness
			• See infectious diseases chapter	

Lambert-Eaton Myasthenic Syndrome	• Ab against voltage-gated Ca channels decreasing release of ACh	• Up to half of cases are paraneoplastic (most common with lung cancer SCLC) • Proximal weakness of the legs with ptosis and diplopia	• Serum:VGCC Ab • EMG: - Muscle response decreases with repetitive stimulation	• Treatment of underlying cancer

Ab = antibody; Ach = acetylcholine; Ca = calcium; VGCC = voltage-gated calcium channel; SCLC = small cell lung cancer.

Table 19-21

Frequent Causes of Back Pain

CAUSE	CLINICAL	DIAGNOSIS	TREATMENT
Lumbosacral Sprain	• Pain confined to the lower back with no radiation • No neurologic deficits • Paraspinal muscle spasms may cause patients to assume unusual postures • Usually posttraumatic	• No diagnostic tests needed	• Encourage light exercise and return to normal activity • Consider physical therapy referral • NSAIDs or acetaminophen • Careful use of opioids and muscle relaxants
Vertebral Fracture	• Caused by trauma, osteoporosis, or vertebral tumor • Persistent local pain with overlying paraspinal muscle spasm • Neurologic deficit from radiculopathy may be present	• Plain radiographs • Bone scan or MRI if pathologic fracture from tumor suspected	• Ensure adequate pain control • Orthopedic consult • Consider kyphoplasty
Lumbar Disk Disease	• Presents with limitation of spine flexion and radiculopathic features • Most common at L4-L5 and L5-S1 • Exacerbated by Valsalva maneuver	• If no red flags, may manage conservatively for 1 month • MRI is the best diagnostic test • Many patients with herniated disks on MRI do not have back pain	• See lumbosacral sprain • Surgery indicated for progressive motor weakness, abnormal bowel or bladder function, and incapacitating radicular pain with MRI correlation
Spinal Stenosis	• Caused by a narrowed spinal canal • Back and bilateral leg pain provoked by standing or walking (pseudoclaudication) • Usually relieved by sitting	• MRI is the most sensitive diagnostic test	• Conservative treatment includes NSAIDs, and physical therapy • Surgical management indicated if pain is incapacitating or if severe focal deficits

(continued)

Table 19-21

Frequent Causes of Back Pain (continued)

CAUSE	CLINICAL	DIAGNOSIS	TREATMENT
Spondylosis	• Pain usually caused by osteophytes compressing nerve roots • Pain centered in the spine increased by motion and is associated with limitation of motion	• Plain films will show osteophytes and can suggest whether there is narrowing of the intervertebral foramen • MRI and CT useful	• Conservative treatment includes NSAIDs, other pain relievers, and physical therapy • Surgical management may be indicated for severe pain or if focal deficits
Neoplasm	• Pain is usually constant, dull, unrelieved by rest and worse at night	• MRI is the most sensitive study for evaluating epidural disease and vertebral metastases • Bone scan and CT scan also play a role	• Intractable pain from vertebral metastasis may respond to radiation, depending on tumor type • Neurologic deficits from epidural disease demand radiation or surgery
Infection	• Fever and back pain aggravated by palpation or movement • Vertebral osteomyelitis may not present with fever	• MRI	• Antibiotics and surgical management are usually combined

NSAIDs = nonsteroidal anti-inflammatory drugs.

Table 19-22

Neuro-Oncology

TUMOR	KEY POINTS	TREATMENT

Meningioma	• Arises from arachnoid cells
	• Second most common primary brain tumor
	• Often benign and discovered incidentally
	• More common in patients >50 and in women
	• Contains progesterone receptors and may grow during pregnancy
	• Imaging: partially calcified extra-axial mass adherent to the dura
		• Symptomatic:
		  - Surgery
		• Asymptomatic:
		  - Follow with regular
		• CT scan
		  - Prognosis is excellent

Table 19-22

Neuro-Oncology (continued)

TUMOR	KEY POINTS	TREATMENT

Glioblastoma Multiforme	• Subtype of glial tumor (arise from neuroepethelial cells)
	• Most common primary brain tumor, usually high grade
	• Clinical:
	  - Morning headaches, worsened with Valsalva maneuver
	  - Seizures
		• Temozolomide along with XRT may improve survival
		• Median survival: 1–2 years

Primary CNS Lymphoma	• Occurs in immunosuppressed patients (HIV, leukemia, status post transplant) • Related to EBV proliferation • Imaging: solitary or multiple brain masses	• Reverse immunosup-pression if possible • Corticosteroids after biopsy • Methotrexate and XRT prolong survival to >3 years

Metastatic Cancer	• Lung, melanoma, and breast are the most common primary tumors
	• Symptoms
	  - usually are not the first manifestation of the cancer
	  - Parenchymal metastasis: headaches, focal deficits
	  - Leptomeningeal metastasis: weakness, spinal pain, radiculopathy
	• Imaging: MRI better than CT for meningeal involvement
		• Corticosteroids reduce mass effect and vaso-genic edema
		• XRT

EBV = Epstein-Barr virus; XRT = radiotherapy.

Table 19-23

Paraneoplastic Disease of the Nervous System

CONDITION	KEY POINTS	TREATMENT
Cerebellar Degeneration	• Most common autoimmune paraneoplastic disorder • More frequent in women • Initially CT/MRI show normal cerebellum and later develop severe cerebellar atrophy	• Supportive
Encephalomyelitis	• Associated with lung cancer (SCLC) • May present as rapidly progressive dementia and seizures	• Supportive
Sensory Neuropathy	• Associated with lung cancer (SCLC) • Presents as sensory ataxia, sensory loss, and progressive paresthesias	• Supportive
Opsoclonus Myoclonus	• Associated with lung and breast cancer • Progressive cerebellar ataxia, opsoclonus (irregular, conjugate, involuntary eye movements), clonus (involuntary muscle gaze)	• Treatment of underlying cancer

Table 19-24
Summary of Seizures

| FEATURE | GENERALIZED SEIZURE | PARTIAL SEIZURE | |
		SIMPLE	COMPLEX
Cortical Discharge	• Entire cortex	• Regional	• Regional
Alert	• No	• Yes	• No
Initial workup	• Blood work to determine etiology	• Neuroimaging to determine etiology	• Neuroimaging to determine etiology
Examples	• Generalized tonic-clonic • Absence • Tonic • Myoclonic	• Motor (Jacksonian march: focal epilepsy in which the attack usually moves from distal to proximal limb muscles on the same side of the body) • Sensory psychic *(deja vu)* • Autonomic (rising epigastric sensation)	• Temporal lobe seizures • Frontal lobe seizures
Common Causes	• Systemic abnormalities • Fever, genetic epilepsy syndromes, sleep deprivation	• Stroke, neoplasm, head trauma, infection, mesial temporal sclerosis	

Table 19-25
Summary of Brain Death, Vegetative State, and Coma

FEATURE	COMA	LOCKED-IN STATE	VEGETATIVE STATE	BRAIN DEATH
Consciousness	• None	• Full	• None	• None
Sleep/Awake	• Absent	• Present	• Present	• Absent
Motor Function	• Reflex and postural responses only	• Quadriplegic	• Postures or withdrawals from noxious stimuli	• Movements originating from the spinal cord or peripheral nerve may occur • Positive apnea test
Auditory Function	• None	• Preserved	• Startle	• None • Absent oculovestibular reflex
Visual Function	• None	• Preserved	• Startle	• No vision • Absent corneal, pupillary, and oculocephalic reflexes

Table 19-25

Summary of Brain Death, Vegetative State, and Coma (continued)

FEATURE	COMA	LOCKED-IN STATE	VEGETATIVE STATE	BRAIN DEATH
Communication	• None	• Aphonic/anarthic • Vertical eye movement and blinking usually intact	• None	• None • Absent gag and cough reflex
Emotion	• None	• Preserved	• None	• None
Anatomic Lesion	• Bilateral cerebral or upper brain stem	• Pontine base	• Diffuse cerebral hemisphere	• Catastrophic brain injury with permanent absence of cerebral and brainstem functions
Key Points	• Rarely lasts more than 2–4 weeks • Prognosis depends on the cause, severity, and site of neurologic damage	• The majority of cases are irreversible conditions leading to death shortly after onset • Some may regain some function over time • Minority have good functional recovery	• Life expectancy is approximately 2–5 years • Most patients die from infection	• Must rule out confounding factors such as drug intoxication/poisoning, metabolic derangements, and hypothermia • Rarely lasts for more than a few days before somatic death

Psychiatry

Categories of Psychiatric Disorders

- Mood—pathologic affective states
- Psychotic—primarily disorders of cognition and thinking
- Anxiety—including anxiety states and phobias
- Somatoform—involving physical complaints that are without objective medical basis
- Psychoactive substance use—abuse and dependence on psychoactive substances

Psychiatric Medication Management Factors

- Specific diagnosis
- Favorable versus unfavorable side effect profile
- Medical comorbidity
- Drug-drug interactions

Table 20-1

Mood Disorders

	DEFINITION/DSM CRITERIA	EPIDEMIOLOGY	PROGNOSIS/COURSE	TREATMENT/NOTE
Major Depressive Disorder (MDD)	• Depressed mood OR loss of interest/pleasure AND at least five of the following for 2 weeks: - (**S**) Sleep: In/hypersomnia - (**I**) Decreased interest/ pleasure in activities, anhedonia - (**G**) Feelings of worthlessness or excessive or inappropriate guilt - (**E**) Fatigue or loss of energy - (**C**) Diminished ability to think or concentrate, or indecisiveness - (**A**) Change in appetite, weight loss when not dieting, or weight gain - (**P**) Psychomotor agitation or retardation - (**S**) Recurrent thoughts of death, suicidal ideation with or without a plan, or suicide attempt	• Variable age of onset • Occurs in 5–10% of primary care patients • Occurs in 10–20% of patients with chronic illness • F > > M	• Relapsing and remitting • 50% risk of recurrence within 2 years of first episode and 80% recurrence risk after 2 episodes • 50–60% respond to any antidepressant drug • Untreated episodes usually remit in 4–6 months	• Usually treated with SSRIs, SNRIs, and TCAs (see Table 20-2) • ECT used for medica- tion-resistant patients • Combined medica- tion and talk therapy may be better than monotherapy with either alone • All patients with depressive symptoms should be screened for bipolar disorder • Screen for suicidality

(continued)

Table 20-1
Mood Disorders (continued)

	Definition/DSM Criteria	**Epidemiology**	**Prognosis/Course**	**Treatment/Note**

Dysthymic Disorder	• Chronically mild-moderate depressed mood present for >2 years, associated with two of the following:
	  - Poor appetite or overeating
	  - Insomnia or hypersomnia
	  - Low energy or fatigue
	  - Low self-esteem
	  - Poor concentration or difficulty making decisions
	  - Feelings of hopelessness
		• Lifetime prevalence 6%	• Called "double depression" when comorbid with MDD
			• Slow and insidious course
				• Medication treatment same as MDD
				• Response rate < 50%
				• Often requires combined treatment with medication and therapy

Bipolar Disorder, Type 1	• Extreme swings in mood, with mania plummeting into depression
	• Manic episode includes irritable or euphoric mood for ≥1 week with >3 of the following:
	  - **(D)**istractibility
	  - **(I)**mpulsivity
	  - **(G)**randiosity
	  - **(F)**light of ideas
	  - **(A)**Activities. Increased goal-directed activities
	  - **(S)**leep, Decreased need for sleep
	  - **(T)**alkative. Pressured speech, difficult to interrupt
		• Occurs in 1–2% of general population
		• Onset usually in 20–30s
		• M = F
		• Strong genetic component
			• 90% of patients with a manic episode will have another within 5 years
			• Frequency of episodes often increases with age
			• Depressive episodes have same criteria as MDD
				• Mood stabilizers (see Table 20-3)
				• Lifetime prevalence of comorbid substance addiction (60%) and anxiety disorders (50%)
				• Associated with lifetime rate of completed suicide of 15%
				• Bipolar depression rarely treated with antidepressant as monotherapy

Bipolar Disorder, Type 2	• Hypomanic criteria same as mania but symptoms present <4 days without social or occupational dysfunction			

Bereavement/ Grief Reaction		

• Any psychological, physiologic, or behavioral response to significant loss
• As part of their reaction to the loss, some grieving individuals present with symptoms characteristic of a MDE
• The presence of certain symptoms, however, are NOT characteristic of normal grief. Consider MDE instead of bereavement if:
  - Guilt about things unrelated to actions at the time of death
  - Suicidal, with plan, intent, or gesture
  - Prolonged and marked functional impairment
  - Hallucinations
	• Duration varies considerably among different cultural groups	• Support from family and friends is integral
		• Support groups
		• Psychopharmacologic treatment is NOT the primary treatment of grief, but may promote sleep or relieve anxiety
		• Benzodiazepines may be indicated for severe anxiety or insomnia

DSM = The Diagnostic and Statistical Manual of Mental Disorders; F = female; M = male; SSRIs: selective serotonin reuptake inhibitors; SNRIs: serotonin-norepinephrine reuptake inhibitors; TCAs: tricyclic antidepressants; ECT = electroconvulsive therapy; MDE = major depressive episode.

Table 20-2

Antidepressants

DRUG CLASS	METHOD OF ACTION	SELECT SIDE EFFECTS	MONITORING/PEARLS
TCAs: • **Imipramine** • **Desipramine** • **Amitriptyline** • **Nortriptyline**	• Blocks reuptake of serotonin (5-HT) and NE at the synapse	• Antihistaminic effect: sedation and weight gain • Anticholinergic effect: dry mouth, constipation, urinary hesitancy, confusion • Alpha-blockade: orthostatic hypotension • Sexual dysfunction • May lower seizure threshold • QT prolongation, arrhythmia, conduction defects	• Fatal in overdose; usually from dysrhythmias • Caution in patients who are suicidal • Can take 3–6 weeks to reach full effect
SSRIs: • **Fluoxetine** • **Sertraline** • **Paroxetine** • **Fluvoxamine** • **Citalopram** • **Escitalopram**	• Selectively blocks reuptake of 5-HT at the synapse	• Nausea • Reduced appetite • Excessive sweating • Sexual dysfunction • Disruption of sleep architecture	• Relatively safe in overdose • Can take 3–6 weeks to reach full effect • DO NOT combine with MAOI as can lead to serotonin syndrome • Fluoxetine and paroxetine have many drug-drug interactions • Sertraline and citalopram have very few drug-drug interactions • Paroxetine may have more efficacy in anxiety disorders, and is more sedating than the other SSRIs

	Mechanism	Side Effects	Notes
MAOIs: • **Tranylcypromine** • **Phenelzine** • **Selegiline**	• Blocks monoamine oxidase, the enzyme responsible for deamination of neurotransmitters such as 5-HT, DA, NE, leading to increased activity of these neurotransmitters	• Postural hypotensive effects—up to 50% of patients experience dizziness • Anticholinergic effects: dry mouth, urinary hesitancy, gastrointestinal upset • Fatigue • Headache • Peripheral neuropathy • Myoclonic jerks	• Patients MUST avoid tyramine-containing foods (i.e., cheese, wine) as combination can cause a hypertensive crisis • Do NOT combine with opiates; can lead to malignant hyperthermia • Do NOT combine with SSRIs; can lead to serotonin syndrome • Multiple drug-drug interactions with prescribed and OTC meds (i.e., nasal decongestants) • Can be useful for atypical depression or treatment-resistant depression
Bupropion	• Blocks NE and DA uptake	• Lowers seizure threshold • Headache • Insomnia • Appetite suppression • Rare sexual dysfunction	• Mild stimulant • May also be more suitable for overweight patients with depression • Also used for smoking cessation
Venlafaxine	• Blocks 5-HT and NE reuptake	• Can increase diastolic BP • Nausea • Dizziness • Insomnia • Sedation: more prominent at lower doses • Constipation • Sweating	• Combines features of SSRIs and SNRIs, but better side effect profile • Must monitor blood pressure
Mirtazapine	• Releases 5-HT and NE by blocking DA D2 receptors; blocks 5-HT$_2$ and 5-HT$_3$ receptors	• Potent histamine blockade: sedation, weight gain • Dry mouth • Postural hypotension	• Useful in depressed patients with insomnia • May be used as an appetite stimulant
Duloxetine	• Blocks 5-HT and NE reuptake	• Nausea • Mild increase in heart rate • Sweating	• Useful for depressive and physical symptoms • May be used as an appetite stimulant

5-HT = serotonin; MAOIs = monoamine oxidase inhibitors; DA = dopamine; NE = norepinephrine; OTC: over the counter.

Table 20-3

Mood Stabilizers

Drug	Method of Action	Select Side Effects	Monitoring/Pearls
Lithium	• Exact mechanism of action as a mood stabilizer has yet to be elucidated • Works on multiple neurotransmitter and second messenger systems	• Cognitive slowing • Weight gain • Polydipsia • Polyuria • Tremor • Hypothyroidism • ↓ Renal function • Nephrogenic diabetes insipidus	• Treats mania (acute and as prophylaxis) • Contraindicated in patients with renal failure • Obtain BUN/Cr, pregnancy test, and TSH prior to initiation • If platelet count >50,000 or with heart disease check ECG • Frequently check serum lithium level, renal function, TSH • Many medications effect lithium levels: diuretics, NSAIDs, ACEI, calcium channel blockers
Valproic Acid	• Inhibits histone deacetylase, resulting in inactivation of glycogen synthase kinase-3	• Weight gain • Nausea, vomiting • Hair loss • Easy bruising, ↓ platelets • Hepatic failure	• Treats acute mania • Contraindicated in patients with hepatic impairment • Must monitor transaminases, platelets, and drug levels • Teratogen—neural tube defects
Carbamazepine	• Unclear mechanism of action	• Agranulocytosis • Aplastic anemia • Leukopenia (relative) • Neurotoxicity: drowsiness, dizziness, blurred vision, lethargy, headache	• Treats acute mania • Frequent drug-drug interactions by induction of liver enzymes • Must monitor serum carbamazepine level, liver function tests, complete blood count, serum sodium
Lamotrigine	• Decreases glutamate release • Modulates serotonin/monoamine reuptake	• Rash • Stevens-Johnson syndrome • Neurotoxicity: drowsiness, dizziness, double vision, headache	• Maintenance treatment of bipolar disorder • Commonly used in treatment of bipolar depression

ACEI = angiotensin converting enzyme inhibitors; BUN/Cr: blood urea nitrogen/creatinine; ECG = electrocardiogram; NSAIDs = nonsteroidal anti-inflammatory drugs; TSH = thyroid-stimulating hormone.

Table 20-4
Psychotic Disorders

	DEFINITION/DSM CRITERIA	EPIDEMIOLOGY	PROGNOSIS/COURSE	TREATMENT/PEARLS

Schizophrenia	• >2 of the following present for a 1 month period:
	- Positive symptoms:
	  ○ Delusions
	  ○ Hallucinations
	  ○ Disorganized speech
	  ○ Grossly disorganized or catatonic behavior
	- Negative symptoms:
	  ○ Flat affect
	  ○ Alogia
	  ○ Avolition
	• Significant social/occupational dysfunction
	• Duration of at least 6 months
		• Lifetime prevalence 0.5–1.5%
		• Presents earlier in males; age 18–25 vs. 25–35 in females
		• Late-onset cases occur rarely
			• Phasic disorder (i.e., prodrome, acute/active phase, recovery phase, residual phase)
			• Variable course. Better outcomes for patients with higher function premorbidly
			• Negative > positive symptoms, which cause greatest dysfunction
			• Paranoid subtype—best prognosis
				• Most traditional psychotherapies ineffective
				• Family interventions and social skills training may be useful
				• Treated with antipsychotics (see below)

Schizoaffective Disorder	• Must meet criteria for mood disorder (i.e., MDE or bipolar) • During the same period, there must be delusions or hallucinations for at least 2 weeks in the absence of prominent mood symptoms • Note: If mood symptoms consistently concurrent with psychotic symptoms then consider mood disorder with psychotic features	• Not adequately studied	• Outcomes dependent on whether predominant symptoms are affective (better prognosis) or schizophrenic (worse prognosis)	• Treatment based on symptoms; treat mood symptoms with mood stabilizers and antidepressants; treat psychosis with antipsychotic agents
Mood Disorder (Bipolar or Major Depressive) With Psychotic Features	• Patient meets criteria for manic episode or MDE (see Table 20-3) • Delusions or hallucinations present concurrent with mood episode			• Antipsychotic plus antidepressant/mood stabilizer • ECT

Table 20-5

Antipsychotic Medications

Drug	Method of Action	Side Effect	Monitoring/Pearls
Typical • **Haloperidol** • **Fluphenazine** • **Chlorpromazine** • **Trifluoperazine**	• High potency/specificity for D2 receptor blockade • Reduces positive symptoms of psychosis	• High risk for EPS • Fewer autonomic effects • Galactorrhea • Parkinsonism • Anticholinergic effects • Orthostatic hypotension • Neuroleptic malignant syndrome	• May be given IM/IV/PO • Depot preparations available • Low cost • Equal efficacy to atypical antipsychotics but greater side effects
Atypical • **Clozapine** • **Risperidone** • **Olanzapine** • **Quetiapine** • **Ziprasidone** • **Aripiprazole**	• D2/5-HT$_2$ antagonist • Reduces positive and negative symptoms of psychosis and • Stabilizes affective symptoms	• Low risk for EPS • Weight gain • Insulin resistance • ↑ Triglycerides • Agranulocytosis (clozapine) • Orthostatic hypotension • Galactorrhea (risperidone)	• Very expensive • Equal efficacy to typical antipsychotics but less EPS • Used in treatment of schizophrenia, bipolar, depression, eating disorders, and anxiety • Treats negative symptoms of schizophrenia better than typical agents

EPS = extrapyramidal side effects; IM: intramuscular; IV: intravenous; ECT = electroconvulsive therapy.

Table 20-6

Anxiety Disorders

	DEFINITION/DSM CRITERIA	EPIDEMIOLOGY	PROGNOSIS/COURSE	TREATMENT/PEARLS
Panic Attacks, Panic Disorder	• Panic attacks: unexpected intense episodes of terror and fear with somatic symptoms • Panic disorder: the broader behavior and thought pattern of panic attacks plus prolonged apprehension about repeated attacks/ avoidance of certain circumstances or behaviors in an attempt to control recurrence	• Incidence of panic attacks is 7% • Incidence of panic disorder 1% • F:M is 2:1 • Age of onset is mid-20s	• Up to 50% have coexistent major depression • A 60–90% lifetime prevalence of depression • 40% have agora-phobia • 10–50% have social phobia • High suicide rate, especially if with depression • Excellent response to CBT • 50–80% response to SSRIs • 50–70% relapse rate after stopping medications	• Relaxation techniques • Phobic avoidance or apprehension needs CBT • Therapy plus medication is more effective than either alone • Treated with SSRIs, SNRIs, and benzodiazepines • 90% complain to primary care clinics about somatic symptoms (i.e., migraine, atypical chest pain, and headaches)

(continued)

Table 20-6
Anxiety Disorders (continued)

	DEFINITION/DSM CRITERIA	EPIDEMIOLOGY	PROGNOSIS/COURSE	TREATMENT/PEARLS
Generalised Anxiety Disorder (GAD)	• Uncontrolled worry or concern of 6 months' duration that is disproportionate to the likelihood of the feared event • Associated with at least three of the following symptoms: - Feeling on edge - Easily fatigued - Difficulty concentrating - Irritability - Muscle tension - Sleep disturbance	• 5% lifetime prevalence • F:M 2:1	• 40% are concurrently depressed • 20% have social or other phobia • 20% have panic disorder	• Behavior modification, psychotherapy, and medication • Limit caffeine use • Relaxation techniques • SSRIs and NE reuptake inhibitors are first-line pharmacotherapy • Long-acting benzodiazepines • Patients may have somatic symptoms
Obsessive Compulsive Disorder (OCD)	• Chronic anxiety disorder characterized by recurrent, intrusive thoughts (obsessions) and habitual or routine actions (compulsions) which are time consuming and cause distress • Patient recognizes these obsessions and compulsions as excessive or unreasonable	• Affects up to 3% of the general population • Average at of onset is 14.5 years • M = F	• Waxing and waning course • 40–60% response rate to medications	• Relatively resistant to psychodynamic and behavior modification approaches • SSRIs, frequently at higher doses than those used to treat depression • If one SSRI doesn't work, others may still work
Post-traumatic Stress Disorder (PTSD)	• Reaction to a perceived life-threatening event, which must include all of the following for at least 1 month: - Re-experiencing - Avoidance - Increased arousal	• Affects up to 1% of the general population • Must have a perceived life-threatening trauma • M:F is 1:2	• Present in 30% of Vietnam veterans • Acute stress disorder has similar symptoms and often lasts less than 1 month	• Research shows that debriefing may increase likelihood of developing PTSD • Responds well to benzodiazepines, but often needs psychotherapy (individual and group)

CBT: cognitive behavioral therapy.

Table 20-7

Substance Abuse Disorders

	DEFINITION/DSM CRITERIA
Substance Dependence	• A psychological or physiologic need for continuing a substance that includes symptoms of withdrawal without continued use
Substance Abuse	• Pathologic use of a substance or impairment in social and occupational performance secondary to substance use
Substance Intoxication	• The development of a reversible substance-specific syndrome due to recent ingestion • Often accompanied by maladaptive behavior or psychological changes that are due to the effect of the substance on the central nervous system and developed during or shortly after use of the substance
Treatment/Notes	
• 13% lifetime prevalence rates for alcohol dependence and abuse • M:F ratio is 5:1 for alcohol dependence and abuse • 6% lifetime prevalence rates for drug dependence and abuse • Drug abuse/dependence is only slightly more common in men than in women • 30–55% of the mentally ill have a substance use disorder • Cannabis is the most widely abused illicit substance in the United States, and accounts for 75% of all illicit drug use • Tobacco is the leading cause of preventable morbidity and mortality in the United States; 30.2% of Americans (66.8 million) currently use cigarettes • Benzodiazepine abuse is often iatrogenically induced • Treatment includes therapeutic communities (sober houses/residences), self-help organization (AA, NA, etc.), and individual psychotherapy (supportive or CBT). Family support/education is important to patient's overall treatment outcome	

AA = Alcoholics Anonymous; NA = Narcotics Anonymous.

Table 20-8

Substance Abuse Treatment Modalities

DRUG	METHOD OF ACTION	SELECT SIDE EFFECTS	MONITORING/PEARLS
Naltrexone	• Opiate receptor antagonist	• GI upset • Joint pain • Muscle soreness • Nervousness	• Relapse prevention in opiate and EtOH dependence • Helpful in reducing binge drinking
Acamprosate	• Unclear mechanism • Acts at the NMDA receptor to reduce glutamatergic hyperactivity	• Diarrhea • Headache	• Reduces EtOH intake • Reduces relapse drinking • Reduces EtOH cravings
Disulfiram	• Potent reversible inhibitor of aldehyde dehydrogenase	• Fatigue • Metallic taste • Fatal toxic hepatitis • Impotence	• Liver function tests should be performed prior to and during treatment • Can substantially raise level of oral anticoagulants
Buprenorphine	• Mixed opioid agonist–antagonist	• Will cause withdrawal if taken in conjunction with opiates • Less risk of respiratory depression in overdose • Mild elevations in LFTs	• Used to treat opiate withdrawal and maintenance • Taken sublingually
Methadone	• Long-acting opioid agonist	• Constipation • Increases sweating • Sexual dysfunction	• Use for opiate withdrawal and maintenance • Blocks effects of illicit opiates
Ondansetron	• Selective 5-HT$_3$ receptor antagonist	• Headache • Constipation	• Reduces overall alcohol intake

EtOH = ethanol; GI = gastrointestinal; LFTs = liver function tests; NMDA = *N*-methyl-D-aspartic acid.

Table 20-9

Alcohol Withdrawal

CLINICAL/TIME COURSE	TREATMENT/PEARLS
• Minor withdrawal symptoms occur within 6–12 hours of alcohol cessation and resolve within 48 hours: - Insomnia - Tachycardia - Tremor - Headache - Gastrointestinal upset • Risk factors for more severe withdrawal include chronic use, previous difficult withdrawal, age > 30, presence of a concurrent illness • Major withdrawal symptoms include: - Seizures: seen in 3% of chronic alcoholics. Tend to be generalized tonic-clonic and occur within 6–48 hours of withdrawal - Hallucinations: tend to be visual, occur within first 24 hours of alcohol cessation, and resolve within 48 hours - DT <5%. Symptoms are disorientation, hallucinations, tremor, agitation, elevated heart rate and blood pressure, and low-grade fever. Begins several days after last alcohol use and persists for up to 5 days	• Detoxification - Inpatient if moderate to severe withdrawal, history of DT, or unsuccessful attempts at outpatient detoxification • Give thiamine before glucose to prevent Wernicke's encephalopathy • Hydration • Check electrolytes (common changes are ↓Na, ↓K, ↓Mg) • Benzodiazepines improve symptoms and decrease the incidence of seizure and DT - Longer acting benzodiazepines are typically used (diazepam, chlordiazepoxide) - Lorazepam is used in patients with liver disease (limited hepatic clearance) - Symptom triggered dosing is associated with less total medication and shorter duration of therapy (e.g., CIWA scale based)

DT = delirium tremens; CIWA = Clinical Institute Withdrawal Assessment.

Table 20-10

Toxicology

SUBSTANCE	LENGTH OF TIME DETECTED IN URINE
Alcohol	7–12 hours
Amphetamines	48 hours
Barbiturates	24 hours–3 weeks
Benzodiazepines	3 days
THC	3 days to 4 weeks (depending on degree of use)
Cocaine	6 hours–4 days (depending on test used)
Heroin	36–72 hours
Methadone	3 days
PCP	8 days

PCP = phencyclidine; THC = tetrahydrocannabinol.

Table 20-11
Sleep Disorders

	CLINICAL/DIAGNOSIS	EPIDEMIOLOGY	ETIOLOGY	TREATMENT/PEARLS
Insomnia	• Difficulty initiating or maintaining sleep, or nonrestorative sleep for >1 month	• At least 30% of adults have insomnia at some point in any given year • 10–15% of adults report frequent or chronic insomnia	• Situational stress • Anxiety and mood disorders • Poor sleep hygiene • Pain • Sleep apnea • Restless leg syndrome • Substance use/abuse (including caffeine, alcohol, nicotine) • Medications • Substance withdrawal • Aging • PTSD	• Improve sleep hygiene - Set the same wake-up time daily - Keep bedroom quiet and dark - Use bedroom for sleep and sex only - Avoid nicotine, caffeine, alcohol within 6 hours of bedtime - Exercise daily, but not within 3 hours of bedtime - If unable to sleep, leave bedroom and do a quiet activity, return when sleepy - Get exposure to sunlight or bright light daily - Avoid naps • Benzodiazepines, newer seda-tive-hypnotics such as zolpidem, zaleplon can be used in acute/ short-term use • Antihistamines and tricyclic antidepressants may be useful long term in low doses • CBT more effective than medications or relaxation therapy

Table 20-12

Attention Deficit Hyperactivity Disorder (ADHD)

EPIDEMIOLOGY	CLINICAL/DIAGNOSIS	COURSE/PROGNOSIS	TREATMENT/NOTES

• 30–70% of children with ADHD continue to manifest symptoms in adulthood
• 5% of adults have symptoms of the disorder
• Increased risk for developing alcohol and drug dependence
• M:F is 5:1
	• Criteria not well defined for adults
	• Symptoms usually much more subtle than in childhood
	• A history of distractibility, restlessness, and impulsiveness severe enough to disrupt at least two areas of daily life
	• Symptoms persistently present since age 7
	• Utah criteria for ADHD in adults:
	  - Hyperactivity and poor concentration
	  - Two of the following:
	    ◦ Affective labiality
	    ◦ Hot temper
	    ◦ Inability to complete tasks and disorganization
	    ◦ Stress intolerance
	    ◦ Impulsivity
		• Chronic/lifelong condition, continuing from childhood
		• Pharmacotherapy throughout adulthood usually indicated
		• Comorbid psychiatric diagnoses are common, including generalized anxiety disorder, substance abuse, MDD
			• Stimulants: caution in hypertension or history of substance abuse
			  - Methylphenidate
			  - Dextroamphetamine
			• Antidepressants may be effective
			  - TCAs
			  - Bupropion
			  - Atomoxetine

Table 20-13

Somatoform Disorders

DISORDER	DEFINITION/DSM CRITERIA
	• Disorders involved in physical complaints that are without objective medical science. Five major categories (see below). Prevalence is 0.1%. Predominantly found in women
Somatization Disorder	• Recurrent multiple physical complaints that are not fully explained by cofactors and result in medical attention or significant impairment
Conversion Disorder	• Unintentional symptoms over a defect affecting voluntary motor or sensory function not fully explained by a neurologic or general medical condition. Not a culturally sanctioned behavior or experience
Pain Disorder	• Intractable, often multiple pain complaints, which are usually inappropriate to existing somatic problems • Multiple physician contacts and many nonproductive diagnostic procedures; excessive preoccupation with the pain problem • Only somatoform d/o which may respond to antidepressant therapy
Hypochondriasis	• Preoccupation not with symptoms themselves but rather the fear of having a serious disease • Frequently based on the misinterpretation of bodily signs and sensations • Not improved with evidence to the contrary or reassurance from physicians
Body Dysmorphic Disorder	• Preoccupation with imagined defect in appearance or marked concern with a minor physical abnormality • Preoccupation persists even after reassurance

Adolescent Medicine

Table 21-1

Adolescent Medicine

GOAL/TOPIC	NOTES
Provide Support During the Period of Biological, Psychosocial, and Sexual Maturation that Bridges the Period from Childhood to Adulthood	• A gradual separation from parental influence and an increased importance placed on peer groups is characteristic of this age group • Increased reliability on peer groups and desire for independence can result in many positive, healthy lifelong habits, or may provide an environment for accidents, drug use, and suicide • The leading causes of death among teens are accidents, homicide, and suicide
The Adolescent Interview	• Health care encounters between physicians and adolescents are an opportunity to advise, promote, and encourage positive health habits and lifestyles • Adolescents should be interviewed both with their parents and alone during each maintenance health visit • Issues to address in each health care encounter: home, education, diet, depression, drugs, sex, suicide, and violence (HEADDDSSV)
Adolescent Treatment	• Although specific laws vary from state to state, adolescents generally may seek treatment for sexual, mental health, and drug-related matters without permission from a parent - Examples: contraception, pregnancy testing, sexually transmitted disease testing and treatment, substance abuse
Adolescent Confidentiality	• All information the adolescent discloses privately to the health care provider is confidential • Confidentiality may be broken if the teen discloses he/she is at significant risk of harm such as harming themselves (suicidal ideation), harming someone else or is being abused • Whenever confidentiality is to be broken, the teen should be informed about the practitioner's plan
Conditions that Legally Emancipate a Minor, Allowing Him or Her to Consent for and/or Refuse Medical Treatment	• Marriage • Parenthood • Military service • Evidence of self-support

Table 21-2
Eating Disorders

Eating Disorder Epidemiology	• Affects mostly females, of all ethnicities • Approximately 1% of the female adolescent population • 10% of all cases affect males • Adolescents who participate in activities that stress low body weight (i.e., gymnastics, cheerleading, and wrestling) are especially at risk
Etiology	• The etiology of eating disorders is unknown, but is thought to be multifactorial • There is a suspected genetic component • Risk factors include depression, stress, and body changes associated with puberty • Psychiatric comorbidities are common (depression, obsessive-compulsive disorder)
Treatment	• Nutritional rehabilitation is the most important goal in providing care and support for patients with eating disorders • Family and patient counseling is important to help educate and prevent progression of the disease • Antidepressant therapy may help patients with bulimia nervosa and those with associated psychiatric illness • Hospitalization may be warranted for patients with syncope, electrolyte abnormalities, bradycardia, hypotension, hypothermia, uncontrolled binge eating and purging, or who have failed outpatient therapy

Table 21-3
Anorexia Nervosa and Bulimia

	DEFINITION	CLINICAL PRESENTATION	DIAGNOSIS
Anorexia Nervosa	• Insufficient caloric intake (as demonstrated by either failure to gain weight in a normal fashion and/or weight loss) combined with an intense fear of being fat and a desire to be thinner	• Anorexia affects up to 1% of the female adolescent population • Affected patients have a distorted body image, imagining themselves to be overweight, even when they are quite thin • Amenorrhea frequently occurs before significant weight loss • The medical consequences include electrolyte disturbances, cardiac dysrhythmias, prolonged Q-T interval, osteoporosis, anemia, hypercholesterolemia, and a low white blood cell count • Common comorbid conditions include obsessive-compulsive disorder and depression • Anorexics may develop bulimia nervosa in the long term	• Diagnostic criteria: 1. Refusal to maintain or gain weight that is more than 85% of ideal 2. Amenorrhea for three cycles (in postpubertal females) 3. Intense fear of gaining weight, even though underweight 4. Distorted body image

(continued)

Table 21-3

Anorexia Nervosa and Bulimia (continued)

	DEFINITION	CLINICAL PRESENTATION	DIAGNOSIS
Bulimia Nervosa	• The most distinctive feature of bulimia is recurrent binge eating • Binges are followed by an inappropriate compensatory attempt at weight loss	• Patients with bulimia are often of normal weight or slightly overweight • Physical examination may reveal: 　- Salivary gland enlargement (especially parotid and submandibular) 　- Dental enamel erosion (especially the lingual surface) from recurrent vomiting 　- Peripheral edema • Laboratory findings include: 　- Electrolyte disturbances (hypokalemic alkalosis from vomiting, or metabolic acidosis from laxative use) • Comorbid conditions are more frequently associated with bulimia, including depression, drug, and alcohol abuse, delinquency, and personality disorders. Features of anorexia nervosa may also be present at the same time • There are two types: 　- Purging (self-induced vomiting, laxative, or diuretic abuse) 　- Nonpurging (fasting or excessive exercise)	• Diagnostic criteria: 　1. Recurrent episodes of binge eating, with a feeling of loss of control during episodes 　2. Recurrent inappropriate compensatory behavior 　3. Binge eating and compensatory behavior occurring at least twice a week for 3 months 　4. Sense of self disproportionately influenced by weight 　5. Episodes do not occur exclusively at the time as in symptoms of anorexia nervosa

Table 21-4

Adolescent Pregnancy and Emergency Contraception

Adolescent Pregnancy	• There are approximately 1 million adolescent pregnancies in the United States each year • Adolescents often engage in risky sexual behavior because they fail to appreciate the potential consequences of their actions • Contraception should be addressed during each adolescent health visit, even if the patient is not currently sexually active • Abstinence is the most effective method for prevention of both pregnancy and sexually transmitted diseases • Consistent use of two birth control methods protect against both pregnancy and sexually transmitted diseases

Table 21-4

Adolescent Pregnancy and Emergency Contraception (continued)

Emergency Contraception	• Indications include rape, unprotected consensual intercourse, or barrier contraception failure • Oral hormonal methods are the mainstay of treatment and should be started within 72 hours of intercourse • Options include: - Two doses of combined hormonal oral contraception pills with ethinyl estradiol and levonorgestrel administered 12 hours apart - Alternative option commonly known as "the morning after pill" consists of two doses of levonorgestrel administered 12 hours apart, and is available over-the-counter for patients aged 18 and over • Mifepristone (a prostaglandin inhibitor) is not approved in the United States as a means of emergency contraception and can only be used as an abortifacient

Table 21-5

Adolescent Immunizations

DISEASE	VACCINE	NOTES
HPV	• Quadrivalent HPV vaccine prevents genital warts (HPV 6, 11) and cervical cancer (HPV 16, 18)	• The vaccine is most efficacious prior to onset of sexual activity, but can still be administered after the onset of sexual activity • Immunologically similar to the hepatitis B vaccine, it is administered as a series of three intramuscular injections • The recommended age for vaccination is 11–12 years; however, the vaccine is approved for females ages 9–26 years • Use of the vaccination for males is controversial and currently being investigated
Tdap	• The Tdap vaccine has a lower concentration of pertussis components than the DTaP/DTP given in the primary series	• The recommended age of immunization is 11–12 years of age • Adolescents ages 11–18 years who have completed the five shot series of DTP or DTaP prior to age 7 and have not received a booster dose of Td can be given one dose of Tdap • For adolescents who have received both the primary series and a booster dose of Td, a 5-year interval is recommended prior to Tdap immunization

(*continued*)

Table 21-5

Adolescent Immunizations (continued)

DISEASE	VACCINE	NOTES

Meningococcal	• Meningococcal vaccine protects against four sero-types of *Neisseria menin-gitides*; serotype A, C, Y, and W-135
	 • Currently two vaccines are available:
	   1. Polysaccharide vaccine (MPSV4) which is approved for all patients age 2 years and above
	   2. Conjugate vaccine (MCV4) which is approved for ages 11–55 years
		• Current recommendation is to administer one dose of the MCV4 vaccine to all 11–12 year olds or at high school entry (15 years), or to freshmen entering college living in dorms who have not been previously vaccinated
		 • The polysaccharide vaccine is reserved for ages 2–10 years and 56 years+, who have underlying medical conditions that predispose to meningococcal disease (HIV, asplenia, complement deficiencies, diabetes, etc.)

DTP = diphtheria, tetanus, and whole cell pertussis; DTaP = diphtheria, tetanus, and acellular pertussis; HIV = human immunodeficiency virus; HPV = human papilloma virus; Tdap = tetanus, diphtheria, and pertussis

Table 21-6

Summary of Adolescent Substance Abuse and Dependency

General Facts	• Over one-fifth of middle school and one-half of high school students have used illicit substances • Approximately 15% of high school students use tobacco daily • The most frequently abused illicit drug in adolescence is marijuana • Frequent comorbidities include depression, attention deficit-hyperactivity disorder, and personality disorders • Additional risk factors for drug abuse include physical and/or sexual abuse, family history of drug use, and association with family/peers who use drugs • It is unethical to test an adolescent for drugs without his or her consent (except in the emergency setting) • Parental request is not a sufficient reason to perform clandestine screening
Substance Abuse	• Substance abuse definition: user experiences academic, occupational, social, or legal problems due to the use of the drug
Substance Dependency	• Substance dependency results in an inability to control use, increased efforts to obtain the drug, abandonment of social obligations, continued use despite harm or desire to quit, and the development of withdrawal and tolerance (the need for greater amounts of the drug to have the desired effect)

Table 21-7
Frequently Abused Substances

SUBSTANCE	HOW USED/EFFECT	NOTES
Tobacco	• Smoked, chewed (snuff) • Nicotine causes alertness, muscle relaxation, increased memory and attention, and decreased appetite • Most smokers start smoking in adolescence • Cigarette smoking has been linked to early cardiovascular disease, chronic lung disease, ulcers, and cancer	• Potential nicotine replacement modalities include nicotine gum, patches, lozenges, nasal spray, and inhalers • Antidepressant theory (bupropion) and a novel agent (varenicline) that acts as both a nicotine receptor agonist and competitive inhibitor, are also used in nicotine cessation programs • Anticipatory guidance in adolescents is important to prevent initiation of smoking
Marijuana (THC and Cannabinoids)	• Smoked or orally ingested • Causes feelings of euphoria, relaxation, and well-being	• Physiologic addiction is possible
Cocaine/Amphetamines	• Cocaine may be smoked, snorted intranasally, or injected (intravenous "crack-cocaine") • Other amphetamines may be orally ingested, or crushed and taken intranasally • Stimulates release and inhibits reuptake of dopamine and norepinephrine, causing euphoria, and sympathomimetic effects	• "Ecstasy" (MDMA) and crystal meth are derivatives of methamphetamine • Phenylpropanolamine, ephedrine, ma huang, and caffeine all can cause a similar effect if taken in large enough quantities • Nasal septal damage, sinus infections, and nosebleeds can all be consequences of intranasal snorting
Opiates	• Can be taken intranasally (i.e., heroin), intravenously (morphine, heroin), orally (oxycodone, codeine, hydrocodone, dextromethorphan), subcutaneously (morphine), transdermally (fentanyl), or smoked (opium) • Effects include analgesia, sedation, and euphoria	• Dependency can develop quickly (~2 weeks) with use of short-acting opiates • Risk of hepatitis, infectious endocarditis, and HIV from injections

(continued)

Table 21-7

Frequently Abused Substances (continued)

Substance	How Used/Effect	Notes
Sedative Hypnotics	• Can be ingested orally or sublingually • Results in sedation, anxiolysis, and anesthesia • Slurred speech, unsteady gait, and impaired judgment may also occur	• Includes alprazolam (Xanax) and diazepam (Valium) • Highly addictive
Hallucinogens	• Orally ingested • Causes alteration of perception (especially visually), and altered sense of time • Disinhibition, euphoria, and psychosis may also occur	• Agents include hallucinogenic mushrooms, LSD, ketamine (special-K), and PCP • "Ecstasy" (MDMA) also has hallucinogenic properties • "Flashbacks" are possible
Inhalants	• Substance is sniffed from an open container, poured into a bag or on cloth ("huffing") and then inhaled • Causes rapid onset of euphoria, and alteration of mental status	• Frequently used household substances include glue, gasoline, markers, aerosolized products, nitrites, and cleaning fluid • Most frequently used by younger adolescents • Encephalopathy and sudden sniffing death due to cardiac arrhythmias are possible severe effects

THC = delta-9-tetrahydrocannbinol; MDMA = 3,4-methylenedioxymethamphetamine; LSD = lysergic acid diethylamide; PCP = phencyclidine.

Chapter 22

Nutrition

Nutritional Assessment

Table 22-1

Nutritional Assessment Measurements

MEASUREMENT	CALCULATION	REFERENCE RANGE	NOTE
BMI	• Weight (kg)/height (m²)	• Healthy = 18.5–24.9 • Overweight = BMI 25–29.9 • Obese = BMI >30	• More accurate assessment of body fat than weight alone • Not accurate with muscular subjects, short stature, and the elderly • As BMI becomes >25, the greater the risk of health problems

Waist Circumference	• Number of inches around the abdomen at the upper hip bone	• Increased morbidity:
		  - Men: >40 in.
		  - Women: >35 in.
			• Visceral abdominal fat is associated with greatest health risk
			• Independent predictor of morbidity
			• Independently associated with: diabetes, hypertension, heart disease, dyslipidemia

WHR	• Number of inches around the waist (at its narrowest point) divided by the number of inches around widest part of the hip bones	• Increased morbidity:
		  - Men: ≥0.95
		  - Women: ≥0.85
			• Higher WHR associated with increased morbidity and mortality

IBW	• Men: = 50 kg + 2.3 kg for each inch over 5 ft • Women: = 45.5 kg + 2.3 kg for each inch over 5 ft	• Debated	• Formula does apply to people under 5 ft • Frequently used to calculate medication (chemotherapy) dose in the obese

BMI = body mass index; WHR = waist-to-hip ratio; IBW = ideal body weight.

Obesity and Overweight

Table 22-2

The Obese Patient

Category	Definition	Epidemiology	Associated Diseases
Overweight	• BMI 25–29.9	• 34% of U.S. adults are overweight	• Hypertension • Diabetes mellitus
Obese	• BMI >30	• 31% of U.S. adults are obese • Obesity has increased 100% in the last 20 years	• Hyperinsulinemia • Hypertriglyceridemia • Low serum HDL cholesterol concentration • Hypercholesterolemia • Coronary heart disease • Congestive heart failure • Osteoarthritis • Gallstones • Steatohepatitis • Cancer

HDL = high-density-lipoprotein.

Table 22-3

Treatment Options for Excess Weight

Treatment	Indications	Details	Notes
Behavioral Management	• BMI >27	• Decrease energy intake (diet) • Increase energy expenditure (exercise) • Low calorie diet = 800–1200 kcal/day	• Always the first step • A caloric deficit of 500 kcal/day induces a 1 lb/week weight loss

Pharmacotherapy	• BMI >30 OR
	• BMI >27 with comorbidities (hypertension, diabetes, dyslipidemia, etc.)
		• Sibutramine:
		  - Norepinephrine and serotonin reuptake inhibitor
		  - Inhibits appetite and increases thermogenesis
		• Orlistat:
		  - Inhibits pancreatic lipase
		  - 30% reduction in the absorption of fat ingested
			• Sibutramine adverse effects:
			  - Increase in blood pressure and pulse
			• Orlistat adverse effects:
			  - Decreased absorption of fat-soluble vitamins (A, D, E, K)
			  - Diarrhea, anal leakage

(continued)

Table 22-3

Treatment Options for Excess Weight (continued)

TREATMENT	INDICATIONS	DETAILS	NOTES
Surgery	• BMI >40 OR • BMI >35 with medical comorbidities that would improve with weight loss	• Roux-en-Y gastric bypass OR • Lap-Band Adjustable Gastric Banding System	• 0.5–1% mortality

Adapted from: The Practical Guide: Identification, Evaluation, and Treatment of Overweight and Obesity in Adults. Available at: http://www.nhlbi.nih.gov/guidelines/obesity/practgde.htm.

Table 22-4

The Malnourished Patient

DEFINITION	RISK FACTORS	CLINICAL PRESENTATION
• 10% weight loss within 6 months • 20% weight loss within year • BMI <18.5	• Advanced age • Poor dentition • Poverty • Isolation, poor social structure • Alcoholism • Chronic illness (particularly malignancy or GI disease) • GI symptoms (anorexia, nausea, vomiting, diarrhea) • Homebound/bed-bound	• Loss of subcutaneous tissue • Muscle wasting (temporal wasting) • Edema • Ascites • Decreased muscle mass • Associated with increased length of stay in hospital and increased mortality

GI = gastrointestinal.

Table 22-5

Metabolic Markers for Malnutrition

MARKER	HALF-LIFE	NOTES
Albumin	18–20 days	• <2.2 g/dL generally reflects severe malnutrition • Can be inaccurate if cirrhosis, nephrosis, sepsis, cancer, dehydration, or recent trauma
Transferrin	8–9 days	• Some studies suggest clinically significant changes in albumin can be predicted by changes in serum transferrin and prealbumin
Prealbumin	2–3 days	

Table 22-6

Comparison of Starvation and Cachexia

MANIFESTATION	STARVATION	CACHEXIA
Metabolic Rate	↓	=, ↑
Protein Turnover	↓	↑
Glucose Turnover	↓	=, ↑
Liver Metabolic Activity	=, ↓	↑

Table 22-7

Comparison of Marasmus and Kwashiorkor

	DEFINITION	CLINICAL PRESENTATION	DIAGNOSIS	TREATMENT
Marasmus	• Calorie insufficiency	• Alert • Hungry • Dramatic weight loss • Emaciation • Loss of fat • Muscle atrophy	• Clinical history and presentation	• Caloric modification
Kwashiorkor	• Protein-calorie insufficiency	• Lethargic • Pitting edema • Neurologic changes • Recurrent infections • Striped red hair • Dramatic weight loss • Emaciation • Loss of fat • Muscle atrophy	• Low albumin • Low glucose	• Slow advancement of calories and nutrition • Antibiotic prophylaxis

Table 22-8

Summary of Vitamins

VITAMIN	FUNCTION	EXCESS	DEFICIENCY
Water Soluble			
B₁ Thiamine	• Oxidative decarboxylation of alpha-ketoacids and sugars	• Rare	• Beriberi • Cardiomegaly • Wernicke encephalopathy • Korsakoff's psychosis
B₂ Riboflavin	• Oxidative phosphorylation • Electron transfer reactions	• Rare	• Cheilosis • Greasy, scaly facial rash

(*continued*)

Table 22-8

Summary of Vitamins (continued)

VITAMIN	FUNCTION	EXCESS	DEFICIENCY
B₃ Niacin	• NAD, NADPH cofactors	• Skin flushing • Pruritus	• Pellagra • Rash
B₆ Pyridoxine	• Heme synthesis • Neurotransmission	• Sensory neuropathy	• Seizures • Glossitis • Dermatitis • Peripheral neuropathy with INH treatment
B₁₂ Cyanocobalamin	• Methylation of homocysteine to methionine	• Rare	• Pernicious anemia • Common in small bowel disease, celiac disease, irritable bowel disease, fish tapeworm
Folate	• Synthesis of purines, pyrimidines, nucleoproteins	• May mask vitamin B₁₂ deficiency	• Megaloblastic anemia (macrocytic) • Glossitis • Fetal neural tube defect
C Ascorbic acid	• Collagen stability • Aids iron absorption • Antioxidant	• Oxaluria • Renal stones • Diarrhea	• Scurvy • Poor wound healing • Bleeding gums • Infection • Anorexia
Fat Soluble	**Deficiencies more common in cystic fibrosis, pancreatic disease, and cholestatic disease**		
A Retinol Retinal Retinoic acid	• Retinal pigmentation • Vision • Epithelial development • Bone structure	• Pseudotumor cerebri • Hair loss • Liver damage	• Night blindness • Dry eyes • Keratomalacia • Dry skin
D Ergocalciferol Cholecalciferol	• Regulates calcium serum levels • Important for bone mineralization	• Hypercalcemia • Nausea/vomiting	• Rickets (children) • Osteomalacia (adults)
E Tocopherols	• Antioxidant	• Rare	• Neuropathies • Myopathies • Ataxia
K Phylloquinone Menaquinone Menadione	• Procoagulant • Needed to synthesize factors II, VII, IX, and X	• Decreased INR	• Increased INR/bleeding

INH = isoniazid; INR = international normalized ratio; NAD = nicotinamide-adenine dinucleotide; NADPH = nicotinamide-adenine nucleotide, reduced.

Table 22-9
Summary of Minerals

MINERAL	FUNCTION	EXCESS	DEFICIENCY
Calcium	• Important for structure of bones/teeth • Cardiac contractility • Muscle contraction • Nerve conduction • Blood coagulation production	• Nausea/vomiting • Altered mental status • Constipation • Weakness • Abdominal pain • Polyuria • Headache • Short QT • Renal stones • Calcinosis	• Chvostek sign (facial twitch) • Trousseau sign (carpal spasm) • Prolonged QT • Laryngospasm • Seizures • Perioral/hand/foot numbness/tingling
Phosphorus	• Regulates pH • Structure of bones/teeth • ATP precursor	• Abdominal pain • Vomiting • Renal impairment • Neuromuscular impairment	• Muscle weakness/myopathy • Hypercalciuria • Metabolic encephalopathy
Fluoride	• Structure of bones/teeth	• Mottling of teeth	• Cavities
Iron	• Structure of hemoglobin • Structure of myoglobin	• Fatigue • Abdominal pain • Vomiting • Hemachromatosis	• Hypochromic, microcytic anemia • Recurrent infection • Angular stomatitis
Potassium	• Major *intra*cellular ion • Muscle contraction • Nerve conduction • Cardiac rhythm	• Cardiac conduction disturbances • Tall peaked T wave with shortened QT interval on ECG • Muscle weakness	• Muscle weakness • Nausea • Depressed ST segment, flattened T wave and U waves • Cardiac arrhythmias • Cramps, paresthesias, tetany
Sodium	• Major osmotic force • Major *extra*cellular ion • Nerve conduction • Muscle contraction	• Lethargy • Weakness • Irritability • Seizures • Coma	• Cerebral edema and associated neurologic changes (especially if acute hyponatremia) • Nausea • Gait disturbances • Lethargy
Magnesium	• Muscle contraction • Nerve conduction • Protein synthesis • Calcium antagonist	• Bradycardia • Lethargy • Hyporeflexia	• Tetany • Hypocalcemia

(continued)

Table 22-9

Summary of Minerals (continued)

MINERAL	FUNCTION	EXCESS	DEFICIENCY
Copper	• Collagen stability	• Kayser-Fleischer ring • Can be caused by Wilson disease (autosomal recessive defect of cellular copper export) • Nausea/vomiting • Hepatic necrosis	• Rare
Zinc	• Collagen stability	• Rare • Secondary copper deficiency	• Change in hair color • Poor wound healing • Skin changes • Common in patients dependent on chronic TPN

ACTH = adrenocorticotrophic hormone; ATP = adenine triphosphate; PTH = parathyroid hormone; ECG = electrocardiogram; TPN = total parenteral nutrition.

Table 22-10

Enteral and Parenteral Nutritional Support

	INDICATION	METHOD	NOTE/COMPLICATION
Enteral Nutrition	• Preexisting nutritional deprivation • Anticipated prolonged period of NPO	• NG tube if short term • PEG tube long term	• Complications of NG tube: sinus infections • Complications of PEG: entry site infection • Does NOT eliminate aspiration risk • Safer and cheaper than TPN
Total Parenteral Nutrition (TPN)	• Only when enteral feeds are impossible	• Needs to be given via central venous catheter	• Composed of dextrose (carbohydrate), amino acids (protein), and lipids (fat) • Added: electrolytes, minerals, trace elements, and a multivitamin preparation • Complications: sepsis, thrombosis, hyperglycemia

NG = nasogastric; NPO = nothing per os; PEG = percutaneous gastrostomy.

Chapter 23

Basic Statistics and Epidemiology

Table 23-1

Characteristics of a Clinically Useful Screening, Diagnostic, and Monitoring Tests

	DEFINITION	CHARACTERISTIC OF A "GOOD" TEST	EXAMPLE DETAIL
Screening Test	• Detects a condition in asymptomatic persons • Example: mammograms to detect breast cancer in women without a palpable breast mass	• The condition has a high prevalence and is detectable when asymptomatic	• The lifetime risk of a woman developing invasive breast cancer = 1:9. Breast cancer is often asymptomatic until it is advanced
		• The condition has significant mortality and/or morbidity	• The median survival of untreated metastatic breast cancer is 18–24 months
		• Earlier treatment during an asymptomatic stage decreases the morbidity and mortality of the condition	• Early treatment increases the survival rate of women with breast cancer
		• The test has low morbidity and mortality rates	• Mammograms may be uncomfortable, but there are no other significant morbidities (or mortality) associated with the test
		• The test is relatively inexpensive, accurate, and readily available	• Mammograms are widely available and relatively inexpensive
		• The test has few false negatives (high sensitivity)	• Most people who have breast cancer are identified on mammogram. However, a diagnostic test (biopsy) is needed to confirm the diagnosis and to exclude those with a false positive result
Diagnostic Test	• Aids diagnosis of a condition in a symptomatic patient • Example: biopsy of a palpable breast mass	• Rules a diagnosis in or out	• Biopsy of a palpable breast mass can distinguish between a malignant and a benign etiology
		• Few false positives (high specificity)	• Only those patients with breast cancer are diagnosed as having breast cancer. Therefore, patients without breast cancer are not exposed to the risks of breast cancer treatment
Monitoring Test	• Gauges disease progression • Example: hemoglobin A1c in diabetic patients	• Helps prevent disease-associated morbidity and mortality by assessing the success (or failure) of treatment	• Hemoglobin A1c in diabetic patients describes average glycemic control by reflecting the mean blood glucose over the prior 2–3 months

Table 23-2

Evaluation of Test Results

	Positive Test	Negative Test
Patient Has the Disease	True positive (TP)	False negative (FN)
Patient Does NOT Have Disease	False positive (FP)	True negative (TN)

FP = false positive; FN = false negative; TN = true negative; TP = true positive.

Table 23-3

Sensitivity and Specificity*

Term	Definition	Formula	Note
Sensitivity	The proportion of patients with a condition that test positive out of all persons in the population with the condition as determined by the "gold-standard test"	$TP \times 100/(TP + FN)$	• The greater the sensitivity of a test, the more likely people with the disease will have a positive test • A highly sensitive test is useful to rule out a condition
Specificity	The proportion of patients without a condition testing negative out of all person in the population without the condition as determined by the "gold-standard test"	$TN \times 100/(TN + FP)$	• The greater the specificity of a test, the more likely people without the disease will have a negative test • A highly specific test is useful to rule in a disease

*Each test has a unique sensitivity and specificity. Although the best test has a high sensitivity and a high specificity, it is often not possible to maximize both.

Predictive Value of a Test

In order to interpret a test result for an individual patient, the clinician must ask: "What is the likelihood that a given patient with a positive result actually has the condition?" The answer to this question is called the positive predictive value (PPV) of a test and is closely related to the test's specificity. The negative predictive value (NPV) is closely related to the sensitivity of the test and describes the likelihood that a patient with a negative result does not have the condition.

Example: Suppose "Rapid Lyme" is a hypothetical test to detect Lyme disease. Out of 100 people tested with "Rapid Lyme," 40 people are positive. However, of the 40 people with a positive " Rapid Lyme" test, only 35 people actually have Lyme disease as determined by the "gold-standard test." Of the 60 people with a negative "Rapid Lyme" test, 3 people actually have Lyme disease as determined by the "gold-standard test." This data detailed in Table 23-4, is also called a 2 × 2 table. The sensitivity, specificity, PPV, and NPV are calculated in Table 23-5 and 23-6.

Table 23-4
Positive Predictive Value and Negative Predictive Value

TERM	DEFINITION	FORMULA
PPV	The probability that a patient with a positive test result actually has the condition	TP × 100/(TP + FP)
NPV	The probability that a patient with a negative test result actually does not have the condition	TN × 100/(TN + FN)

Table 23-5
Two by Two Table for "Rapid Lyme" Hypothetical Example

	POSITIVE "RAPID LYME" TEST	NEGATIVE "RAPID LYME" TEST
Patient Has Lyme Disease	TP = 35	FN = 3
Patient Does NOT Have Lyme Disease	FP = 5	TN = 57

Table 23-6
Sensitivity, Specificity, PPV, and NPV for "Rapid Lyme" Hypothetical Example

	FORMULA	CALCULATION	MEANING
Sensitivity	TP × 100/(TP + FN)	35/(35 + 3) × 100 = 92.1%	92.1% of people who truly have Lyme disease have a positive "Rapid Lyme" test
Specificity	TN × 100/(TN + FP)	57/(57 + 5) × 100 = 91.9%	91.9% of people who truly do *not* have Lyme disease have a negative "Rapid Lyme" test
PPV	TP × 100/(TP + FP)	35/(35 + 5) × 100 = 87.5%	87.5% of people with a positive "Rapid Lyme" test truly have Lyme disease
NPV	TN × 100/(TN + FN)	57/(57 + 3) × 100 = 95%	95% of people with a negative "Rapid Lyme" test truly do *not* have Lyme disease

Table 23-7
Other Statistical Terms: Definitions and Comments

Term	Definition	Comment	Example
Null Hypothesis	• The hypothesis that we accept as true unless the study disproves it • Often states that there is *no difference* in a specified outcome between an experimental group and a control group	• The null hypothesis can be disproved, but it cannot be proved	• Null hypothesis: there is *no* difference in the number of emergency department visits between asthmatic patients taking an experimental drug and those who are not
Alternative Hypothesis	• The "opposite" of the null hypothesis • Often states that there is a difference between an experimental group and a control group	• Accepted as true when the null hypothesis is disproven	• Alternative hypothesis: there is a difference in the number of emergency department visits between asthmatic patients taking an experimental drug and those who are not
Type I Error	• Occurs if the null hypothesis is rejected when, in fact, the null hypothesis is true	• Similar to a "false positive" • More likely to occur in unblinded studies	• A researcher concludes that there is a difference in the number of emergency department visits between the experimental and the control groups when, in fact, there is *no* difference
Type II Error	• Occurs if the null hypothesis is not rejected when, in fact, the null hypothesis is false	• Similar to a "false negative" • More likely to occur with small sample sizes	• A researcher concludes that there is *no* difference in the number of emergency department visits between experimental and the control groups when, in fact, there is a difference
The *P*-Value	• Describes the probability that the same (or more extreme) results would occur again if the same study were performed an infinite number of times and the null hypothesis is true	• If the data would be very unlikely to occur again if the null hypothesis were true, then the alternative hypothesis is accepted as true	• Although results must always be interpreted with knowledge of the strengths and weakness of the study, a $P \leq 0.05$ is classically considered significant enough to accept the alternative hypothesis and reject the null hypothesis • If the null hypothesis is not a prospectively defined primary endpoint, then the result should be considered exploratory and should be verified prospectively
Confounding	• A variable is associated both with the intervention being studied and the outcome of interest	• Randomization can help control for confounding	• In a nonrandomized study of a surgical intervention, older patients may not be sent to surgery as often as younger patients. Therefore, the surgical mortality rate outcome may be confounded by age
Bias	• Errors in the execution of the study may distort the results and affect the conclusions	• Less likely to occur in blinded studies	• The physician who determines if a rash has improved because of an experimental pill knows if the patient was using the experimental pill or the control cream

Appendix

References and Suggested Readings

In addition to using this book to study for the internal medicine boards, we suggest reviewing high-yield topics in a general textbook. For topics on which additional information is needed, a subspecialty textbook or a picture atlas may be useful.

Suggested books:

Braunwald E, Fauci AS, Kasper DL, et al: *Harrison's Principles of Internal Medicine*. New York, NY: McGraw-Hill, 2001.

Braunwald E, ed: *Heart Disease: A Textbook of Cardiovascular Medicine*, 5th ed. Philadelphia, PA: W.B. Saunders, 1997.

Dawson-Saunder B, Trapp RG: *Basic and Clinical Biostatistics*. East Norwalk, CT: Appleton & Lange, 1994.

Fitzpatrick T, Johnson R, Wolff K, et al: *Color Atlas and Synopsis of Clinical Dermatology*, 4th ed. New York, NY: McGraw-Hill, 2000.

Hall JB, Schmidt GA, Wood LDH: *Principles of Critical Care*, 3rd ed. New York, NY: McGraw Hill, 2005.

Rose BD, Post TW: *Clinical Physiology of Acid-Base and Electrolyte Disorders*, 5th ed. New York, NY: McGraw-Hill, 2001.

Yamada T, Alpers D, Laine L, et al: *Textbook of Gastroenterology*, 4th ed. Philadelphia, PA: Lippincott, Williams & Wilkins, 2003.

For additional details, we recommend the following references (please note the Internet-based references may change after publication of this book):

Adolescent Medicine

Centers for Disease Control and Prevention: Quadrivalent human papillomavirus vaccine: Recommendations of the Advisory Committee on Immunization Practices. *MMWR Morb Mortal Wkly Rep* 2007;56(RR-2):1–23.

Centers for Disease Control and Prevention: Preventing, tetanus, diphtheria, and pertussis among adolescents. Use of tetanus toxoid, reduced diphtheria toxoid and acellular pertussis vaccines: Recommendations of the Advisory Committee on Immunization Practices 2006;55(RR-3):1–43.

Centers for Disease Control and Prevention: Prevention and control of meningococcal vaccine: Recommendations of the Advisory Committee on Immunization Practices 2005;54(RR-7):1–21.

Emans SJ, Laufer MR, Goldstein DP, eds: *Pediatric and Adolescent Gynecology*, 5th ed. Philadelphia, PA: Lippincott, Williams & Wilkins, 2004.

Goldenring JM, Rosen DS: Getting into adolescent heads: an essential update. *Contemp Pediatr* 2004;21:64–80.

Greene JP, Ahrendt D, Stafford EM. In: Strasburger VC, Greydaynus DE (series eds) and Schydlower M, Arredondo RM (vol. eds): *Adolescent Medicine Clinics: Vol. 17.2. Substance Abuse Among Adolescents*. Philadelphia, PA: W.B. Saunders, 2006.

Greydaynus DE, Patel DR: The adolescent substance abuse: current concepts. *Curr Probl Pediatr Adolesc Health Care* 2005;51:78–98.

Hatcher RA, Trussell J, Stewart F, et al: *Contraceptive Technology*, 18th ed. New York, NY: Ardent Media, 2004.

Kahn JA, Hillard PJ: Cervical cytology screening and management of abnormal cytology in adolescent girls. *J Pediatr Adolesc Gynecol* 2003;16:167–171.

Middleman AB: Immunization update: pertussis, meningococcus and human papillomavirus. In: Strasburger VC, Greydaynus DE (series eds) and O'brien RF, Kulig J (vol. eds): *Adolescent Medicine Clinics: Vol. 17.3. Hot Topics in Adolescent Medicine*. Philadelphia, PA: W.B. Saunders, 2006.

Neinstein LS, ed: *Adolescent Health Care*. Philadelphia, PA: Lippincott Williams and Wilkins, 2002.

Allergy and Immunology

Adkinson NF, Yunginger JW, Busse WW, et al: *Middleton's Allergy: Principles and Practice*, 6th ed. St. Louis, MO: Mosby, 2003.

American Academy of Allergy, Asthma and Immunology: The Allergy Report. Available at: http://www.theallergyreport.com.

Cardiology

Antman EM, Anbe DT, Armstrong PW, et al: ACC/AHA guidelines for the management of patients with ST-elevation myocardial infarction: executive summary: a report of the American College of Cardiology/American Heart Association Task Force on Practice Guidelines (Committee to Revise the 1999 Guidelines on the Management of Patients With Acute Myocardial Infarction). *J Am Coll Cardiol* 2004;44:671–719. Available at: http://www.acc.org/qualityandscience/clinical/guidelines/stemi/Guideline1/index.htm.

Chobanian AV, Bakris GL, Black HR, et al: The Seventh Report of the Joint National Committee on Prevention, Detection, Evaluation, and Treatment of High Blood Pressure: the JNC 7 report. *JAMA* 2003;289(19):2560–2572.

Fuster V, Ryden LE, Cannom DS, et al: ACC/AHA/ESC 2006 guidelines for the management of patients with atrial fibrillation: a report of the American College of Cardiology/American Heart Association Task Force on Practice Guidelines and the European Society of Cardiology Committee for Practice Guidelines (Writing Committee to Revise the 2001 Guidelines for the Management of Patients with Arial Fibrillation). *J Am Coll Cardiol* 2006;48:e149–e246.

Smith SC, Allen J, Blair SN, et al: AHA/ACC guidelines for secondary prevention for patients with coronary and other atherosclerotic vascular disease: 2006 update. *J Am Coll Cardiol* 2006;47:2130–2139. DOI: 10.1016/j.jacc.2006.04.026. Available at: http://content.onlinejacc.org/cgi/content/full/47/10/2130.

The Third Report of the Expert Panel on Detection, Evaluation, and Treatment of High Blood Cholesterol in Adults (ATP III). Available at: http://www.nhlbi.nih.gov/guidelines/cholesterol/index.htm.

Dermatology

Fitzpatrick J, Aeling J, eds: *Dermatology Secrets in Color*, 2nd ed. Philadelphia, PA: Hanley & Belfus, 2000.

Freedberg I, Eisen A, Wolff K, et al: *Fitzpatrick's Dermatology in General Medicine*, 6th ed. New York, NY: McGraw-Hill, 2003.

Odom R, James W, Berger T: *Andrews' Diseases of the Skin: Clinical Dermatology*, 9th ed. Philadelphia, PA: W.B. Saunders, 2000.

Geriatrics

American Geriatrics Society, British Geriatrics Society and American Academy of Orthopaedic Surgeons Panel on Falls Prevention: Guideline for the Prevention of Falls in Older Persons. *JAGS* 2001;49:664–672.

American Geriatrics Society Panel on Persistent Pain in Older Persons: The management of persistent pain in older persons. *JAGS* 2002;50:S205–S224.

Marcincuk MC, Roland PS: Geriatric hearing loss. Understanding the causes and providing appropriate treatment. *Geriatrics* 2002;57(4):44, 48–50, 55–56.

Hematology

DaVita VT, Hellman S, Rosenberg SA, eds: *Cancer: Principles and Practice of Oncology*, 7th ed. Philadelphia, PA: Lippincott, Williams and Wilkins, 2005.

Lichtman AL, Ernest BE, Kaushansky K, et al: *Williams Hematology*, 7th ed. New York, NY: McGraw-Hill, 2005.

Infectious Disease

American Thoracic Society Documents and Infectious Diseases Society of America: Guidelines for the management of adults with hospital-acquired, ventilator-associated, and healthcare-associated pneumonia. *Am J Respir Crit Care* 2005;171:388–416.

Baird JK: Effectiveness of antimalarial drugs. *N Engl J Med* 2005;352:1565–1577.

Bartlett JG: Antibiotic-associated diarrhea. *N Engl J Med* 2002;346:334–339.

Bratton RL, Corey GR: Tick-borne disease. *Am Fam Physician* 2005;71(12):2323–2330.

Centers for Disease Control and Prevention: Viral hepatitis fact sheets. Available at: http://www.cdc.gov/Ncidod/diseases/hepatitis.

Cheung MC, Pantanowitz L, Dezube BJ: AIDS-related malignancies: emerging challenges in the era of highly active antiretroviral therapy. *Oncologist* 2005;10:412–426.

Cooper MA, Pommering TL, Koranyi K: Primary immunodeficiencies. *Am Fam Physician* 2003;68:2001–2008.

Drebot MA, Artsob H: West Nile virus: update for family physicians. *Can Fam Physician* 2005;51:1094–1099.

Ghislaine PD, Roujeau JC: Treatment of severe drug reactions: Stevens-Johnson syndrome, toxic epidermal necrolysis and hypersensitivity syndrome. *Dermatol Online J* 2002;8(1):5.

Gilbert DN, Moellering RC, Eliopoulos GM, et al: *The Sanford Guide to Antimicrobial Therapy*, 35th ed. Hyde Park, VT: Antimicrobial Therapy, 2005.

Golden MP, Vikram HR: Extrapulmonary tuberculosis: an overview. *Am Fam Physician* 2005;72(9):1761–1768.

Golpe R, Marin B, Alonso M: Lemierre's syndrome (necrobacillosis). *Postgrad Med J* 1999;75:141–144.

Goodyear PWA, Firth AL, Strachan DR, et al: Periorbital swelling: the important distinction between allergy and infection. *Emerg Med J* 2004;21:240–242.

Jerant AF, Bannon M, Rittenhouse S: Identification and management of tuberculosis. *Am Fam Physician* 2000;61(9):2667–2678, 81–82.

Kauffman CA: Fungal infections. *Proc Am Thorac Soc* 2006;3(1):35–40.

Kovacs JA, Masur H: Prophylaxis against opportunistic infections in patients with human immunodeficiency virus infection. *N Engl J Med* 2000;342(19):1416–1429.

Kurowski R, Ostapchuk M: Overview of histoplasmosis. *Am Fam Physician* 2002;66(12):2247–2252.

Lauer GM, Walker BD: Hepatitis C virus infection. *N Engl J Med* 2001;345:41–52.

Lee WM: Hepatitis B virus infection. *N Engl J Med* 1997;337:1733–1745.

Light RW: Parapneumonic effusions and empyema. *Proc Am Thorac Soc* 2006;3(1):75–80.

Lowy FD: Medical progress: *Staphylococcus aureus* infections. *N Engl J Med* 1998;339:520–532.

Lutfiyya MN, Henley E, Chang LF, et al: Diagnosis and treatment of community-acquired pneumonia. *Am Fam Physician* 2006;73(3):442–450.

Lynch JP: Hospital-acquired pneumonia: risk factors, microbiology, and treatment. *Chest* 2001;119:373S–384S.

Melles DC, de Marie S: Prevention of infections in hyposplenic and asplenic patients: an update. *Neth J Med* 2004;62(2):45–52.

Miller KE: Diagnosis and treatment of *Chlamydia trachomatis* infection. *Am Fam Physician* 2006;73(8):1411–1416.

Miller KE: Diagnosis and treatment of *Neisseria gonorrhoeae* infections. *Am Fam Physician* 2006;73(10):1779–1784.

Morrow GL, Abbott RL: Conjunctivitis. *Am Fam Physician* 1998;57(4):735–746.

O'Brien KK, Higdon ML, Halverson JJ: Recognition and management of bioterrorism infections. *Am Fam Physician* 2003;67:1927–1934.

Panlilio AL, Cardo DM, Grohskopf LA, et al: U.S. Public Health Service: Updated U.S. Public Health Service guidelines for the management of occupational exposures to HIV and recommendations for postexposure prophylaxis. *MMWR Recomm Rep* 2005;54(RR-9):1–17.

Potter B, Kraus CK: Management of active tuberculosis. *Am Fam Physician* 2005;72(11):2225–2232.

Ramakrishnan K, Scheid DC: Diagnosis and management of acute pyelonephritis in adults. *Am Fam Physician* 2005;71:933–942.

Saifeldeen K, Evans R: Ludwig's angina. *Emerg Med J* 2004;21:242–243.

Scheid DC, Hamm RM: Acute bacterial rhinosinusitis in adults: part I. Evaluation. *Am Fam Physician* 2004;70:1685–1692.

Scheid DC, Hamm RM: Acute bacterial rhinosinusitis in adults: part II. Treatment. *Am Fam Physician* 2004;70:1697–1704, 1711–1712.

Schroeder MS: *Clostridium difficile*-associated diarrhea. *Am Fam Physician* 2005;71(5):921–928.

Singh N, Paterson D: *Aspergillus* infections in transplant recipients. *Clin Micro Rev* 2005;18(1):44–69.

Singh AE, Romanowski B: Syphilis: review with emphasis on clinical, epidemiologic, and some biologic features. *Clin Microbiol Rev* 1999;12(2):187–209.

Stevens, DA: Coccidioidomycosis. *N Engl J Med* 1995; 332(16):1077–1082.

Swartz MN: Cellulitis. *N Engl J Med* 2004;350:904–912.

Swygard H, Sena AC, Hobbs MM, et al: Trichomoniasis: clinical manifestations, diagnosis, and management. *Sex Transm Infect* 2004;80(2):91–95.

Taylor GH: Cytomegalovirus. *Am Fam Physician* 2003; 67:519–524.

Thibodeau KP, Viera AJ: Atypical pathogens and challenges in community-acquired pneumonia. *Am Fam Physician* 2004;69(7):1699–1706.

Thielman NM, Guerrant RL: Acute infectious diarrhea. *N Engl J Med* 2004;350:38–47.

Ward RP, Kugelmas M: Using pegylated interferon and ribavirin to treat patients with chronic hepatitis C. *Am Fam Physician* 2005;72(4):655–662.

Wheat J: Endemic mycoses in AIDS: a clinical review. *Clin Microbiol Rev* 1995;8(1):146–159.

Nephrology

Delvecchio FC, Preminger GM: Medical management of stone disease. *Curr Opin Urol* 2003;13:229–233.

Massry S, Glassock R, eds: *Textbook of Nephrology*, 3rd ed. Baltimore, MD: Williams & Wilkins, 1995.

K/DOQI Clinical Practice Guidelines on Chronic Kidney Disease: Evaluation, classification, and stratification. National Kidney Foundation Kidney Disease Outcomes Quality Initiative Clinical Practice Guidelines on Chronic Kidney Disease Work Group. Part I. *Am J Kidney Dis* 2002;39(2 Suppl 1):S17–S31. Available at: http://www.kidney.org/professionals/kdoqi/guidelines_ckd/p4_class_g1.htm.

Kashtan CE: Alport syndrome and thin glomerular basement membrane disease. *J Am Soc Nephrol* 1998;9:1736–1750.

Palmer BF, Alpern RJ: Liddle's syndrome. *Am J Med* 1998;104:301–309.

Parivar F, Low RK, Stoller ML: The influence of diet on urinary stone disease. *J Urol* 1996;155:432–440.

Portis AJ, Sundaram CP: Diagnosis and initial management of kidney stones. *Am Fam Physician* 2001; 63:1329–1338.

Rivers K, Shetty S, Menon M: When and how to evaluate a patient with nephrolithiasis. *Urol Clin North Am* 2000;27:203–213.

Rizk D, Chapman AB: Cystic and inherited kidney diseases. *Am J Kidney Dis* 2003;42:1305–1317.

Neurology

Adams H, Adams R, Del Zoppo G, et al: Guidelines for the early management of patients with ischemic stroke: 2005 guidelines update a scientific statement from the Stroke Council of the American Heart Association/American Stroke Association. *Stroke* 2005;36(4):916–923.

Albers GW: A review of published TIA treatment recommendations. *Neurology* 2004;62(8 Suppl 6):S26–S28.

Alagiakrishnan K, Wiens CA: An approach to drug induced delirium in the elderly. *Postgrad Med J* 2004;80(945):388–393.

Alter M: The epidemiology of Guillain-Barré syndrome. *Ann Neurol* 1990;27(Suppl):S7–S12.

American Psychiatric Association: *Diagnostic and Statistical Manual of Mental Disorders*, 4th ed. Washington, DC: American Psychiatric Press, 2000.

American Psychiatric Association: *Diagnosis and Statistical Manual of Mental Disorders*, 4th ed. Washington, DC: American Psychiatric Press, 1994.

American Psychiatric Association: Practice guideline for the treatment of patients with Alzheimer's disease and other dementias of late life. *Am J Psychiatry* 1997;154(5 Suppl):1–39.

Ashwal S: Brain death in the newborn. Current perspectives. *Clin Perinatol* 1997;24:859–882.

Barker RA: Disorders of movement excluding Parkinson's disease. In: Warrell DA, Cox TM, Firth JD, et al., eds: *Oxford Textbook of Medicine*. Oxford: Oxford University Press, 2005.

Benbadis SR, Luders HO: Epileptic syndromes: an underutilized concept. *Epilepsia* 1996;37(11):1029–1034.

Bernat JL: Practice parameters for determining brain death in adults (summary statement). The Quality Standards Subcommittee of the American Academy of Neurology. *Neurology* 1999;45:1012.

Brodie MJ, Dichter MA: Antiepileptic drugs. *N Engl J Med* 1996;334(3):168–175.

Brott T, Bogousslavsky J: Treatment of acute ischemic stroke. *N Engl J Med* 2000;343(10):710–722.

Bussone G, Grazzi L, D'Amico D, et al: Acute treatment of migraine attacks: efficacy and safety of a nonsteroidal anti-inflammatory drug, diclofenac-potassium, in comparison to oral sumatriptan and placebo. The Diclofenac-K/Sumatriptan Migraine Study Group. *Cephalalgia* 1999;19(4):232–240.

Caesar R: Acute headache management: the challenge of deciphering etiologies to guide assessment and treatment. *Emerg Med Rep* 1995;16(13): 117–128.

Chisholm N, Gillett G: The patient's journey: living with locked-in syndrome. *BMJ* 2005;331:94–97.

Cocho D, Belvis R, Marti-Fabregas J, et al: Reasons for exclusion from thrombolytic therapy following acute ischemic stroke. *Neurology* 2005;64(4): 719–720.

Culebras A, Kase CS, Masdeu JC, et al: Practice guidelines for the use of imaging in transient ischemic attacks and acute stroke: a report of the Stroke Council, American Heart Association. *Stroke* 1997; 28(7):1480–1497.

Dichter MA, Brodie MJ: New antiepileptic drugs. *N Engl J Med* 1996;334(24):1583–1590.

Dyck PJ, Dyck JB, Grant IA, et al: Ten steps in characterizing and diagnosing patients with peripheral neuropathy. *Neurology* 1996;47:10–17.

England JD, Gronseth GS, Franklin G, et al: Distal symmetric polyneuropathy: a definition for clinical research. Report of the American Academy of Neurology, the American Association of Electrodiagnostic Medicine, and the American Academy of Physical Medicine and Rehabilitation. *Neurology* 2005;64:199–207.

Evans RW: Diagnostic testing for the evaluation of headaches. *Neurol Clin* 1996;14(1):1–26.

Gasser T, Bressman S, Durr A, et al: State of the art review: molecular diagnosis of inherited movement disorders. Movement Disorders Society task force on molecular diagnosis. *Mov Disord* 2003;18(1): 3–18.

Glauser T, Ben-Menachem E, Bourgeois B, et al: International league against epilepsy treatment guidelines: evidence-based analysis of antiepileptic drug efficacy and effectiveness as initial monotherapy for epileptic seizures and syndromes. *Epilepsia* 2006;47(7):1094–1120.

Gubitz G, Sandercock P, Counsell C. Anticoagulants for acute ischaemic stroke. *Cochrane Database Syst Rev* 2004;(3). Art. No.: CD000024. DOI: 10.1002/ 14651858.CD000024.pub2.

Hacke W, Donnan G, Fieschi C, et al: Association of outcome with early stroke treatment: pooled analysis of ATLANTIS, ECASS, and NINDS rt-PA stroke trials. *Lancet* 2004;363(9411):768–774.

Inouye SK, Bogardus ST, Charpentier PA, et al: A multicomponent intervention to prevent delirium in hospitalized older patients. *N Engl J Med* 1999;340(9):669–676.

Inwald D, Jakobovits I, Petros A: Brain stem death: managing care when accepted medical guidelines and religious beliefs are in conflict. Consideration and compromise are possible. *BMJ* 2000;320: 1266–1268.

Jones MM, Nogajski JH, Faulder K, et al: Intra-arterial thrombolysis in acute ischaemic stroke. *Intern Med J* 2005;35(5):300–302.

Karceski S, Morrell MJ, Carpenter D: Treatment of epilepsy in adults: expert opinion. *Epilepsy Behav* 2005;7(Suppl 1):S1–S64; quiz S65–S67.

Karceski S, Morrell M, Carpenter D: The Expert Consensus Guideline Series: treatment of epilepsy. *Epilepsy Behav* 2001;2:A1–A50.

Kase CS, Wolf PA, Chodosh EH, et al: Prevalence of silent stroke in patients presenting with initial stroke: the Framingham Study. *Stroke* 1989;20(7): 850–852.

Kasner SE, et al: Emergency identification and treatment of acute ischemic stroke. *Ann Emerg Med* 1997;30(5):642–653.

Kishore A, Calne DB: Approach to the patient with a movement disorder and overview of movement disorders. In: Watts RL, Koller WC, eds: *Movement Disorders: Neurologic Principles and Practice*. New York, NY: McGraw Hill, 2004.

Lance JW: Current concepts of migraine pathogenesis. *Neurology* 1993;43(6 Suppl 3):S11–S15.

Lauria G: Small fibre neuropathies. *Curr Opin Neurol* 2005;18:591–597.

Lees AJ: Odd and unusual movement disorders. *J Neurol Neurosurg Psychiatry* 2002;72(Suppl 1):I17–I21.

Lewandowski C, Barsan W: Treatment of acute ischemic stroke. *Ann Emerg Med* 2001;37(2):202–216

Lipowski ZJ: Delirium (acute confusional states). *JAMA* 1987;258(13):1789–1792.

Martyn CN, Hughes RA: Epidemiology of peripheral neuropathy. *J Neurol Neurosurg Psychiatry* 1997; 62:310–318.

Nagata K, Maruya H, Yuya H, et al: Can PET data differentiate Alzheimer's disease from vascular dementia? *Ann N Y Acad Sci* 2000;903:252–261.

National Institute of Neurological Disorders Stroke rt-PA Stroke Study Group: Recombinant tissue plasminogen activator for minor strokes: the National Institute of Neurological Disorders and Stroke rt-PA Stroke

Study experience. *Ann Emerg Med* 2005;46(3): 243–252.

Paolin A, Manuali A, Di Paola F, et al: Reliability in diagnosis of brain death. *Intensive Care Med* 1995; 21:657–662.

Partanen J, Niskanen L, Lehtinen J, et al: Natural history of peripheral neuropathy in patients with non-insulin dependent diabetes mellitus. *N Engl J Med* 1995; 333:89–94.

Patterson JR, Grabois M: Locked-in syndrome: a review of 139 cases. *Stroke* 1986;17:758–764.

Rees JH, Soudain SE, Gregson NA, et al: *Campylobacter jejuni* infection and Guillain-Barré syndrome. *N Engl J Med* 1995;333:1374–1379.

Salloway S, Ferris S, Kluger A, et al: Donepezil 401 Study Group. Efficacy of donepezil in mild cognitive impairment: a randomized placebo-controlled trial. *Neurology* 2004;63(4):651–657.

Saper JR: Diagnosis and symptomatic treatment of migraine. *Headache* 1997;37(Suppl 1):S1–S14.

Scheuer ML, Pedley TA: The evaluation and treatment of seizures. *N Engl J Med* 1990;323(21): 1468–1474.

Schwamm LH, Pancioli A, Acker JE, et al: Recommendations for the establishment of stroke systems of care: recommendations from the American Stroke Association's Task Force on the Development of Stroke Systems. *Circulation* 2005;111(8): 1078–1091.

Shorvon S: We live in the age of the clinical guideline. *Epilepsia* 2006;47(7):1091–1093.

Silberstein SD: Evaluation and emergency treatment of headache. *Headache* 1992;32(8):396–407.

Skoog I: Status of risk factors for vascular dementia. *Neuroepidemiology* 1998;17(1):2–9.

Skre H: Genetic and clinical aspects of Charcot-Marie-Tooth disease. *Clin Genet* 1974;6:98–118.

Solomon GD, Cady RK, Klapper JA, et al: Standards of care for treating headache in primary care practice. National Headache Foundation. *Cleve Clin J Med* 1997; 64(7):373–383.

Thomas SH, Stone CK: Emergency department treatment of migraine, tension, and mixed-type headache. *J Emerg Med* 1994;12(5):657–664.

Tomson J, Lip GY: Blood pressure changes in acute haemorrhagic stroke. *Blood Press Monit* 2005;10(4):197–199.

Trzepacz PT: Delirium: advances in diagnosis, pathophysiology, and treatment. *Psychiatr Clin North Am* 1996;19(3):429–448.

Veld BA, Ruitenberg A, Hofman A: Antihypertensive drugs and incidence of dementia: the Rotterdam Study. *Neurobiol Aging* 2001;22(3):407–412.

Wechsler LR, Roberts R, Furlan AJ, et al: Factors influencing outcome and treatment effect in PROACT II. *Stroke* 2003;34(5):1224–1229.

Wijdicks EFM: *Brain Death.* Philadelphia, PA: Lippincott Williams and Wilkins, 2001.

Wijdicks EFM: Brain death worldwide: accepted fact but no global consensus in diagnostic criteria. *Neurology* 2002;58:20–25.

Wijdicks EFM: Determining brain death in adults. *Neurology* 1995;45:1003–1011.

Wijdicks EFM: The diagnosis of brain death. *N Engl J Med* 2001;344:1215–1221.

Nutrition

The Practical Guide: Identification, Evaluation, and Treatment of Overweight and Obesity in Adults. Available at: http://www.nhlbi.nih.gov/guidelines/ obesity/practgde.htm.

Oncology

A predictive model for aggressive non-Hodgkin's lymphoma. The International Non-Hodgkin's Lymphoma Prognostic Factors Project. *N Engl J Med* 1993;329:987–994.

Arnold A, Ayoub J, Douglas L, et al: Phase II trial of 13-cis-retinoic acid plus interferon alpha in non-small-cell lung cancer. The National Cancer Institute of Canada Clinical Trials Group. *J Natl Cancer Inst* 1994;86(4):306–309.

Attal M, Harousseau JL, Stoppa AM, et al: A prospective, randomized trial of autologous bone marrow transplantation and chemotherapy in multiple myeloma. Intergroupe Francais du Myélome. *N Engl J Med* 1996;335:91–97.

Autier P, Dore JF, Negrier S, et al: Sunscreen use and duration of sun exposure: a double-blind, randomized trial. *J Natl Cancer Inst* 1999;91:1304–1309.

Barry MJ: Clinical practice. Prostate-specific-antigen testing for early diagnosis of prostate cancer. *N Engl J Med* 2001;344:1373–1377.

Birkmeyer JD, Siewers AE, Finlayson EVA, et al: Hospital volume and surgical mortality in the United States. *N Engl J Med* 2002;346:1128–1137.

Burris HA 3rd, Moore MJ, Andersen J, et al: Improvements in survival and clinical benefit with gemcitabine as first-line therapy for patients with advanced pancreas cancer: a randomized trial. *J Clin Oncol* 1997;15:2403–2413.

Burstein HJ, Winer EP: Primary care for survivors of breast cancer. *N Engl J Med* 2000;343:1086–1094.

Canellos GP, Anderson JR, Propert KJ, et al: Chemotherapy of advanced Hodgkin's disease with MOPP, ABVD, or MOPP alternating with ABVD. *N Engl J Med* 1992;327:1478–1484.

Chu KC, Tarone RE, Kessler LG, et al: Recent trends in U.S. breast cancer incidence, survival, and mortality rates. *J Natl Cancer Inst* 1996;88:1571–1579.

Coiffier B, Lepage E, Briere J, et al: CHOP chemotherapy plus rituximab compared with CHOP alone in elderly patients with diffuse large-B-cell lymphoma. *N Engl J Med* 2002;346:235–242.

Criteria for the classification of monoclonal gammopathies, multiple myeloma and related disorders: a report of the International Myeloma Working Group. *Br J Haematol* 2003;121:749–757.

Darnell RB, Posner JB: Paraneoplastic syndromes involving the nervous system. *N Engl J Med* 2003; 349:1543–1554.

DaVita VT, Hellman S, Rosenberg SA, eds: *Cancer: Principles and Practice of Oncology*, 7th ed. Philadelphia, PA: Lippincott, Williams and Wilkins, 2005.

Desch CE, Benson AB 3rd, Smith TJ, et al: Recommended colorectal cancer surveillance guidelines by the American Society of Clinical Oncology. *J Clin Oncol* 1999;17:1312–1321.

Donegan WL: Evaluation of a palpable breast mass. *N Engl J Med* 1992;327:937–942.

Eisenberger MA, De Wit R, Berry W, et al: A multi-center phase III comparison of docetaxel + prednisone and mitoxantrone + prednisone in patients with hormone-refractory prostate cancer. *Proc Am Soc Clin Oncol* 2004 (22:2 abstr).

Fisher B, Anderson S, Bryant J, et al: Twenty-year follow-up of a randomized trial comparing total mastectomy, lumpectomy, and lumpectomy plus irradiation for the treatment of invasive breast cancer. *N Engl J Med* 2002;347:1233–1241.

Fisher B, Costantino JP, Wickerham DL, et al: Tamoxifen for prevention of breast cancer: report of the National Surgical Adjuvant Breast and Bowel Project P-1 Study. *J Natl Cancer Inst* 1988;90:1371–1388.

Hoffman PC, Mauer AM, Vokes EE: Lung cancer. *Lancet* 2000;355:479–485.

Hruban RH, Petersen GM, Goggins M, et al: Familial pancreatic cancer. *Ann Oncol* 1999;4(10 Suppl):69–73.

Jorenby DE, Leischow SJ, Nides MA, et al: A controlled trial of sustained-release bupropion, a nicotine patch, or both for smoking cessation. *N Engl J Med* 1999;340(9):685–691.

Lindor NM, Green MH, and the Mayo Familial Cancer Program: The concise handbook of family cancer syndromes. *J Natl Cancer Inst* 1998;90:1039–1071.

Steinbach G, Lynch PM, Phillips RK, et al: The effect of celecoxib, a cyclooxygenase-2 inhibitor, in familial adenomatous polyposis. *N Engl J Med* 2000;342(26): 1946–1952.

Swerdlow AJ, Douglas AJ, Hudson GV, et al: Risk of second primary cancers after Hodgkin's disease by type of treatment: analysis of 2846 patients in the British National Lymphoma Investigation. *BMJ* 1992;304:1137–1143.

Truewing JP, Hartge P, Wacholder S, et al: The risk of cancer associated with specific mutations of BRCA1 and BRCA2 among Ashkenazi Jews. *N Engl J Med* 1997;336:1401–1408.

Vogelstein B, Fearon ER, Hamilton SR, et al: Genetic alterations during colorectal tumor development. *N Engl J Med* 1988;319:525–532.

Wingo PA, Ries LAG, Giovino GA, et al: Annual report to the nation on the status of cancer, 1973–1996, with a special section on lung cancer and tobacco smoking. *J Natl Cancer Inst* 1999;91: 675–690.

Opthalmology

Tierney L, McPhee S, Papadakis M: *Current Medical Diagnosis & Treatment, 2005*, 44th ed. New York, NY: McGraw-Hill, 2004.

Perioperative Care

Eagle KA, Berger PB, Calkins H, et al: ACC/AHA guideline update for perioperative cardiovascular evaluation for noncardiac surgery—executive summary: a report of the American College of Cardiology/American Heart Association Task Force on Practice Guidelines (Committee to Update the 1996 Guidelines on Perioperative Cardiovascular Evaluation for Noncardiac Surgery). *J Am Coll*

Cardiol 2002;39:542–543. Available at: http://www. acc.org/clinical/guidelines/perio/update/periup-date_index.htm.

Fleisher LA: American College of Cardiology/American Heart Association 2006 Guideline. *Circulation* 2006; 113(22):2662–2674.

Fletcher GF, Froelicher VF, Hartley LH, et al: Exercise standards: a statement for health professionals from the American Heart Association. *Circulation* 1990;82:2288–2322.

Hlatky MA, Boineau RE, Higginbotham MB, et al: A brief self-administered questionnaire to determine functional capacity (the Duke Activity Status Index). *Am J Cardiol* 1989;64:651–654.

Jacober SJ, Sowers JR. An update on perioperative management of diabetes. *Arch Intern Med* 1999; 159:2405–2411.

Smetana GW: Preoperative pulmonary evaluation. *N Engl J Med* 1999;340:937–944.

Pulmonary

American Thoracic Society. Standards for Diagnosis and Care of Patients with COPD. *Am J Respir Crit Care Med* 1995;152:S77–S120.

Light RW: *Pleural Diseases*, 4th ed. Philadelphia, PA: Williams and Wilkins, 2001.

National Institutes of Health: Practical Guide for the Diagnosis and Management of Asthma. NIH Publication Number 97-4053, 1997.

Psychiatry

Kaplan H, Sadock B: *Synopsis of Psychiatry*, 7th ed. Baltimore, MD: Williams and Wilkins, 1996.

Schatzberg AF, Cole JO, DeBattista C: *Manual of Clinical Psychopharmacology*, 5th ed. Arlington, VA: American Psychiatric Publishing, Inc, 2005.

Stahl SM: *Essential Psychopharmacology: The Prescriber's Guide*. New York, NY: Cambridge University Press, 2005.

Rheumatology:

Hochberg MC, Silman AJ, Smolen JS: *Rheumatology*, 3rd ed. St. Louis, MO: Mosby, 2003.

Klippel JH, Crofford LJ, Stone JH: *Primer on the Rheumatic Diseases*. Atlanta, GA: Arthritis Foundation, 2001.

Paget SA, Gibofsky A, Beary JF: *Manual of Rheumatology and Outpatient Orthopedic Disorders*, 4th ed. Philadelphia, PA: Lippincott, Williams and Wilkins, 2000.

Yee A, Paget SA, eds: *American College of Physicians Expert Guide to Rheumatology*. Peoria, IL: Versa Press, 2004.

Sports Medicine

Birrer RB: *Sports Medicine for the Primary Care Physician*. Boca Raton, FL: CRC Press, 1994.

DeLee JC: *DeLee and Drez's Orthopaedic Sports Medicine: Principles and Practice*. Philadelphia, PA: Elsevier, 2003.

Fu FH, Stone DA: *Sports Injuries: Mechanisms, Prevention, Treatment*. Baltimore, MD: Williams & Wilkins, 1994.

Reider B: *The Orthopaedic Physical Examination*. Philadelphia, PA: W.B. Saunders, 1999.

Stiell IG, McKnight RD, Greenberg GH, et al: Implementation of the Ottawa ankle rules. *JAMA* 1994;271:827–832.

Statistics/Epidemiology

Hunink M, Glasziou P, Siegel J, et al: *Decision Making in Health and Medicine*. Cambridge, UK: Cambridge University Press, 2004.

Urology

Kursh ED, Ulchaker JC, eds: *Office Urology: The Clinician's Guide*. Totowa, NJ: Humana Press, 2001.

Macfarlane MT, ed: *Urology House Officers Series*. Philadelphia, PA: Lippincott, Williams, and Wilkins, 2001.

Tanagho EA, McAninch JW, eds: *Smith's General Urology*. New York, NY: McGraw-Hill, 2000.

Walsh PC, Retick AB, Vaughan ED, et al, eds: *Campbell's Textbook of Urology*, 8th ed. New York, NY: W.B. Saunders, 2002.

Women's Health

Epstein FH: Pregnancy in renal disease (editorial). *N Engl J Med* 1996;35:277–278.

Hou S: Pregnancy in chronic renal insufficiency and end-stage renal disease. *Am J Kidney* 1999;33:235–252.

Lindheimer MD, Davison JM, Katz AI: The kidney and hypertension in pregnancy: twenty exciting years. *Semin Nephrol* 2001;21:173–189.

Jones DC, Hyslett JP: Outcome of pregnancy in women with moderate or severe renal insufficiency. *N Engl J Med* 1996;35:226–232.

Siu SC, Sermer M, Colman JM, et al: Prospective multicenter study of pregnancy outcomes in women with heart disease. *Circulation* 2001;104(5):515–521.

Index

Page numbers followed by italic *f* or *t* denote figures or tables, respectively.

A

AAT. *See* Alpha 1-antitrypsin
ABCs (airway control, breathing, circulation), 72*t*–73*t*
Abdominal aortic aneurysm
  clinical presentations of, 36*t*–37*t*
  diagnosis of, 36*t*–37*t*
  management of, 36*t*–37*t*
  pathophysiology/risk factors of, 36*t*–37*t*
  types of, 36*t*–37*t*
ABPA. *See* Allergic bronchopulmonary aspergillosis
Abscesses, 135*t*
  retropharyngeal, 212*t*–213*t*
Absolute neutrophil count (ANC), 294*t*
Acamprosate, 482*t*
ACEs. *See* Angiotensin-converting enzyme inhibitors
Acetaminophen, 90*t*–92*t*, 332*t*
Acetic acids, 230*t*, 389*t*–391*t*
Achalasia
  clinical presentations of, 100*t*
  definition of, 100*t*
  diagnosis of, 100*t*
  etiology of, 100*t*
  radiologic features of, 100*t*
  treatments for, 100*t*
Achilles tendonitis, 401*t*–402*t*
Acid base disorders
  approaches to, 164*t*
  compensated, 164*t*
Acidosis, 256*t*
Acne, 384*t*–385*t*
Acquired clotting factor abnormalities, 286*t*
Acquired immunodeficiency syndrome. *See* AIDS
Acquired melanocytic nevi, 374*t*–375*t*
Acromegaly, 248*t*
Acromioclavicular joint sprain, 399*t*–400*t*
ACS. *See* Acute coronary syndrome
ACTH. *See* Adrenocorticotropic hormone
Actinic keratosis, 376*t*–378*t*
Acute bacterial sinusitis, 212*t*–213*t*
Acute chest syndrome, 280*t*
Acute complicated cystitis, 196*t*–197*t*

Acute coronary syndrome (ACS), 8*t*
  definition of, 8*t*
  epidemiology of, 8*t*
  etiology of, 8*t*, 11*t*
  other clinical conditions of, 11*t*
  treatments for, 8*t*
  with clinical instability, 11*t*
Acute diarrhea
  clinical presentations of, 104*t*
  diagnostic tests for, 104*t*
  etiology of, 104*t*
  infectious, 104*t*
  toxin mediated, 104*t*
  treatments for, 104*t*
  types of, 104*t*
Acute fatty liver pregnancy (AFLP), 299*t*–300*t*
Acute heart failure
  definition of, 28*t*
  medical management of, 29*t*
  prognosis for, 29*t*
  treatment options for, 28*t*
  valve surgery and, 29*t*
  worldwide epidemiology of, 29*t*
Acute hemolytic reactions, 292*t*–293*t*
Acute hypercarbic respiratory failure (type 2)
  definition of, 83*t*–84*t*
  etiology of, 83*t*–84*t*
  pathophysiology of, 83*t*–84*t*
  presentations of, 83*t*–84*t*
  treatments for, 83*t*–84*t*
Acute hypoxemic respiratory failure (type I)
  definition of, 83*t*–84*t*
  etiology of, 83*t*–84*t*
  pathophysiology of, 83*t*–84*t*
  presentations of, 83*t*–84*t*
  treatments for, 83*t*–84*t*
Acute leukemias, 303*t*–304*t*
Acute lung injury (ALI)
  definition of, 83*t*–84*t*
  etiology of, 83*t*–84*t*
  pathophysiology of, 83*t*–84*t*
  presentations of, 83*t*–84*t*
  treatments for, 83*t*–84*t*
Acute lymphoid leukemia (ALL), 303*t*–304*t*
Acute mesenteric ischemia

clinical presentations of, 114*t*
  diagnosis of, 114*t*
  etiology of, 114*t*
  location of, 114*t*
  risk factors of, 114*t*
  treatments for, 114*t*
Acute myeloid leukemia (AML), 303*t*–304*t*
Acute pericarditis
  diagnosis of, 38*t*–40*t*
  etiology of, 38*t*–40*t*
  findings on, 38*t*–40*t*
  pathophysiology of, 38*t*–40*t*
  signs/symptoms of, 38*t*–40*t*
  treatments for, 38*t*–40*t*
Acute poisonings
  antidotes/treatments for, 90*t*–92*t*
  by cocaine, 90*t*–92*t*
  common, 90*t*–92*t*
  diagnosis of, 90*t*–92*t*
  digitalis by, 90*t*–92*t*
  oxygen for, 90*t*–92*t*
  presentations of, 90*t*–92*t*
Acute promyelocytic leukemia (APL), 303*t*–304*t*
Acute renal failure
  categories of, 144*t*–146*t*
  clinical, 144*t*–146*t*
  etiology of, 144*t*–146*t*
  management of, 144*t*–146*t*
Acute respiratory distress syndrome (ARDS)
  definition of, 83*t*–84*t*
  etiology of, 83*t*–84*t*
  pathophysiology of, 83*t*–84*t*
  presentations of, 83*t*–84*t*
  treatments for, 83*t*–84*t*
Acute rheumatic fever, 353*t*
Acute uncomplicated cystitis, 196*t*–197*t*
Acute visual loss, 362, 363*t*–364*t*
Acyclovir, 217*t*–219*t*
Addison disease, 249*t*, 250*t*
Adefovir, 209*t*
Adenocarcinoma, 317*t*, 322*t*–323*t*
  clinical presentations of, 98*t*
  diagnosis of, 98*t*, 135*t*–136*t*
  epidemiology of, 98*t*, 135*t*–136*t*
  etiology/risk factors of, 98*t*
  treatments for, 98*t*, 135*t*–136*t*

534 • Index